T0093881

Machine Learning in Medicine – A Complete Overview

Ton J. Cleophas • Aeilko H. Zwinderman

Machine Learning in Medicine – A Complete Overview

Second Edition

With the help from Henny I. Cleophas-Allers, BChem

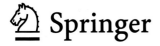 Springer

Ton J. Cleophas
Department Medicine
Albert Schweitzer Hospital
Dordrecht, The Netherlands

Aeilko H. Zwinderman
Academic Medical Center
Department Biostatistics and Epidemiology
Amsterdam, The Netherlands

Additional material to this book can be downloaded from http://extras.springer.com

ISBN 978-3-030-33972-2   ISBN 978-3-030-33970-8   (eBook)
https://doi.org/10.1007/978-3-030-33970-8

This Springer imprint is published by the registered company Springer Nature Switzerland AG.
The registered company address is: Gewerbestrasse 11, 6330 Cham, Switzerland

Preface to the Second Edition

In the second edition, the authors will remove the textual errors from the first edition. Also, the improved tables from the first edition will be replaced with the original tables from the software programs as applied. This is, because, unlike the former, the latter were without error and the readers were better familiar with them.

The main purpose of the first edition was to provide stepwise analyses of the novel methods from data examples, but background information and clinical relevance information may have been somewhat lacking. Therefore, each chapter will now contain a section entitled "Background Information."

Machine learning may be more informative and may provide better sensitivity of testing than traditional analytic methods may do. In the second edition, a place will be given for the use of machine learning not only to the analysis of observational clinical data but also to that of controlled clinical trials.

Unlike the first edition, the second edition will have drawings in full color, providing a helpful extra dimension to the data analysis.

Several machine learning methodologies not yet covered in the first edition, but increasingly important today, will be included in this updated edition, for example, negative binomial and Poisson regressions, sparse canonical analysis, Firth's bias adjusted logistic analysis, omics research, eigenvalues, and eigenvectors.

Lyon, France   Ton J. Cleophas
Lyon, France   Aeilko H. Zwinderman
May 2019

v

Preface to First Edition

The amount of data stored in the world's databases doubles every 20 months, as estimated by Usama Fayyad, one of the founders of machine learning and co-author of the book "Advances in knowledge discovery and data mining" (ed. by the American Association for Artificial Intelligence, Menlo Park, CA, USA, 1996), and clinicians, familiar with traditional statistical methods, are at a loss to analyze them.

Traditional methods have, indeed, difficulty to identify outliers in large datasets, and to find patterns in big data and data with multiple exposure / outcome variables. In addition, analysis-rules for surveys and questionnaires, which are currently common methods of data collection, are, essentially, missing. Fortunately, the new discipline, machine learning, is able to cover all of these limitations.

So far medical professionals have been rather reluctant to use machine learning. Ravinda Khattree, co-author of the book "Computational methods in biomedical research" (ed. by Chapman & Hall, Baton Rouge, LA, USA, 2007) suggests that there may be historical reasons: technological (doctors are better than computers (?)), legal, cultural (doctors are better trusted). Also, in the field of diagnosis making, few doctors may want a computer checking them, are interested in collaboration with a computer or with computer engineers.

Adequate health and health care will, however, soon be impossible without proper data supervision from modern machine learning methodologies like cluster models, neural networks, and other data mining methodologies. The current book is the first publication of a complete overview of machine learning methodologies for the medical and health sector, and it was written as a training companion, and as a must-read, not only for physicians and students, but also for any one involved in the process and progress of health and health care.

Some of the 80 chapters have already appeared in Springer's Cookbook Briefs, but they have been rewritten and updated. All of the chapters have two core characteristics. First, they are intended for current usage, and they are, particularly, concerned with improving that usage. Second, they try and tell what readers need to know in order to understand the methods.

In a nonmathematical way stepwise analyses of the underneath three most important classes of machine learning methods will be reviewed:

cluster and classification models (Chaps. 1–18),
(log) linear models (Chaps. 19–49),
rules models (Chaps. 50–80).

The book will include basic methodologies like "typology of medical data, quantile-quantile plots for making a start with your data, rate analysis and trend analysis as more powerful alternatives to risk analysis and traditional tests, probit models for binary effects on treatment frequencies, higher order polynomes for circadian phenomena, contingency tables and its myriad applications. Particularly, the Chaps. 9, 14, 15, 18, 45, 48, 49, 79, and 80 will review these methodologies.

The Chap. 7 describes the use of visualization processes instead of calculus methods for data mining. The Chap. 8 describes the use of trained clusters, a scientifically more appropriate alternative to traditional cluster analysis. The Chap. 69 describes evolutionary operations (evops), and the evop calculators, already widely used for chemical and technical process improvement.

Various automated analyses and simulation models are in the Chaps. 4, 29, 31, and 32. The Chaps. 67, 70, 71 review spectral plots, Bayesian networks, support vector machines. A first description of several methods already employed by technical and market scientists, and of their suitabilities for clinical research is given in the Chaps. 37–39, 56 (ordinal scalings for inconsistent intervals, loglinear models for varying incident risks, iteration methods for crossvalidations).

Modern methodologies like interval censored analyses, exploratory analyses using pivoting trays, repeated measures logistic regression, doubly multivariate analyses for health assessments, and gamma regression for best fit prediction of health parameters, are reviewed in the Chaps. 10–13, 16, 17, 42, 46, 47.

In order for the readers to perform their own analyses, SPSS data files of the examples are given in extras.springer.com, as well as XML (eXtended Markup Language), SPS (Syntax), and ZIP (compressed) files for outcome predictions in future patients. Furthermore, 4 csv type excel files are available for data analysis in the Konstanz information miner (Knime) and Weka (Waikato University New Zealand) miner, widely approved free machine learning software packages on the internet since 2006. Also a first introduction is given to SPSS modeler (SPSS' data mining workbench, the Chaps. 61, 64, 65), and to SPSS Amos, the graphical and non-graphical data analyzer for the identification of cause effect relationships as principle goal of research (the Chaps. 48 and 49). The free Davidwees polynomial grapher is used in the Chap.79.

The current book will demonstrate that machine learning performs sometimes better than traditional statistics does. For example, if the data perfectly fit the cut-offs for node splitting, because, e.g., ages >55 years give an exponential rise in infarctions, then decision trees, optimal binning, and optimal scaling will be better analysis-methods than traditional regression methods with age as continuous predictor. Machine learning may have little options for adjusting confounding and interaction, but you can add propensity scores and interaction variables to almost any machine learning method.

Each chapter will start with purposes and scientific questions. Then, step-by-step analyses, using both real data and simulated data examples, will be given. Finally, a paragraph with conclusion, and references to the corresponding sites of three introductory textbooks previously written by the same authors, is given.

Lyon, France   Ton J. Cleophas
Lyon, France   Aeilko H. Zwinderman
December 2015

Contents

Part I
Cluster and Classification Models

Chapter 1
Hierarchical Clustering and K-Means Clustering to Identify Subgroups in Surveys (50 Patients)

General Purpose

Clusters are subgroups in a survey estimated by the distances between the values needed to connect the patients, otherwise called cases. It is an important methodology in explorative data mining.

Background

Cluster analysis involves grouping of sets of objects in such a way, that objects in the same group are more similar to one another than to those in other groups (clusters). It is a main task of exploratory data mining, and a common technique for statistical data analysis, used in many fields, including machine learning, pattern recognition, image analysis, information retrieval, bioinformatics, data compression, and computer graphics. Cluster analysis itself can be achieved by various algorithms that differ in their understanding of what constitutes a cluster and how to find them. Popular characteristics of clusters are groups with small distances between cluster

This chapter was previously published in "Machine learning in medicine-cookbook 1" as Chap. 1, Springer Heidelberg Germany, 2013.

Electronic Supplementary Material The online version of this chapter (https://doi.org/10.1007/978-3-030-33970-8_1) contains supplementary material, which is available to authorized users.

members, dense areas of the data space, intervals or particular statistical distribu tions. Cluster analysis is sometimes called multi-objective optimization. The appropriate clustering algorithm and parameter settings (including parameters such as the distance function to use, a density threshold or the number of expected clusters) depend on the individual data set and intended use of the results. Cluster analysis as such is not an automatic task, but an iterative process of knowledge discovery or interactive multi-objective optimization that involves trial and failure. Besides the term cluster analysis, there are a number of terms with similar meanings, including automatic classification, numerical taxonomy, botryology (from Greek βότρυς "grape"), typological analysis, and community detection. The subtle differences are often in the use of the results: while in data mining, the resulting groups are the matter of interest, in automatic classification the resulting discriminative power is of interest. Cluster analysis was originated in anthropology by Driver and Kroeber in 1932 and introduced to psychology by Zubin and Tryon in 1939 and famously used by Cattell beginning in 1943 for trait theory classification in personality psychology. In the Chaps. 1, 2, 3 and 4 of this edition four classes of cluster analysis will be addressed:

(1) hierarchical and k-means clustering for subgroup identification,
(2) density-based clustering for outlier group identification,
(3) two step clustering for predicting future subgroup members,
(4) nearest neighbors classification of, e.g., demographic data.

Specific Scientific Question

This chapter will address hierarchical and k-means clustering will use a 50 patient survey for the purpose. In patients with mental depression of different ages and depression scores, we will show how hierarchical and k-means clustering perform in identifying outlier groups in otherwise homogeneous data.

Var1	Var2	Var3
20,00	8,00	1
21,00	7,00	2
23,00	9,00	3
24,00	10,00	4
25,00	8,00	5
26,00	9,00	6
27,00	7,00	7
28,00	8,00	8
24,00	9,00	9
32,00	9,00	10
30,00	1,00	11
40,00	2,00	12
50,00	3,00	13
60,00	1,00	14
70,00	2,00	15
76,00	3,00	16
65,00	2,00	17
54,00	3,00	18

Var = variable

Var 1 age

Var 2 depression score (0 = very mild, 10 = severest)

Var 3 patient number (called cases here)

Only the first 18 patients are given, the entire data file is entitled "hierkmeansdensity" and is in extras.springer.com.

Hierarchical Cluster Analysis

SPSS 19.0 and up can be used for data analysis. Start by opening the data file.

Command
Analyze....Classify....Hierarchical Cluster Analysis....enter variables....Label Case by: case variable with the values 1-50....Plots: mark Dendrogram....Method ....Cluster Method: Between-group linkage....Measure: Squared Euclidean Distance....Save: click Single solution....Number of clusters: enter 3....Continue ....OK.

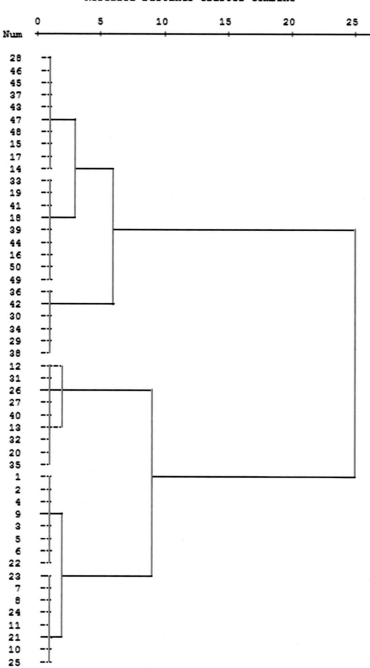

In the output a dendrogram of the results is given. The actual distances between the cases are rescaled to fall into a range of 0–25 units (0 = minimal distance, 25 = maximal distance). The cases no. 1–11, 21–25 are clustered together in cluster 1, the cases 12, 13, 20, 26, 27, 31, 32, 35, 40 in cluster 2, both at a rescaled distance from 0 at approximately 3 units, the remainder of the cases is clustered at approximately 6 units. And so, as requested, three clusters have been indentified with cases more similar to one another than to the other clusters. When minimizing the output, the data file comes up and it now shows the cluster membership of each case. We will use SPSS again to draw a Dotter graph of the data.

Command
Analyze....Graphs....Legacy Dialogs: click Simple Scatter....Define....Y-axis: enter Depression Score....X-axis: enter Age....click OK.

The graph (with age on the x-axis and severity score on the y-axis) produced by SPSS shows the cases. Using Microsoft's drawing commands we can encircle the clusters as identified. All of them are oval and even, approximately, round, because variables have similar scales, but they are different in size.

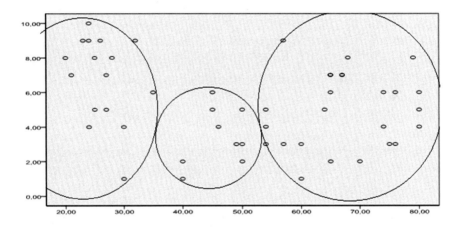

K-Means Cluster Analysis

Command
Analyze....Classify....K-means Cluster Analysis....Variables: enter Age and Depression score....Label Cases by: patient number as a string variable....Number of clusters: 3 (in our example chosen for comparison with the above method)....
click Method: mark Iterate....click Iterate: Maximal Iterations: mark 10....

Convergence criterion: mark 0....click Continue....click Save: mark Cluster Membership....click Continue....click Options: mark Initiate cluster centers.... mark ANOVA table....mark Cluster information for each case....click Continue....click OK.

The output shows that the three clusters identified by the k-means cluster model were significantly different from one another both by testing the y-axis (depression score) and the x-axis variable (age). When minimizing the output sheets, the data file comes up and shows the cluster membership of the three clusters.

ANOVA

	Cluster		Error			
	Mean Square	df	Mean Square	df	F	Sig.
Age	8712,723	2	31,082	47	280,310	,000
Depression Score	39,102	2	4,593	47	8,513	,001

We will use SPSS statistical software again to draw a Dotter graph of the data.

Command

Analyze....Graphs....Legacy Dialogs: click Simple Scatter....Define....Y-axis: enter Depression Score....X-axis: enter Age....click OK.

The graph (with age on the x-axis and severity score on the y-axis) produced by SPSS shows the cases. Using Microsoft's drawing commands we can encircle the clusters as identified. All of them are oval and even approximately round because variables have similar scales, and they are approximately equal in size.

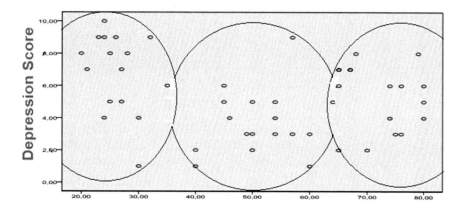

Conclusion

Clusters are estimated by the distances between the values needed to connect the cases. It is an important methodology in explorative data mining. Hierarchical clustering is adequate if subgroups are expected to be different in size, k-means clustering if approximately similar in size. Density-based clustering is more appropriate if small outlier groups between otherwise homogenous populations are expected. The latter method is in the Chap. 2.

Note

More background, theoretical and mathematical information of the two methods is given in Machine learning in medicine part two, Chap. 8 Two-dimensional Clustering, pp. 65–75, Springer Heidelberg Germany 2013. Density-based clustering will be reviewed in the next chapter.

Chapter 2
Density-Based Clustering to Identify Outlier Groups in Otherwise Homogeneous Data (50 Patients)

General Purpose

Clusters are subgroups in a survey estimated by the distances between the values needed to connect the patients, otherwise called cases. It is an important methodology in explorative data mining. Density-based clustering is used.

Background

Cluster analysis involves grouping of sets of objects in such a way, that objects in the same group are more similar to one other than to those in other groups (clusters). It is a main task of exploratory data mining, and a common technique for statistical data analysis, used in many fields, including machine learning, pattern recognition, image analysis, information retrieval, bioinformatics, data compression, and computer graphics. Cluster analysis itself can be achieved by various algorithms that differ in their understanding of what constitutes a cluster and how to find them. Popular characteristics of clusters are groups with small distances between cluster members, dense areas of the data space, intervals or particular statistical distributions. Cluster analysis is sometimes called multi-objective optimization. The appropriate clustering algorithm and parameter settings (including parameters such as the distance function to use, a density threshold or the number of expected clusters) depend on the individual data set and intended use of the results. Cluster analysis as such is not an automatic task, but an iterative process of knowledge discovery or interactive

This chapter was previously published in "Machine learning in medicine-cookbook 1" as Chap. 2, Springer Heidelberg Germany, 2013.

Electronic Supplementary Material The online version of this chapter (https://doi.org/10.1007/978-3-030-33970-8_2) contains supplementary material, which is available to authorized users.

T. J. Cleophas, A. H. Zwinderman, *Machine Learning in Medicine – A Complete Overview*, https://doi.org/10.1007/978-3-030-33970-8_2

multi-objective optimization that involves trial and failure. Besides the term cluster analysis, there are a number of terms with similar meanings, including automatic classification, numerical taxonomy, botryology (from Greek βότρυς "grape"), typological analysis, and community detection. The subtle differences are often in the use of the results: while in data mining, the resulting groups are the matter of interest, in automatic classification the resulting discriminative power is of interest. Cluster analysis was originated in anthropology by Driver and Kroeber in 1932 and introduced to psychology by Zubin and Tryon in 1939 and famously used by Cattell beginning in 1943 for trait theory classification in personality psychology. In the Chaps. 1, 2, 3 and 4 of this edition four classes of cluster analysis will be addressed:

1. hierarchical and k-means clustering for subgroup identification
2. density-based clustering for outlier group identification
3. two step clustering for predicting future subgroup members
4. nearest neighbors classification of, e.g., demographic data.

Specific Scientific Question

This chapter will apply the same data example as that of the previous chapter. In 50 patients with mental depression of different ages and depression scores, we will show how density-based clustering performs in identifying outlier groups in otherwise homogeneous data.

1	2	3
20,00	8,00	1
21,00	7,00	2
23,00	9,00	3
24,00	10,00	4
25,00	8,00	5
26,00	9,00	6
27,00	7,00	7
28,00	8,00	8
24,00	9,00	9
32,00	9,00	10
30,00	1,00	11
40,00	2,00	12
50,00	3,00	13
60,00	1,00	14
70,00	2,00	15
76,00	3,00	16
65,00	2,00	17
54,00	3,00	18

Var = variable
Var 1 age
Var 2 depression score (0 = very mild, 10 = severest)
Var 3 patient number (called cases here)

Only the first 18 patients are given, the entire data file is entitled "hierk-meansdensity" and is in extras.springer.com.

Density-Based Cluster Analysis

The DBSCAN method was used (density based spatial clustering of application with noise). As this method is not available in SPSS, an interactive JAVA Applet freely available at the Internet was used [Data Clustering Applets. http://webdocs.cs. ualberts.ca/~yaling/Cluster/applet]. The DBSCAN connects points that satisfy a density criterion given by a minimum number of patients within a defined radius (radius = Eps; minimum number = Min pts).

Command
User Define....Choose data set: remove values given....enter you own x and y values....Choose algorithm: select DBSCAN....Eps: mark 25....Min pts.: mark 3....Start....Show.

Three cluster memberships are again shown. We will use SPSS 19.0 again to draw a Dotter graph of the data.

Command
Analyze....Graphs....Legacy Dialogs: click Simple Scatter....Define....Y-axis: enter Depression Score....X-axis: enter Age....click OK.

The graph (with age on the x-axis and severity score on the y-axis) shows the cases. Using Microsoft's drawing commands we can encircle the clusters as identified. Two very small ones, one large one. All of the clusters identified are non-circular and, are, obviously, based on differences in patient-density.

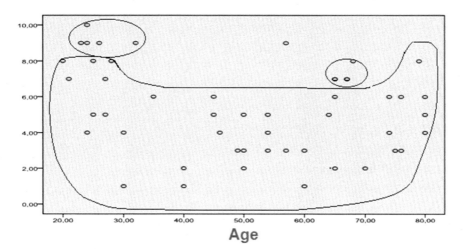

Conclusion

Clusters are estimated by the distances between the values needed to connect the cases. It is an important methodology in explorative data mining. Density-based clustering is suitable if small outlier groups between otherwise homogeneous populations are expected. Hierarchical and k-means clustering are more appropriate if subgroups have Gaussian-like patterns (Chap. 1).

Note

More background, theoretical and mathematical information of the three methods is given in Machine learning in medicine part two, Chap. 8 Two-dimensional clustering, pp. 65–75, Springer Heidelberg Germany 2013. Hierarchical and k-means clustering are reviewed in the previous chapter.

Chapter 3
Two Step Clustering to Identify Subgroups and Predict Subgroup Memberships in Individual Future Patients (120 Patients)

General Purpose

To assess whether two step clustering of survey data can be trained to identify subgroups and subgroup membership.

Background

Cluster analysis involves grouping of sets of objects in such a way, that objects in the same group are more similar to one other than to those in other groups (clusters). It is a main task of exploratory data mining, and a common technique for statistical data analysis, used in many fields, including machine learning, pattern recognition, image analysis, information retrieval, bioinformatics, data compression, and computer graphics. Cluster analysis itself can be achieved by various algorithms that differ in their understanding of what constitutes a cluster and how to find them. Popular characteristics of clusters are groups with small distances between cluster members, dense areas of the data space, intervals or particular statistical distributions. Cluster analysis is sometimes called multi-objective optimization. The appropriate clustering algorithm and parameter settings (including parameters such as the distance function to use, a density threshold or the number of expected clusters) depend on the individual data set and intended use of the results. Cluster analysis as such is not an automatic task, but an iterative process of knowledge discovery or interactive multi-objective optimization that involves trial and failure. Besides the term cluster

This chapter was previously published in "Machine learning in medicine-cookbook 1" as Chap.3, Springer Heidelberg Germany, 2013.

Electronic Supplementary Material The online version of this chapter (https://doi.org/10.1007/978-3-030-33970-8_3) contains supplementary material, which is available to authorized users.

analysis, there are a number of terms with similar meanings, including automatic classification, numerical taxonomy, botryology (from Greek βότρυς "grape"), typological analysis, and community detection. The subtle differences are often in the use of the results: while in data mining, the resulting groups are the matter of interest, in automatic classification the resulting discriminative power is of interest. Cluster analysis was originated in anthropology by Driver and Kroeber in 1932 and introduced to psychology by Zubin and Tryon in 1939 and famously used by Cattell beginning in 1943 for trait theory classification in personality psychology. In the Chaps. 1, 2, 3 and 4 of this edition four classes of cluster analysis will be addressed:

1. hierarchical and k-means clustering for subgroup identification
2. density-based clustering for outlier group identification
3. two step clustering for predicting future subgroup members
4. nearest neighbors classification of, e.g., demographic data.

Specific Scientific Question

This chapter will address two step clustering. In 120 patients with mental depression, can the item scores of depression severity be used to classify subgroups and to predict subgroup membership of future patients.

Var 1	Var 2	Var 3	Var 4	Var 5	Var 6	Var 7	Var 8	Var 9
9,00	9,00	9,00	2,00	2,00	2,00	2,00	2,00	2,00
8,00	8,00	6,00	3,00	3,00	3,00	3,00	3,00	3,00
7,00	7,00	7,00	4,00	4,00	4,00	4,00	4,00	4,00
4,00	9,00	9,00	2,00	2,00	6,00	2,00	2,00	2,00
8,00	8,00	8,00	3,00	3,00	3,00	3,00	3,00	3,00
7,00	7,00	7,00	4,00	4,00	4,00	4,00	4,00	4,00
9,00	5,00	9,00	9,00	2,00	2,00	2,00	2,00	2,00
8,00	8,00	8,00	3,00	3,00	3,00	3,00	3,00	3,00
7,00	7,00	7,00	4,00	6,00	4,00	4,00	4,00	4,00
9,00	9,00	9,00	2,00	2,00	2,00	2,00	2,00	2,00
4,00	4,00	4,00	9,00	9,00	9,00	3,00	3,00	3,00
3,00	3,00	3,00	8,00	8,00	8,00	4,00	4,00	4,00

Var = variable
Var 1-9 = depression score 1-9

Only the first 12 patients are given, the entire data file is entitled "twostepclustering" and is in extras.springer.com.

The Computer Teaches Itself to Make Predictions

SPSS 19.0 and up will be used for data analysis. It will use XML (eXtended Markup Language) files to store data. Now start by opening the data file.

Command

Click Transform....click Random Number Generators....click Set Starting Point ....click Fixed Value (2000000)....click OK....click Analyze....Classify.... TwoStep Cluster....Continuous Variables: enter depression 1-9....click Output: in Working Data File click Create cluster membership....in XML Files click Export final model....click Browse....File name: enter "export2step"....click Save.... click Continue....click OK.

Returning to the data file we will observe that 3 subgroups have been identified and for each patient the subgroup membership is given as a novel variable, and the name of this novel variable is TSC (two step cluster). The saved XML file will now be used to compute the predicted subgroup membership in five future patients. For convenience the XML file is given in extras.springer.com.

Var 1	Var 2	Var 3	Var 4	Var 5	Var 6	Var 7	Var 8	Var 9
4,00	5,00	3,00	4,00	6,00	9,00	8,00	7,00	6,00
2,00	2,00	2,00	2,00	2,00	2,00	2,00	2,00	2,00
5,00	4,00	6,00	7,00	6,00	5,00	3,00	4,00	5,00
9,00	8,00	7,00	6,00	5,00	4,00	3,00	2,00	2,00
7,00	7,00	7,00	3,00	3,00	3,00	9,00	9,00	9,00

Var 1-9 = Depression score 1-9

Enter the above data in a new SPSS data file.

Command

Utilities....click Scoring Wizard....click Browse....click Select....Folder: enter the export2step.xml file....click Select....in Scoring Wizard click Next....click Use value substitution....click Next....click Finish.

The above data file now gives subgroup memberships of the 5 patients as computed by the two step cluster model with the help of the XML file.

Var 1	Var 2	Var 3	Var 4	Var 5	Var 6	Var 7	Var 8	Var 9	Var 10
4,00	5,00	3,00	4,00	6,00	9,00	8,00	7,00	6,00	2,00
2,00	2,00	2,00	2,00	2,00	2,00	2,00	2,00	2,00	2,00
5,00	4,00	6,00	7,00	6,00	5,00	3,00	4,00	5,00	3,00
9,00	8,00	7,00	6,00	5,00	4,00	3,00	2,00	2,00	1,00
7,00	7,00	7,00	3,00	3,00	3,00	9,00	9,00	9,00	2,00

Var 1-9 Depression score 1-9
Var 10 predicted value

Conclusion

Two step clustering can be readily trained to identify subgroups in patients with mental depression, and, with the help of an XML file, it can, subsequently, be used to identify subgroup memberships in individual future patients.

Note

More background, theoretical and mathematical information of two step and other methods of clustering is available in Machine learning in medicine part two, Chaps. 8 and 9, entitled "Two-dimensional clustering" and "Multidimensional clustering", pp 65–75 and 77–91, Springer Heidelberg Germany 2013.

Chapter 4
Nearest Neighbors for Classifying New Medicines (2 New and 25 Old Opioids)

General Purpose

Nearest neighbor methodology has a long history, and has, initially, been used for data imputation in demographic data files. This chapter is to assess whether it can also been used for classifying new medicines.

Background

Cluster analysis involves grouping of sets of objects in such a way, that objects in the same group are more similar to one other than to those in other groups (clusters). It is a main task of exploratory data mining, and a common technique for statistical data analysis, used in many fields, including machine learning, pattern recognition, image analysis, information retrieval, bioinformatics, data compression, and computer graphics. Cluster analysis itself can be achieved by various algorithms that differ in their understanding of what constitutes a cluster and how to find them. Popular characteristics of clusters are groups with small distances between cluster members, dense areas of the data space, intervals or particular statistical distributions. Cluster analysis is sometimes called multi-objective optimization. The appropriate clustering algorithm and parameter settings (including parameters such as the distance

This chapter was previously published in "Machine learning in medicine-cookbook 2" as Chap.1, Springer Heidelberg Germany. 2014.

Electronic Supplementary Material The online version of this chapter (https://doi.org/10.1007/978-3-030-33970-8_4) contains supplementary material, which is available to authorized users.

T. J. Cleophas, A. H. Zwinderman, *Machine Learning in Medicine – A Complete Overview*, https://doi.org/10.1007/978-3-030-33970-8_4

function to use, a density threshold or the number of expected clusters) depend on the individual data set and intended use of the results. Cluster analysis as such is not an automatic task, but an iterative process of knowledge discovery or interactive multi-objective optimization that involves trial and failure. Besides the term cluster analysis, there are a number of terms with similar meanings, including automatic classification, numerical taxonomy, botryology (from Greek βότρυς "grape"), typological analysis, and community detection. The subtle differences are often in the use of the results: while in data mining, the resulting groups are the matter of interest, in automatic classification the resulting discriminative power is of interest. Cluster analysis was originated in anthropology by Driver and Kroeber in 1932 and introduced to psychology by Zubin and Tryon in 1939 and famously used by Cattell beginning in 1943 for trait theory classification in personality psychology. In the Chaps. 1, 2, 3 and 4 of this edition four classes of cluster analysis will be addressed:

1. hierarchical and k-means clustering for subgroup identification
2. density-based clustering for outlier group identification
3. two step clustering for predicting future subgroup members
4. nearest neighbors classification of, e.g., demographic data.

Specific Scientific Question

This chapter will address nearest neighbors cluster analysis. For most diseases a whole class of drugs rather than a single compound is available. Nearest neighbor methods can be used for identifying the place of a new drug within its class.

Example

Two newly developed opioid compounds are assessed for their similarities with the standard opioids in order to determine their potential places in therapeutic regimens. Underneath are the characteristics of 25 standard opioids and two newly developed opioid compounds.

Example   21

Drugname	analgesia score	antitussive score	constipation score	respiratory score	abuse score	eliminate time	duration time
buprenorphine	7,00	4,00	5,00	7,00	4,00	5,00	9,00
butorphanol	7,00	3,00	4,00	7,00	4,00	2,70	4,00
codeine	5,00	6,00	6,00	5,00	4,00	2,90	7,00
heroine	8,00	6,00	8,00	8,00	10,00	9,00	15,00
hydromorphone	8,00	6,00	6,00	8,00	8,00	2,60	5,00
levorphanol	8,00	6,00	6,00	8,00	8,00	11,00	20,00
mepriridine	7,00	2,00	4,00	8,00	6,00	3,20	14,00
methadone	9,00	6,00	6,00	8,00	6,00	25,00	5,00
morphine	8,00	6,00	8,00	8,00	8,00	3,10	5,00
nalbuphine	7,00	2,00	4,00	7,00	4,00	5,10	4,50
oxycodone	6,00	6,00	6,00	6,00	8,00	5,00	4,00
oxymorphine	8,00	5,00	6,00	8,00	8,00	5,20	3,50
pentazocine	7,00	2,00	4,00	7,00	5,00	2,90	3,00
propoxyphene	5,00	2,00	4,00	5,00	5,00	3,30	2,00
nalorphine	2,00	3,00	6,00	8,00	1,00	1,40	3,20
levallorphan	3,00	2,00	5,00	4,00	1,00	11,00	5,00
cyclazocine	2,00	3,00	6,00	3,00	2,00	1,60	2,80
naloxone	1,00	2,00	5,00	8,00	1,00	1,20	3,00
naltrexone	1,00	3,00	5,00	8,00	,00	9,70	14,00
alfentanil	7,00	6,00	7,00	4,00	6,00	1,60	,50
alphaprodine	6,00	5,00	6,00	3,00	5,00	2,20	2,00
fentanyl	6,00	5,00	7,00	5,00	4,00	3,70	,50
meptazinol	4,00	3,00	5,00	5,00	3,00	1,60	2,00
nor propoxyphene	8,00	6,00	8,00	5,00	7,00	6,00	4,00
sufentanil	7,00	6,00	8,00	6,00	8,00	2,60	5,00
newdrug1	5,00	5,00	4,00	3,00	6,00	5,00	12,00
newdrug2	8,00	6,00	3,00	4,00	5,00	7,00	16,00

Var = variable
Var 1 analgesia score (0-10)
Var 2 antitussive score (0-10)
Var 3 constipation score (0-10)
Var 4 respiratory depression score (1-10)
Var 5 abuse liability score (1-10)
Var 6 elimination time ($t_{1/2}$ in hours)
Var 7 duration time analgesia (hours)

The data file is entitled "nearestneighbor" and is in extras.springer.com.

SPSS statistical software is used for data analysis. Start by opening the data file. The drug names included, eight variables are in the file. A ninth variable entitled "partition" must be added with the value 1 for the opioids 1–25 and 0 for the two new compounds (cases 26 and 27).

Then Command:

Analyze....Classify....Nearest Neighbor Analysis....enter the variable "drugsname" in Target....enter the variables "analgesia" to "duration of analgesia" in Features....click Partitions....click Use variable to assign cases....enter the variable "Partition"....click OK.

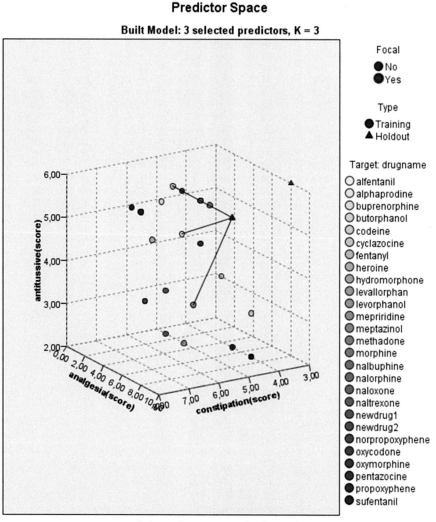

Predictor Space

Built Model: 3 selected predictors, K = 3

Select points to use as focal records

This chart is a lower-dimensional projection of the predictor space, which contains a total of 7 predictors.

Example   23

The above figure shows as an example the place of the two new compounds (the small triangles) as compared with those of the standard opioids. Lines connect them to their 3 nearest neighbors. In SPSS' original output sheets the graph can by double-clicking be placed in the "model viewer", and, then, (after again clicking on it) be interactively rotated in order to improve the view of the distances. SPSS uses 3 nearest neighbors by default, but you can change this number if you like. The names of the compounds are given in alphabetical order. Only three of 7 variables are given in the initial figure, but if you click on one of the small triangles in this figure, an auxiliary view comes up right from the main view. Here are all the details of the analysis. The upper left graph of it shows that the opioids 21, 3, and 23 have the best average nearest neighbor records for case 26 (new drug 1). The seven figures alongside and underneath this figure give the distances between these three and case 26 for each of the seven features (otherwise called predictor variables).

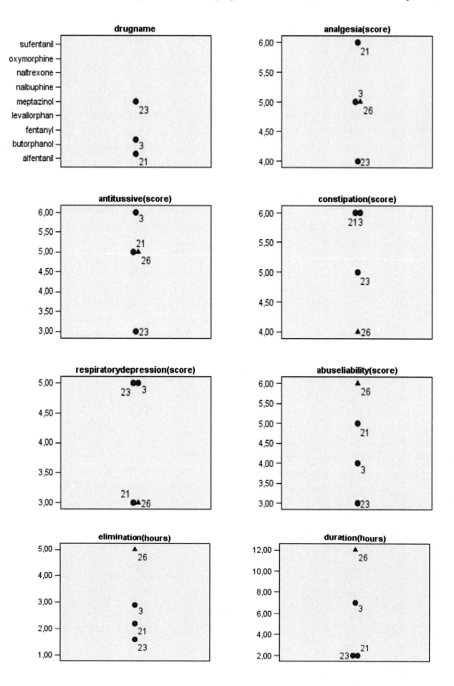

Example   25

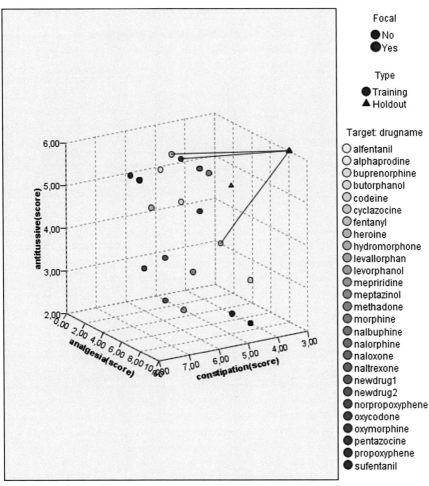

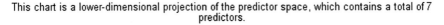

Select points to use as focal records

This chart is a lower-dimensional projection of the predictor space, which contains a total of 7 predictors.

If you click on the other triangle (representing case 27 (newdrug 2) in the initial figure, the connecting lines with the nearest neighbors of this drug comes up. This is shown in the above figure, which is the main view for drug 2. Using the same manoeuvre as above produces again the auxiliary view showing that the opioids 3, 1, and 11 have the best average nearest neighbor records for case 27 (new drug 2). The seven figures alongside and underneath this figure give again the distances between these three and case 27 for each of the seven features (otherwise called predictor variables). The auxiliary view is shown underneath.

Peers Chart

Focal Records and Nearest Neighbors

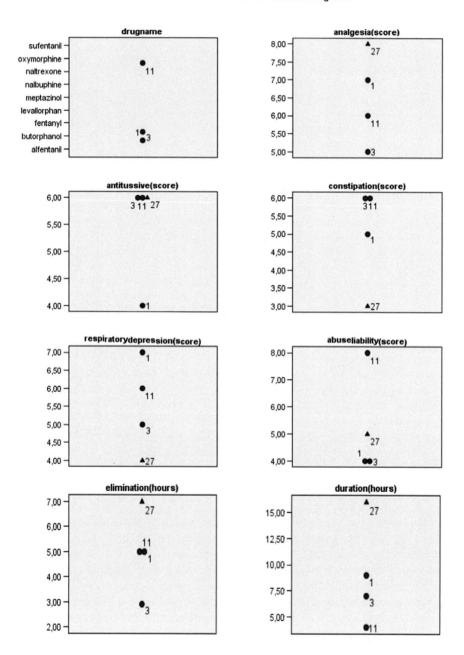

Conclusion

Nearest neighbor methodology enables to readily identify the places of new drugs within their classes of drugs. For example, newly developed opioid compounds can be compared with standard opioids in order to determine their potential places in therapeutic regimens.

Note

Nearest neighbor cluster methodology has a long history and has initially been used for missing data imputation in demographic data files (see Statistics applied to clinical studies 5th edition, 2012, Chap. 22, Missing data, pp. 253–266, Springer Heidelberg Germany, from the same authors).

Chapter 5
Predicting High-Risk-Bin Memberships (1445 Families)

General Purpose

Optimal bins describe continuous predictor variables in the form of best fit categories for making predictions, e.g., about families at high risk of' bank loan defaults. In addition, it can be used for, e.g., predicting health risk cut-offs about families, based on their characteristics (Chap. 61).

Background

Bins are equally-spaced intervals that are used to sort data. If on graphs, it will usually be called histograms. By default, the number of values in each bin is represented by bars on histograms or by stacks of dots on dotplots. For example, on the underneath histogram, the height of each bar represents the frequency of observations within the corresponding range of values. On the underneath dotplot, the height of each stack of dots represents the frequency of observations within the corresponding range of values.

This chapter was previously published in "Machine learning in medicine-cookbook 2" as Chap. 2, Springern Heidelberg Germany, 2014.

Electronic Supplementary Material The online version of this chapter (https://doi.org/10.1007/978-3-030-33970-8_5) contains supplementary material, which is available to authorized users.

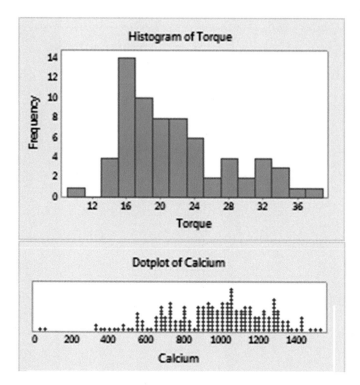

The optimal binning procedure discretizes a scale variable, such that bin formation will be optimal. Bin formation will be optimal, if it is according to a categorical variable that "supervises" the binning process. Bins can then be used as consecutive intervals of one (or more) variables. Examples include (1) categorical variables of crosstabs, (2) binned values instead of actual values safeguarding the privacy of your data sources, (3) reduced bin numbers instead of distinct values for improved process efficiencies. Histograms are an example of a method using binning. To construct a histogram, the first step is to "bin" (or "bucket") the range of values, that is, divide the entire range of values into a series of intervals, and, then, count how many values fall into different intervals.

Specific Scientific Question

Can optimal binning also be applied for other medical purposes, e.g., for finding high risk cut-offs for overweight children in particular families?

Example

A data file of 1445 families was assessed for learning the best fit cut-off values of unhealthy lifestyle estimators to maximize the difference between low and high risk of overweight children. These cut-off values were, subsequently, used to determine the risk profiles (the characteristics) in individual future families.

Var 1	Var 2	Var 3	Var 4	Var 5
0	11	1	8	0
0	7	1	9	0
1	25	7	0	1
0	11	4	5	0
1	5	1	8	1
0	10	2	8	0
0	11	1	6	0
0	7	1	8	0
0	7	0	9	0
0	15	3	0	0

Var = variable
Var 1 fruitvegetables (times per week)
Var 2 unhealthysnacks (times per week)
Var 3 fastfoodmeal (times per week)
Var 4 physicalactivities (times per week)
Var 5 overweightchildren (0 = no, 1 = yes)

Only the first 10 families of the original learning data file are given, the entire data file is entitled "optimalbinning1" and is in extras.springer.com.

Optimal Binning

SPSS 19.0 is used for analysis. Start by opening the data file.

Command
Transform....Optimal Binning....Variables into Bins: enter fruitvegetables, unhealthysnacks, fastfoodmeal, physicalactivities....Optimize Bins with Respect to: enter "overweightchildren"....click Output....Display: mark Endpoints.... mark Descriptive statistics....mark Model Entropy....click Save: mark Create variables that contain binned data....Save Binning Rules in a Syntax file: click Browse....open appropriate folder....File name: enter, e.g., "exportoptimalbinning"....click Save....click OK.

fruitvegetables/wk

Bin	End Point		Number of Cases by Level of overweight children		
	Lower	Upper	No	Yes	Total
1	a	14	802	340	1142
2	14	a	274	29	303
Total			1076	369	1445

unhealthysnacks/wk

Bin	End Point		Number of Cases by Level of overweight children		
	Lower	Upper	No	Yes	Total
1	a	12	830	143	973
2	12	19	188	126	314
3	19	a	58	100	158
Total			1076	369	1445

fastfoodmeal/wk

Bin	End Point		Number of Cases by Level of overweight children		
	Lower	Upper	No	Yes	Total
1	a	2	896	229	1125
2	2	a	180	140	320
Total			1076	369	1445

physicalactivities/wk

Bin	End Point		Number of Cases by Level of overweight children		
	Lower	Upper	No	Yes	Total
1	a	8	469	221	690
2	8	a	607	148	755
Total			1076	369	1445

Each bin is computed as Lower <= physicalactivities/wk < Upper.

a. Unbounded

In the output sheets the above tables are given. It shows the high risk cut-offs for overweight children of the four predicting factors. E.g., in 1142 families scoring under 14 units of (1) fruit/vegetable per week, are put into bin 1 and 303 scoring over 14 units per week, are put into bin 2. The proportion of overweight children in bin 1 is much larger than it is in bin 2: 340/1142 = 0.298 (30%) and 29/303 = 0.096 (10%). Similarly high risk cut-offs are found for (2) unhealthy snacks less than

12, 12–19, and over 19 per week, (3) fastfood meals less than 2, and over 2 per week, (4) physical activities less than 8 and over 8 per week. These cut-offs will be used as meaningful recommendation limits to eleven future families.

fruit	snacks	fastfood	physical
13	11	4	5
2	5	3	9
12	23	9	0
17	9	6	5
2	3	3	3
10	8	4	3
15	9	3	6
9	5	3	8
2	5	2	7
9	13	5	0
28	3	3	9

Var = variable
Var 1 fruitvegetables (times per week)
Var 2 unhealthysnacks (times per week)
Var 3 fastfoodmeal (times per week)
Var 4 physicalactivities (times per week)

The saved syntax file entitled "exportoptimalbinning.sps" will now be used to compute the predicted bins of some future families. Enter the above values in a new data file, entitled, e.g., "optimalbinning2", and save in the appropriate folder in your computer. Then open up the data file "exportoptimalbinning.sps" ....subsequently click File....click Open....click Data....Find the data file entitled "optimalbinning2"....click Open....click "exportoptimalbinning.sps" from the file palette at the bottom of the screen....click Run....click All.

When returning to the Data View of "optimalbinning2", we will find the underneath overview of all of the bins selected for our eleven future families.

fruit	snacks	fastfood	physical	fruit_bin	snacks_bin	fastfood_bin	physical_bin
13	11	4	5	1	1	2	1
2	5	3	9	1	1	2	2
12	23	9	0	1	3	2	1
17	9	6	5	2	1	2	1
2	3	3	3	1	1	2	1
10	8	4	3	1	1	2	1
15	9	3	6	2	1	2	1
9	5	3	8	1	1	2	2
2	5	2	7	1	1	2	1
9	13	5	0	1	2	2	1
28	3	3	9	2	1	2	2

This overview is relevant, since families in high risk bins would particularly qualify for counseling.

Conclusion

Optimal bins describe continuous predictor variables in the form of best fit categories for making predictions, and SPSS statistical software can be used to generate a syntax file, called SPS file, for predicting risk cut-offs in future families. In this way families highly at risk for overweight can be readily identified. The nodes of decision trees can be used for similar purposes (Machine learming in medicine Cookbook One, Chap. 16, Decision trees for decision analysis, pp. 97–104, Springer Heidelberg Germany, 2014), but it has subgroups of cases, rather than multiple bins for a single case.

Note

More background, theoretical and mathematical information of optimal binning.
   is given in Machine Learning in Medicine Part Three, Chap. 5, Optimal binning, pp. 37–48, Springer Heidelberg Germany 2013, and Machine learning in medicine Cookbook One, Optimal binning, Chap.19, pp. 101–106, Springer Heidelberg Germany, 2014, both from the same authors.

Chapter 6
Predicting Outlier Memberships (2000 Patients)

General Purpose

With large data files, outlier recognition requires a more sophisticated approach than the traditional data plots and regression lines. This chapter is to examine whether BIRCH (balanced iterative reducing and clustering using hierarchies) clustering is able to predict outliers in future patients from a known population.

Background

Graphs like data plots and regression lines are convenient for visualizing outliers in therapeutic data patterns, and have been successfully used for that purpose for centuries. They are, however, arbitrary, and, with large data files, both data pattern and outlier recognition require a more sophisticated approach. Also, the number of outliers, generally, tends to rise linearly with the sample size. BIRCH is the abbreviation of "balanced iterative reducing and clustering using hierarchies". It was introduced by 3 computer scientists from Wisconsin University in 1996, and is available in SPSS's module Classify, under "two-step cluster analysis", since 2001. It is an unsupervised data mining methodology suitable for very large datasets, but can also be applied for small data. It is, currently, mainly used by econo- and sociometrists, and, like other machine learning methods, little used in therapeutic research. This is, probably, due to the traditional belief of clinicians in clinical trials where outliers are assumed to be equally balanced by the randomization process and

---

This chapter was previously published in "Machine learning in medicine-cookbook 2" as Chap. 3, Springer Heidelberg Germany, 2014.

Electronic Supplementary Material The online version of this chapter (https://doi.org/10.1007/978-3-030-33970-8_6) contains supplementary material, which is available to authorized users.

T. J. Cleophas, A. H. Zwinderman, *Machine Learning in Medicine – A Complete Overview*, https://doi.org/10.1007/978-3-030-33970-8_6

are not further taken into account. In contrast, modern computer data files often involve large uncontrolled data files, and arbitrary methods like scatter plots do not adequately detect outliers in the data.

The current chapter, using a real data example, examines whether BIRCH clustering is able to detect previously unrecognized outlier data. Step by step analyses were performed for the convenience of investigators. This chapter was also written as a hand-hold presentation accessible to clinicians and a must read publication for those new to the method.

We will use 2-dimensional data for simplicity, but multidimensional data can be applied as well. With traditional clustering methods like hierarchical and k-means clustering (see Chap. 1) clusters are identified by computing their data distances, taking their differences along the x and y-axes. BIRCH clustering uses sums of squares of the x- and y-values to summarize the data of the clusters. It also uses repeated binary partitions of the data to form clusters with each cluster having its own metrics, in terms of size and sum of squares. By iteration the software tries and finds the best fit metrics for the data given, meaning, that clusters can be split and thresholds for forming new clusters are chosen. The computation is rather complex, because all possible combinations of the data are checked by the computer. For example, with only 4 data 6 clusters of two are possible, with 100 data five thousand are possible, etc. Large clusters, generally, produce large metrics, small clusters produce small metrics, and it not only depends on the size of the metrics, but also on the investigators' preferences, which numbers of clusters will ultimately be chosen for further data interpretation. The split clusters can be viewed as the branches of a tree and binary partitioning of the branches increases the height of the tree. The higher the tree, the more time the clustering operation takes.

A major problem of clustering analysis is that it is time-costly and may run out of computer memory. Sometimes, memory allocation, using additional computers, is the only solution. As an example, a tree with binary branches can contain $2^0 + 2^1 + 2^2 + 2 \ldots = 2^{h+1} - 1$ branches on top of one another, where h = the number of branch layers. If we neglect the "1"terms, we will find $h > {}^2\log (n)$. With n = number of branches = 1000, a tree of 10 branch layers would be mostly cost-efficient in terms of computing time / required computer memory. BIRCH clustering manages to keep the height of the tree small, and uses for that purpose cluster rotation by moving branches with multiple clusters up and those with few clusters down.

For the identification of outliers BIRCH applies a-priori given tree capacities. If the tree is full, and cannot further accept any patients, then the patients with the worst fit to the formed clusters will be moved into a so-called noise cluster, otherwise called outlier cluster.

SPSS also offers advanced options: tree capacities can be somewhat improved by changing metrics. This should, however, be handled with care, as it can easily lead to loose and meaningless clusters, and loss of system performance.

Example   37

Specific Scientific Question

Is the XML (eXtended Markup Lamguage) file from a 2000 patient sample capable of making predictions about cluster memberships and outlierships in future patients from the target population.

Example

In a 2000 patient study of hospital admissions 576 possibly iatrogenic admissions were identified. Based on age and numbers of co-medications a two step BIRCH cluster analysis will be performed. SPSS version 19 and up can be used for the purpose. Only the first 10 patients' data are shown underneath. The entire data file is in extras.springer.com, and is entitled "outlierdetection".

age	gender	admis	duration	mort	iatro	comorb	comed
1939,00	2,00	7,00	,00	,00	1,00	2,00	1,00
1939,00	2,00	7,00	2,00	1,00	1,00	2,00	1,00
1943,00	2,00	11,00	1,00	,00	1,00	,00	,00
1921,00	2,00	9,00	17,00	,00	1,00	3,00	3,00
1944,00	2,00	21,00	30,00	,00	1,00	3,00	3,00
1977,00	2,00	4,00	1,00	,00	1,00	1,00	1,00
1930,00	1,00	20,00	7,00	,00	1,00	2,00	2,00
1932,00	1,00	3,00	2,00	,00	1,00	4,00	4,00
1927,00	1,00	9,00	13,00	1,00	1,00	1,00	2,00
1920,00	2,00	23,00	8,00	,00	1,00	3,00	3,00

admis = admission indication code
duration = days of admission
mort = mortality
iatro = iatrogenic admission
comorb = number of comrbidities
comed = number of comedications

Start by Opening the File. Then Command

click Transform....click Random Number Generators....click Set Starting Point....click Fixed Value (2000000)....click OK....click Analyze.... Classify....Two Step Cluster Analysis ....Continuous Variables: enter age and co-medications....Distance Measure: mark Euclidean....Clustering Criterion: mark Schwarz's Bayesian Criterion....click Options: mark Use noise handling ....percentage: enter 25....Assumed Standardized: enter age and co-medications ....click Continue....mark Pivot tables....mark Charts and tables in Model Viewer....Working Data File: mark Create Cluster membership variable....XML

Files: mark Export final model....click Browse....select the appropriate folder in your computer....File Name: enter, e.g., "exportanomalydetection"....click Save....click Continue....click OK.

In the output sheets the underneath distribution of clusters is given.

Cluster Distribution

		N	% of Combined	% of Total
Cluster	1	181	31,4%	9,1%
	2	152	26,4%	7,6%
	3	69	12,0%	3,5%
	Outlier (-1)	174	30,2%	8,7%
	Combined	576	100,0%	28,8%
Excluded Cases		1424		71,2%
Total		2000		100,0%

Additional details are given in Machine learning in medicine Part Two, Chap. 10, Anomaly detection, pp. 93–103, Springer Heidelberg Germany, 2013. The large outlier category consisted mainly of patients of all ages and extremely many co-medications. When returning to the Data View screen, we will observe that SPSS has created a novel variable entitled "TSC_5980" containing the patients' cluster memberships. The patients given the value -1 are the outliers.

With Scoring Wizard and the exported XML (eXtended Markup Language) file entitled "exportanomalydetection" we can now try and predict from age and number of co-medications of future patients the best fit cluster membership according to the computed XML model.

age	comed
1954,00	1,00
1938,00	7,00
1929,00	8,00
1967,00	1,00
1945,00	2,00
1936,00	3,00
1928,00	4,00

comed = number of co-medications

Enter the Above Data in a Novel Data File and Command:
Utilities....click Scoring Wizard....click Browse....Open the appropriate folder with the XML file entitled "exportanomalydetection"....click on the latter and click

Select. . . .in Scoring Wizard double-click Next. . . .mark Predicted Value . . . .click Finish.

age	comed	PredictedValue
1954,00	1,00	3,00
1938,00	7,00	-1,00
1929,00	8,00	-1,00
1967,00	1,00	3,00
1945,00	2,00	-1,00
1936,00	3,00	1,00
1928,00	4,00	-1,00

PredictedValue = predicted cluster membership

In the above novel data file SPSS has provided the new variable as requested. One patient is in cluster 1, two are in cluster 3, and 4 patients are in the outlier cluster.

Conclusion

With the help of BIRCH clustering an XML (eXtended Markup Language) file from a 2000 patient sample is capable of making predictions about cluster memberships and outlierships in future patients from the same target population.

Note

More background theoretical and mathematical information of outlier detection.
     is available Machine learning in medicine part two, Chap. 10, Anomaly detection, pp. 93–103, Springer Heidelberg Germany, 2013, from the same authors.

Chapter 7
Data Mining for Visualization of Health Processes (150 Patients)

General Purpose

Computer files of clinical data are often complex and multi-dimensional, and they are, frequently, hard to statistically test. Instead, visualization processes can be successfully used as an alternative approach to traditional statistical data analysis.

Background

KNIME, the Konstanz Information Miner, is a free and open-source data analytics, reporting and integration platform. KNIME integrates various components for machine learning and data mining through its modular data pipelining. It has a GNU (General Public License) licence, and has been written in Java. It operates in Linux, OS X, Windows, and has a stable release since 2006. Knime (Konstanz information miner) software has been developed by computer scientists from Silicon Valley in collaboration with technicians from Konstanz University at the Bodensee in Switzerland, and it pays particular attention to visual data analysis. It is used since 2006 as a package through the Internet. So far, it is mainly used by chemists and pharmacists, but not by clinical investigators. This chapter is to assess, whether visual processing of clinical data may, sometimes, perform better than traditional statistical analysis.

This chapter was previously published in "Machine learning in medicine-cookbook 3" as Chap. 1, Springer Heidelberg Germany, 2014.

Electronic Supplementary Material The online version of this chapter (https://doi.org/10.1007/978-3-030-33970-8_7) contains supplementary material, which is available to authorized users.

T. J. Cleophas, A. H. Zwinderman, *Machine Learning in Medicine – A Complete Overview*, https://doi.org/10.1007/978-3-030-33970-8_7

Primary Scientific Question

Can visualization processes of clinical data provide insights that remained hidden with traditional statistical tests?

Example

Four inflammatory markers (CRP (C-reactice protein), ESR (erythrocyte sedimentation rate), leucocyte count (leucos), and fibrinogen) were measured in 150 patients with pneumonia. Based on x-ray chest clinical severity was classified as A (mild infection), B (medium severity), C (severe infection). One scientific question was to assess whether the markers could adequately predict the severity of infection.

CRP	leucos	fibrinogen	ESR	x-ray severity
120,00	5,00	11,00	60,00	A
100,00	5,00	11,00	56,00	A
94,00	4,00	11,00	60,00	A
92,00	5,00	11,00	58,00	A
100,00	5,00	11,00	52,00	A
108,00	6,00	17,00	48,00	A
92,00	5,00	14,00	48,00	A
100,00	5,00	11,00	54,00	A
88,00	5,00	11,00	54,00	A
98,00	5,00	8,00	60,00	A
108,00	5,00	11,00	68,00	A
96,00	5,00	11,00	62,00	A
96,00	5,00	8,00	46,00	A
86,00	4,00	8,00	60,00	A
116,00	4,00	11,00	50,00	A
114,00	5,00	17,00	52,00	A

CRP = C-reactive protein (mg/l)
leucos = leucyte count (*10^9/l)
fibrinogen = fibrinogen level (mg/l
ESR = erythrocyte sedimentation rate (mm)
x-ray severity = x-chest severity pneumonia score (A - C = mild to severe)

Example   43

The data file is entitled "decisiontree", and is available in extras.springer.com. Data analysis of these data in SPSS is rather limited. Start by opening the data file in SPSS statistical software.

Command click Graphs....Legacy Dialogs....Bar Charts....click Simple.... click Define....Category Axis: enter "severity score"....Variable: enter CRP.... mark Other statistics....click OK.

After performing the same procedure for the other variables four graphs are produced as shown underneath. The mean levels of all of the inflammatory markers consistently tended to rise with increasing severities of infection. Univariate multinomial logistic regression with severity as outcome gives a significant effect of all of the markers. However, this effect is largely lost in the multiple multinomial logistic regression, probably due to interactions.

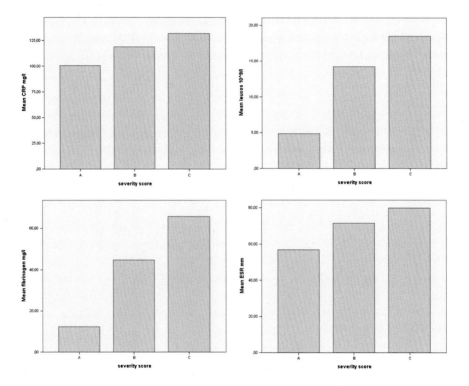

We are interested to explore these results for additional effects, for example, hidden data effects, like different predictive effects and frequency distributions for different subgroups. For that purpose Knime data miner will be applied. SPSS data files can not be downloaded directly in the Knime software, but excel files can, and SPSS data can be saved as an excel file (the cvs file type available in your computer must be used).

Command in SPSS
click File. . . .click Save as. . . .in "Save as" type: enter Comma Delimited (∗.csv). . . . click Save.

Knime Data Miner

In Google enter the term "knime". Click Download and follow instructions. After completing the pretty easy download procedure, open the knime workbench by clicking the knime welcome screen. The center of the screen displays the workflow editor like the canvas in SPSS modeler. It is empty, and can be used to build a stream of nodes, called workflow in knime. The node repository is in the left lower angle of the screen, and the nodes can be dragged to the workflow editor simply by left-clicking. The nodes are computer tools for data analysis like visualization and statistical processes. Node description is in the right upper angle of the screen. Before the nodes can be used, they have to be connected with the "file reader" node, and with one another by arrows drawn again simply by left clicking the small triangles attached to the nodes. Right clicking on the file reader enables to configure from your computer a requested data file. . . .click Browse. . . .and download from the appropriate folder a csv type Excel file. You are set for analysis now. For convenience an CSV file entitled "decisiontree" has been made available at extras. springer.com.

Knime Workflow

A knime workflow for the analysis of the above data example will be built, and the final result is shown in the underneath figure.

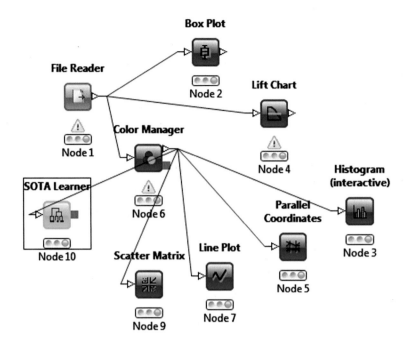

Box and Whiskers Plots

In the node repository find the node Box Plot. First click the IO option (import/ export option nodes). Then click "Read", then the File Reader node is displayed, and can be dragged by left clicking to the workflow editor. Enter the requested data file as described above. A Node dialog is displayed underneath the node entitled Node 1. Its light is orange at this stage, and should turn green before it can be applied. If you right click the node's center, and then left click File Table a preview of the data is supplied.

Now, in the search box of the node repository find and click Data Views....then "Box plot"....drag to workflow editor....connect with arrow to File reader....right click File reader....right click execute....right click Box Plot node....right click Configurate....right click Execute and open view....

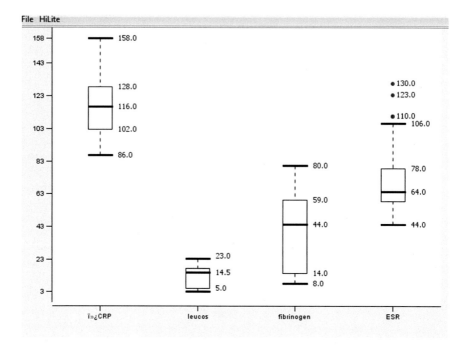

The above box plots with 95% confidence intervals of the four variable are displayed. The ESR plot shows that also outliers have been displayed The smallest confidence interval has the leucocyte count, and it may, thus, be the best predictor.

Lift Chart

In the node repository....click Lift Chart and drag to workflow editor.... connect with arrow to File reader....right click execute Lift Chart node....right click Configurate....right click Execute and open view....

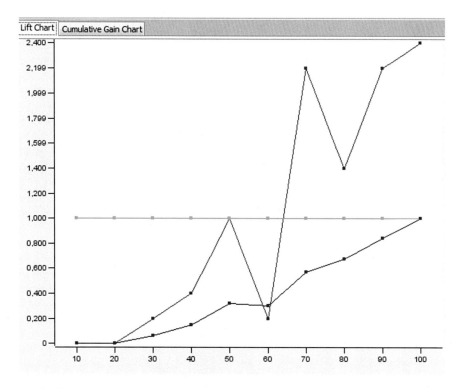

The lift chart shows the predictive performance of the data assuming that the four inflammatory markers are predictors and the severity score is the outcome. If the predictive performance is no better than random, the ratio successful prediction with/ without the model = 1.000 (the green line) The x-axis give dociles (1 = 10 = 10% of the entire sample etc). It can be observed that at 7 or more dociles the predictive performance start to be pretty good (with ratios of 2.100–2.400. Logistic regression (here multinomial logistic regression) is being used by Knime for making predictions.

Histogram

In the node repository click type color. . . .click the color manager node and drag to workflow editor. . . .in node repository click color. . . .click the Esc button of your computer. . . .click Data Views. . . .select interactive histogram and transfer to workflow editor. . . .connect color manager node with File Reader. . .connect color manager with "interactive histogram node". . . .right click Configurate. . . .right click Execute and open view. . . .

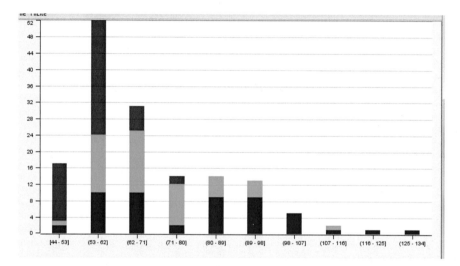

Interactive histograms with bins of ESR values are given. The colors provide the proportions of cases with mild severity (A, red), medium severity (B, green), and severe pneumonias (C, blue). It can be observed that many mild cases (red) are in the ESR 44–71 mm cut-off. Above ESR of 80 mm blue (severe pneumonia) is increasingly present. The software program has selected only the ESR values 44–134. Instead of histograms with ESR, those with other predictor variables can be made.

Line Plot

In the node repository click Data Views. . . .select the node Line plots and transfer to workflow editor. . . .connect color manager with "Line plots". . . .right click Configurate. . . .right click Execute and open view. . . .

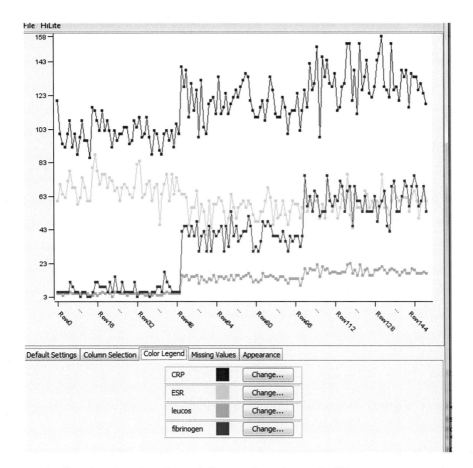

The line plot gives the values of all cases along the x-axis. The upper curve are the CRP values, The middle one the ESR values. The lower part are the leucos and fibrinogen values. The rows 0–50 are the cases with mild pneumonia, the rows 51–100 the medium severity cases, and the rows 101–150 the severe cases. It can be observed that particularly the CRP-, fibrinogen-, and leucos levels increase with increased severity of infection. This is not observed with the ESR levels.

Matrix of Scatter Plots

In the node repository click Data Views....select "Matrix of scatter plots" and transfer to workflow editor....connect color manager with "Matrix of scatter plots" ....right click Configure....right click Execute and open view....

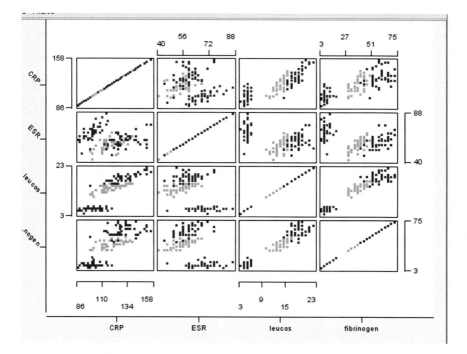

The above figure gives the results. The four predictors variables are plotted against one another. by the colors (blue for severest, red for mildest pneumonias) the fields show that the severest pneumonias are predominantly in the right upper quadrant, the mildest in the left lower quadrant.

Parallel Coordinates

In the node repository click Data Views. . . .select "Parallel coordinates" and transfer to workflow editor. . . .connect color manager with "Parallel coordinates" . . . .right click Configurate. . . .right click Execute and open view. . . .click Appearance. . . . click Draw (spline) Curves instead of lines. . . .

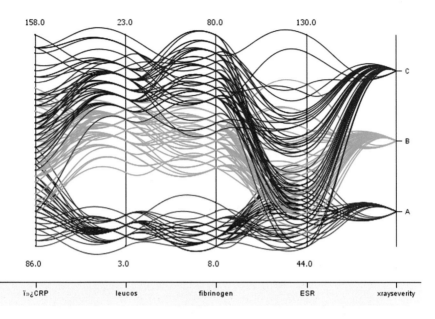

The above figure is given. It shows that the leucocyte count and fibrinogen level are excellent predictors of infection severities. CRP and ESR are also adequate predictors of infections with mild and medium severities, however, poor predictors of levels of severe infections.

Hierarchical Cluster Analysis with SOTA (Self Organizing Tree Algorithm)

In the node repository click Mining. . . .select the node SOTA (Self Organizing tree Algorithm) Learner and transfer to workflow editor. . . .connect color manager with "SOTA learner". . . .right click Configurate. . . .right click Execute and open view. . . .

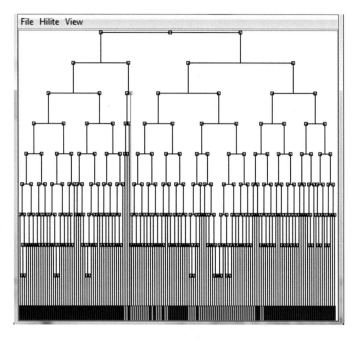

SOTA learning is a modified hierarchical cluster analysis, and it uses in this example the between-case distances of fibrinogen as variable. On the y-axis the standardized distances of the cluster combinations. Clicking the small squares interactively demonstrates the row numbers of the individual cases. It can be observed at the bottom of the figure that the severity classes very well cluster, with the mild cases (red) left, medium severity (green) in the middle, and severe cases (blue) right.

Conclusion

Clinical computer files are complex, and hard to statistically test. Instead, visualization processes can be successfully used as an alternative approach to traditional statistical data analysis. For example, Knime (Konstanz information miner) software developed by computer scientists at Konstanz University Technical Department at the Bodensee, although mainly used by chemists and pharmacists, is able to visualize multidimensional clinical data, and this approach may, sometimes, perform better than traditional statistical testing. In the current example it was able to demonstrate the clustering of inflammatory markers to identify different classes of pneumonia severity. Also to demonstrate that leucocyte count and fibrinogen were the best markers, and that ESR was a poor marker. In all of the markers the best predictive performance was obtained in the severest cases of disease. All of these observations were unobserved in the traditional statistical analysis in SPSS statistical software.

Note

More background, theoretical and mathematical information of splines and hierarchical cluster modeling are in Machine learning in medicine part one, Chap. 11, Non-linear modeling, pp. 127–143, and Chap. 15, Hierarchical cluster analysis for unsupervised data, pp. 183–195, Springer Heidelberg Germany, from the same authors.

Chapter 8
Trained Decision Trees for a More Meaningful Accuracy (150 Patients)

General Purpose

Traditionally, decision trees are used for finding the best predictors of health risks and improvements (Chap. 58). However, this method is not entirely appropriate, because a decision tree is built from a data file, and, subsequently, the same data file is applied once more for computing the health risk probabilities from the built tree. Obviously, the accuracy must be close to 100%, because the test sample is 100% identical to the sample used for building the tree, and, therefore, this accuracy does not mean too much. With neural networks this problem of duplicate usage of the same data is solved by randomly splitting the data into two samples, a training sample and a test sample (Chap. 12 in Machine learning in medicine part one, pp. 145–156, Artificial intelligence, multilayer perceptron modeling, Springer Heidelberg Germany, 2013, from the same authors). The current chapter is to assess whether the splitting methodology, otherwise called partitioning, is also feasible for decision trees, and to assess its level of accuracy. Decision trees are both appropriate for data with categorical and continuous outcome (Chap. 58).

Background

In machine learning the construction of algorithms to make predictions from data is common. The data used to build an analysis model often comes from three datasets. The first one is the training dataset, that, usually, consists of predictor and outcome

This chapter was previously published in "Machine learning in medicine-cookbook 3" as Chap. 2, 2014.

Electronic Supplementary Material The online version of this chapter (https://doi.org/10.1007/978-3-030-33970-8_8) contains supplementary material, which is available to authorized users.

© Springer Nature Switzerland AG 2020
T. J. Cleophas, A. H. Zwinderman, *Machine Learning in Medicine – A Complete Overview*, https://doi.org/10.1007/978-3-030-33970-8_8

variable. This model is run in an analytical model, like regression model, neural network, naive Bayes classifier. The result produces best fit parameters for the model applied. The second dataset is the validation dataset. This dataset uses the parameters of the best fit model from the first dataset and assesses accuracy, reliability, precision of the validation dataset as compared to the best fit model estimated. The third dataset is the test dataset, the values of which should be independent of the training dataset, but, otherwise, follows the same probability distribution as that of the training dataset. If you wish to increase validity of your data, then you may repeat the training and validation procedure, and this is called cross-validation. The problem of invalidated data is, that no information of accuracy, reliability and precision is in your data, and that your analytical model is, therefore, pretty much worthless. Data validation is the most important part of your analytical work, and according to many scientists consumes over 50% of the time spent on it (Efficacy analysis in clinical trials an update, Chap. 20, entitled Validating big data a big issue, 2019, Springer Heidelberg from the same authors).

Primary Scientific Question

Can inflammatory markers adequately predict pneumonia severities wit the help of a decision tree. Can partitioning of the data improve the methodology and is sufficient accuracy of the methodology maintained.

Example

Four inflammatory markers (CRP (C-reactice protein), ESR (erythrocyte sedimentation rate), leucocyte count (leucos), and fibrinogen) were measured in 150 patients. Based on x-ray chest clinical severity was classified as A (mild infection), B (medium severity), C (severe infection). A major scientific question was to assess what markers were the best predictors of the severity of infection.

Example 57

CRP	leucos	fibrinogen	ESR	x-ray severity
120,00	5,00	11,00	60,00	A
100,00	5,00	11,00	56,00	A
94,00	4,00	11,00	60,00	A
92,00	5,00	11,00	58,00	A
100,00	5,00	11,00	52,00	A
108,00	6,00	17,00	48,00	A
92,00	5,00	14,00	48,00	A
100,00	5,00	11,00	54,00	A
88,00	5,00	11,00	54,00	A
98,00	5,00	8,00	60,00	A
108,00	5,00	11,00	68,00	A
96,00	5,00	11,00	62,00	A
96,00	5,00	8,00	46,00	A
86,00	4,00	8,00	60,00	A
116,00	4,00	11,00	50,00	A
114,00	5,00	17,00	52,00	A

CRP = C-reactive protein (mg/l)
leucos = leucyte count ($*10^9$ /l)
fibrinogen = fibrinogen level (mg/l)
ESR = erythrocyte sedimentation rate (mm)
x-ray severity = x-chest severity pneumonia score (A - C = mild to severe)

The first 16 patients are in the above table, the entire data file is in "decisiontree" and can be obtained from "extras.springer.com"on the internet. We will start by opening the data file in SPSS.

Command
click Classify....Tree....Dependent Variable: enter severity score....Independent Variables: enter CRP, Leucos, fibrinogen, ESR....Growing Method: select CHAID....click Output: mark Tree in table format....Criteria: Parent Node type 50, Child Node type 15....click Continue........click OK.

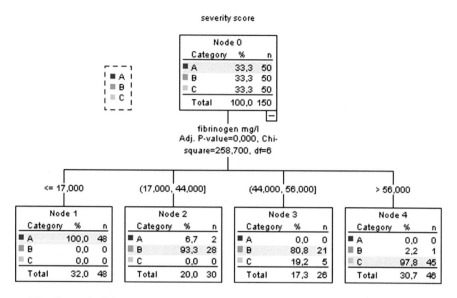

The above decision tree is displayed. A fibrinogen level < 17 is 100% predictor of severity score A (mild disease). Fibrinogen 17–44 gives 93% chance of severity B, fibrinogen 44–56 gives 81% chance of severity B, and fibrinogen >56 gives 98% chance of severity score C. The output also shows that the overall accuracy of the model is 94.7%, but we have to account that this model is somewhat flawed, because all of the data are used twice, one, for building the tree, and, second, for using the tree for making predictions.

Downloading the Knime Data Miner

In Google enter the term "knime". Click Download and follow instructions. After completing the pretty easy download procedure, open the knime workbench by clicking the knime welcome screen. The center of the screen displays the workflow editor. Like the canvas in SPSS Modeler, it is empty., and can be used to build a stream of nodes, called workflow in knime. The node repository is in the left lower angle of the screen, and the nodes can be dragged to the workflow editor simply by left-clicking. The nodes are computer tools for data analysis like visualization and statistical processes. Node description is in the right upper angle of the screen. Before the nodes can be used, they have to be connected with the "file reader" node, and with one another by arrows, drawn, again, simply by left clicking the small triangles attached to the nodes. Right clicking on the file reader enables to configure from your computer a requested data file. . . .click Browse. . . .and download from the appropriate folder a csv type Excel file. You are set for analysis now.

Note: the above data file cannot be read by the file reader, and must first be saved as csv type Excel file. For that purpose command in SPSS: click File. . . .click Save as....in "Save as type: enter Comma Delimited (∗.csv)....click Save. For your convenience it has been made available in extras.springer.com, and entitled "decisiontree".

Knime Workflow

A knime workflow for the analysis of the above data example is built, and the final result is shown in the underneath figure.

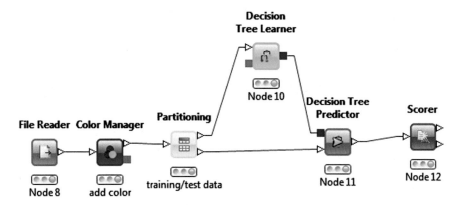

In the node repository click and type color....click the color manager node and drag to workflow editor....in node repository click again color....click the Esc button of your computer....in the node repository click again and type partitioning....the partitioning node is displayed....drag it to the workflow editor....perform the same actions and type respectively Decision Tree Learner, Decision Tree Predictor, and Scorer....Connect, by left clicking, all of the nodes with arrows as indicated above....Configurate and execute all of the nodes by right clicking the nodes and then the texts "Configurate" and "Execute"....the red lights will successively turn orange and then green....right click the Decision Tree Predictor again....right click the text "View: Decision Tree View".

The underneath decision tree comes up. It is pretty much similar to the above SPSS tree, although it does not use 150 cases but only 45 cases (the test sample from which 100 were resampled). Fibrinogen is again the best predictor. A level < 29 mg/l gives you 100% chance of severity score A. A level 29–57.5 gives 92.1% chance of Severity B, and a level over 57.5 gives 100% chance of severity C.

Right clicking the scorer node gives you the accuracy statistics, and shows that the sensitivity of A, B, an C are respectively 100, 93.3, and 90.5%, and that the overall accuracy is 94%, slightly less than that of the SPSS tree (94.7%), but still pretty good. In addition, the current analysis is appropriate, and does not use identical data twice.

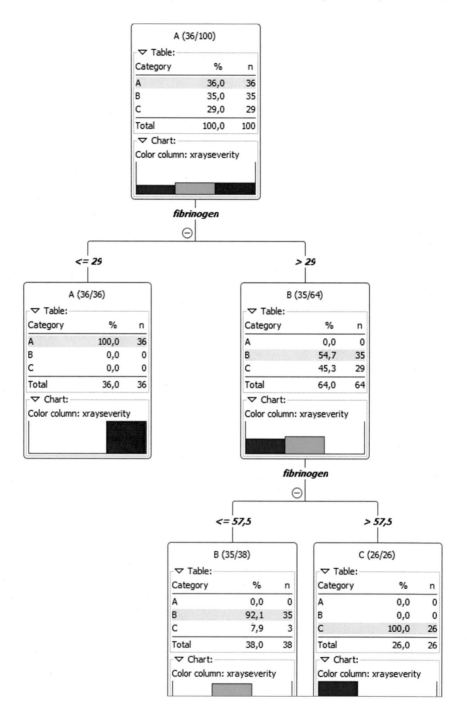

Conclusion

Traditionally, decision trees are used for finding the best predictors of health risks and improvements. However, this method is not entirely appropriate, because a decision tree is built from a data file, and, subsequently, the same data file is applied once more for computing the health risk probabilities from the built tree. Obviously, the accuracy must be close to 100%, because the test sample is 100% identical to the sample used for building the tree, and, therefore, this accuracy does not mean too much. A decision tree with partitioning of a training and a test sample provides similar results, but is scientifically less flawed, because each datum is used only once. In spite of this, little accuracy is lost.

Note

More background, theoretical and mathematical information of decision trees and neural networks are in Chap. 58, and in Machine learning in medicine part one, Chap. 12, pp. 145–156, Artificial intelligence, multilayer perceptron modeling, Springer Heidelberg Germany, 2013, both from the same authors.

Chapter 9
Typology of Medical Data (51 Patients)

General Purpose

Apart from histograms (see Chap. 1, Statistics applied to clinical studies 5th edition, "Hypotheses, data, stratification". pp. 1–14, Springer Heidelberg Germany, 2012), and Q-Q plots (Chap. 43 of current work), the typology of data and frequency procedures (to be reviewed in the Chaps. 10 and 11 of the current work) are a good way to start looking at your data. First, we will address the typology of the data.

Background

Nominal data
Nominal data are discrete data without a stepping pattern, like genders, age classes, family names. They can be assessed with pie charts, frequency tables and bar charts.
Ordinal data
Ordinal data are also discrete data, however, with a stepping pattern, like severity scores, intelligence levels, physical strength scores. They are usually assessed with frequency tables and bar charts.
Scale data
Scale data also have a stepping pattern, but, unlike ordinal data, they have steps with equal intervals. With small steps they are called continuous data. They are sometimes called quantitative data, while nominal and ordinal data are traditionally called qualitative data. The scale data are assessed with summary tables and histograms.

Electronic Supplementary Material The online version of this chapter (https://doi.org/10.1007/978-3-030-33970-8_9) contains supplementary material, which is available to authorized users.

T. J. Cleophas, A. H. Zwinderman, *Machine Learning in Medicine – A Complete Overview*, https://doi.org/10.1007/978-3-030-33970-8_9

Having understanding of different data types, also called measurement scales, is a prerequisite for doing exploratory data analysis (EDA), since you can use certain statistical measurements only for specific data types. You also need to know which data type you are dealing with to choose the right visualization method. Think of data types as a way to categorize different types of variables. We will discuss the main types of variables and look at examples for the purpose.

The typology of the data values becomes particularly important, when it comes to statistical analyses. E.g.:

1. Means and standard deviations makes no sense with nominal data.
2. The problem with ordinal data is, that the steps are usually not equal, like with scale data. With ordinal data, you will usually have a mix-up of larger and smaller steps.
3. This will bias the outcome, if you use a scale data test for their analysis. The Chap. 37 of the current book, entitled "Ordinal scaling for clinical scores with inconsistent intervals", shows how this problem can mathematically be largely solved by complementary log-log transformations.

Primary Scientific Question

In econometrics and marketing research (Foroni, Econometric models for mixed-frequency data, edited by European University of Economics, Florence, 2012), frequency procedures are routinely used for the assessment of nominal, ordinal and scale data. Can they also be adequately applied for assessing medical data?

Example

The patients of an internist's outpatient clinic are reviewed.

Example   65

nominal variable	ordinal variable	scale variable
agegroup	severity	time
2,00	2,00	2,50
2,00	1,00	6,00
2,00	1,00	2,50
1,00	3,00	2,00
1,00	1,00	5,00
2,00	1,00	4,00
2,00	3,00	,50
1,00	1,00	2,50
2,00	3,00	4,00
2,00	2,00	1,50

agegroup: 1 = senior, 2 = adult, 3 = adolescent, 4 = child
severity: complaint severity scores 1-4
time: consulting time (minutes)

The first 10 patients are in the above table. The entire file (51 patients) is entitled "frequencies", and is available at extras.springer.com. We will start by opening the file in SPSS statistical software.

Nominal Variable

Command
click   Analyze....Descriptive   Statistics....Frequencies....Variable(s):   enter agegroups....mark   Display   frequency   tables....click   Charts....click   Pie charts....click OK.

The underneath pie chart shows that seniors and adults predominate and that children are just a small portion of the outpatient clinic population.

age group

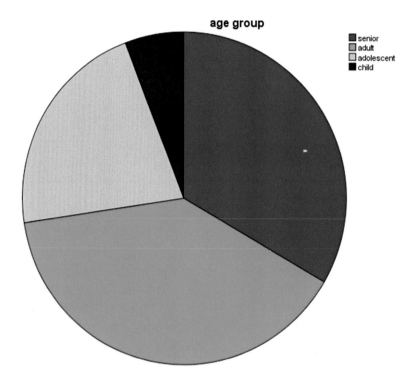

The frequency table shows precise frequencies of the nominal categories.

age group

		Frequency	Percent	Valid Percent	Cumulative Percent
Valid	senior	17	33,3	33,3	33,3
	adult	20	39,2	39,2	72,5
	adolescent	11	21,6	21,6	94,1
	child	3	5,9	5,9	100,0
	Total	51	100,0	100,0	

If you wish, you could present your data in the form of descending or ascending frequencies.

Command
click   Analyze....Descriptive   Statistics....Frequencies....Variable(s):   enter agegroups ....mark Display frequency tables....click Charts....click Bar charts....click Continue ....click Format....click Descending counts....click Continue.......click OK.

Example   67

The underneath graph is in the output sheet. It shows an ordered bar chart with adults as largest category.

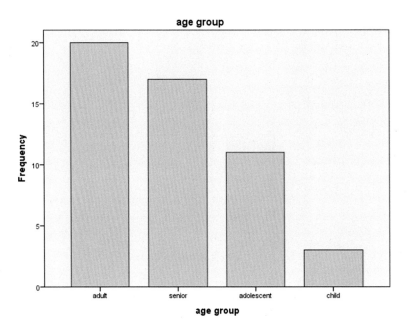

Ordinal Variable

Command
click Analyze....Descriptive Statistics....Frequencies....Variable(s): enter severity ....mark Display frequency tables....click Charts....click Bar charts....click Continue ....click Format....click Ascending counts....click Continue....... click OK.

According to the severity score count the underneath graph shows the percentages of patients. Most of them are in the score one category, least of them in the score five category.

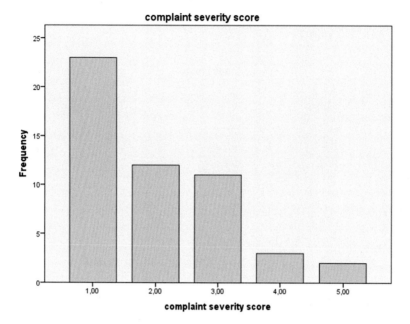

The table gives the precise numbers of patients in each category as well as the percentages. If we have missing values, the valid percent column will give the adjusted percentages, while the cumulative percentage gives the categories one and two, one and two and three etc. percentages.

complaint severity score

		Frequency	Percent	Valid Percent	Cumulative Percent
Valid	1,00	23	45,1	45,1	45,1
	2,00	12	23,5	23,5	68,6
	3,00	11	21,6	21,6	90,2
	4,00	3	5,9	5,9	96,1
	5,00	2	3,9	3,9	100,0
	Total	51	100,0	100,0	

Example   69

Scale Variable

Command

click Analyze....Descriptive Statistics....Frequencies....Variable(s): enter time ....remove mark from "Display frequency tables"....click Statistics....mark Quartiles....Std.deviations....Minimum....Maximum.... Mean....Median .... Skewness....Kurtosis....click   Continue....then   click   Charts.... Histograms...mark Show normal curve on histogram....click Continue.... click OK.

The statistics table tells us that the consulting time is 3,42 min on average, and 50% of the consults are between 2 and 4 min. The most extreme consults took 0,5 and 15,0 min.

Statistics

consulting time (min)

N	Valid		51
	Missing		0
Mean			3,4216
Median			2,5000
Std. Deviation			2,99395
Skewness			2,326
Std. Error of Skewness			,333
Kurtosis			5,854
Std. Error of Kurtosis			,656
Minimum			,50
Maximum			15,00
Percentiles	25		2,0000
	50		2,5000
	75		4,0000

The histogram shows the frequency distribution of the data and suggests skewness to the right. Most of the consults took as little as less than 5 min but some took no less than 5–15 min. This means that the data are not very symmetric and means, and that standard deviation are not very accurate to summarize these data.

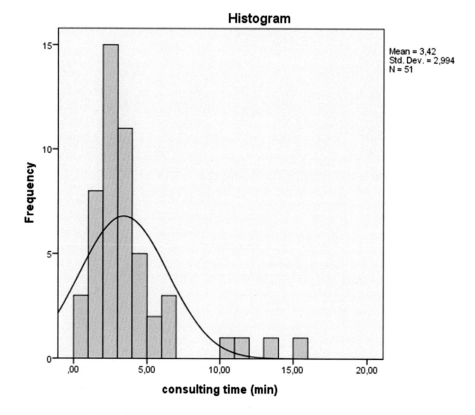

Indeed, a significant level of skewness to the right is in the data, because 2326/0,333 = 6985 is much larger than 1,96 (see the above table). We will try and use a logarithmic transformation of these skewed data. Because this often "normalizes" the skewness.

Command
click Transform. . . .Compute Variable. . . .type logtime in Target Variable. . . .type ln (time) in Numeric Expression. . . .click OK.

In the main screen it can be observed that SPSS now has produced a novel variable entitled "logtime". We will perform the scale variable analysis again, and replace the variable "time" with "logtime".

Command
click   Analyze. . . .Descriptive   Statistics. . . .Frequencies. . . .Variable(s):   enter logtime. . . .click   Charts. . . .Histograms. . .mark   Show   normal   curve   on histogram. . . .click Continue. . . .click OK.

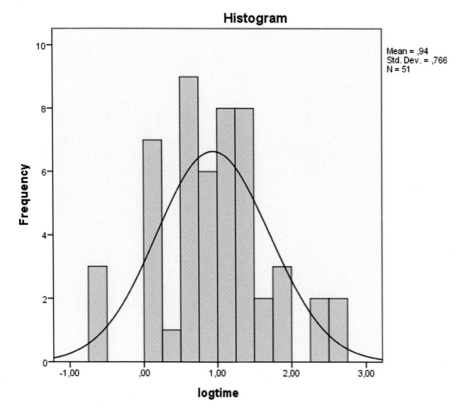

In the output sheets the underneath graph is shown. The data distribution looks less skewed and much closer to a normal distribution now. The logtime data can now be used for data analysis using normal statistical tests.

Conclusion

Data can be classified as nominal, ordinal and scale. For each type frequencies and frequency distributions can readily be calculated, and they enable an unbiased view of their patterns. Nominal data have no mean value. Ordinal data are tricky, because, although they have a stepping pattern, they offer a mix-up of larger and smaller steps. Ordinal regression can largely adjust this irregularity. Skewed scale data often benefit from log-data transformations.

Note

More background, theoretical and mathematical information of ordinal data is given in Chap. 37 of the current book, entitled "Ordinal scaling for clinical scores with inconsistent intervals".

Chapter 10
Predictions from Nominal Clinical Data (450 Patients)

General Purpose

In Chap. 9 the typology of medical data was reviewed. Nominal data are discrete data without a stepping function like genders, age classes, family names. They can be assessed with pie charts, frequency tables and bar charts. Statistical testing is not of much interest. Statistical testing becomes, however, interesting, if we want to know whether two nominal variables like treatment modality and treatment outcome are differently distributed between one another. An interaction matrix of these two nominal variables could, then, be used to test, whether one treatment performs better than the other.

Background

Nominal data

Nominal data are discrete data without a stepping pattern, like genders, age classes, family names. They can be assessed with pie charts, frequency tables and bar charts.

Ordinal data

Ordinal data are also discrete data, however, with a stepping pattern, like severity scores, intelligence levels, physical strength scores. They are usually assessed with frequency tables and bar charts.

Scale data

Scale data also have a stepping pattern, but, unlike ordinal data, they have steps with equal intervals. With small steps they are called continuous data. They are

Electronic Supplementary Material The online version of this chapter (https://doi.org/10.1007/978-3-030-33970-8_10) contains supplementary material, which is available to authorized users.

T. J. Cleophas, A. H. Zwinderman, *Machine Learning in Medicine – A Complete Overview*, https://doi.org/10.1007/978-3-030-33970-8_10

sometimes called quantitative data, while nominal and ordinal data are traditionally called qualitative data. The scale data are assessed with summary tables and histograms.

Having understanding of different data types, also called measurement scales, is a prerequisite for doing exploratory data analysis (EDA), since you can use certain statistical measurements only for specific data types. You also need to know which data type you are dealing with to choose the right visualization method. Think of data types as a way to categorize different types of variables. We will discuss the main types of variables and look at examples for the purpose.

The typology of the data values becomes particularly important, when it comes to statistical analyses. E.g.:

1. Means and standard deviations makes no sense with nominal data.
2. The problem with ordinal data is, that the steps are usually not equal, like with scale data. With ordinal data you will usually have a mix-up of larger and smaller steps.
3. This biases the outcome, if you use a scale data test for their analysis. The Chap. 37 of the current book, entitled "Ordinal scaling for clinical scores with inconsistent intervals", shows how this problem can mathematically be largely solved by complementary log-log transformations.

Primary Scientific Question

This chapter assesses the relationship between four treatment modalities, and, as outcome, five levels of quality of life (qol). Can an interaction matrix, otherwise called contingency table or crosstab, be used to assess whether some treatment modalities are associated with a better qol score than others, and to assess the directions of the differences in distribution of the variables.

Example

In 450 patients with coronary artery disease four complementary treatment modalities, including cardiac fitness, physiotherapy, wellness, and hydrotherapy, were assessed for quality of life scores. The first 10 patients are in the table underneath. The entire data file is entitled "qol", and is in extras.springer.com. The example is also used in the Chap. 11. SPSS is applied for analysis.

Example   75

treatment	counseling	qol	sat doctor
3	1	4	4
4	0	2	1
2	1	5	4
3	0	4	4
2	1	2	1
2	0	1	4
4	0	4	1
3	0	4	1
4	1	4	4
2	1	3	4

treatment	= treatment modality (1 = cardiac fitness, 2 = physiotherapy, 3 = wellness, 4 = hydrotherapy, 5 = nothing)
counseling	= counseling given (0 = no, 1 = yes)
qol	= quality of life score (1 = very low, 5 = vey high)
sat doctor	= satisfaction with doctor (1 = very low, 5 = very high)

Start by opening the data file in SPSS statistical software.

Command

Analyze....Descriptive Statistics....Crosstabs....Rows: enter "treatment".... Columns: enter "qol score"....click Statistics....mark Chi-square....click Continue....click OK.

In the output sheets the underneath tables are given.

treatment * qol score Crosstabulation

Count

		qol score					
		very low	low	medium	high	very high	Total
treatment	cardiac fitness	21	21	16	24	36	118
	physiotherapy	22	20	18	20	20	100
	wellness	23	14	12	30	25	104
	hydrotherapy	20	18	25	35	30	128
Total		86	73	71	109	111	450

Both hydrotherapy and cardiac fitness produce highest qol scores.

Chi-Square Tests

	Value	df	Asymp. Sig. (2-sided)
Pearson Chi-Square	12,288[a]	12	,423
Likelihood Ratio	12,291	12	,423
Linear-by-Linear Association	,170	1	,680
N of Valid Cases	450		

a. 0 cells (,0%) have expected count less than 5. The minimum expected count is 15,78.

However, the cells are not significantly different from one another, and so the result is due to chance. We have clinical arguments that counseling may support the beneficial effects of treatments, and, therefore, perform an analysis with two layers, one in the patients with and one in those without counseling.

Command

Analyze. . . .Descriptive Statistics. . . .Crosstabs. . . .Rows: enter "treatment". . . . Columns: enter "qol score". . . .Layer 1 of 1: enter "counseling". . . .click Statistics . . . . mark Chi-square. . . .mark Contingency coefficient. . . .mark Phi and Cramer's V. . . . mark Lambda. . . .mark Uncertainty coefficient. . . .click Continue. . . .click OK.

The underneath tables are in the output sheets.

treatment * qol score * counseling Crosstabulation

Count

counseling			qol score					Total
			very low	low	medium	high	very high	
No	treatment	cardiac fitness	19	16	8	8	14	65
		physiotherapy	8	8	7	7	15	45
		wellness	23	8	6	15	9	61
		hydrotherapy	15	14	9	10	11	59
	Total		65	46	30	40	49	230
Yes	treatment	cardiac fitness	2	5	8	16	22	53
		physiotherapy	14	12	11	13	5	55
		wellness	0	6	6	15	16	43
		hydrotherapy	5	4	16	25	19	69
	Total		21	27	41	69	62	220

Example   77

Chi-Square Tests

counseling		Value	df	Asymp. Sig. (2-sided)
No	Pearson Chi-Square	14,831[a]	12	,251
	Likelihood Ratio	14,688	12	,259
	Linear-by-Linear Association	,093	1	,760
	N of Valid Cases	230		
Yes	Pearson Chi-Square	42,961[b]	12	,000
	Likelihood Ratio	44,981	12	,000
	Linear-by-Linear Association	,517	1	,472
	N of Valid Cases	220		

Obviously, if we assess the subjects who received counseling, then the high scores appear to appear very significantly more often in the hydrotherapy and cardiac fitness patients than in the physiotherapy and wellness groups.

Symmetric Measures

counseling			Value	Approx. Sig.
No	Nominal by Nominal	Phi	,254	,251
		Cramer's V	,147	,251
		Contingency Coefficient	,246	,251
	N of Valid Cases		230	
Yes	Nominal by Nominal	Phi	,442	,000
		Cramer's V	,255	,000
		Contingency Coefficient	,404	,000
	N of Valid Cases		220	

Also the phi value, which is the ratio of the computed Pearson chi-square value and the number of observations, are statistically significant. They support that the differences observed in the yes-counseling group are real findings, not chance findings. Cramer's V and contingency coefficient are rescaled phi values, and furthermore support this conclusion.

Directional Measures

counseling				Value	Asymp. Std. Error[a]	Approx. T[b]	Approx. Sig.
No	Nominal by Nominal	Lambda	Symmetric	,061	,038	1,570	,116
			treatment Dependent	,079	,061	1,238	,216
			qol score Dependent	,042	,028	1,466	,143
		Goodman and Kruskal tau	treatment Dependent	,021	,011		,277[c]
			qol score Dependent	,018	,009		,182[c]
		Uncertainty Coefficient	Symmetric	,022	,011	1,933	,259[d]
			treatment Dependent	,023	,012	1,933	,259[d]
			qol score Dependent	,020	,010	1,933	,259[d]
Yes	Nominal by Nominal	Lambda	Symmetric	,093	,050	1,806	,071
			treatment Dependent	,132	,054	2,322	,020
			qol score Dependent	,053	,063	,818	,414
		Goodman and Kruskal tau	treatment Dependent	,065	,019		,000[c]
			qol score Dependent	,042	,013		,000[c]
		Uncertainty Coefficient	Symmetric	,071	,018	3,839	,000[d]
			treatment Dependent	,074	,019	3,839	,000[d]
			qol score Dependent	,067	,017	3,839	,000[d]

The lambda value is also given. It shows the percentages of misclassifications in the row if you would know the column values, is also statistically significant in the yes-counseling subgroup at p = 0.020. The value of 0.132 would mean 1.32% reduction of misclassification, which is, however, not very much. Goodman and uncertainty coefficients serve similar purpose and are also statistically significant.

Conclusion

In conclusion, many high qol levels are in the hydrotherapy and physiotherapy groups, and, correspondingly, very few low qol levels are a major factor for the overall result of this study assessing the effects of treatment modalities on qol scores. The interaction matrix can be used to assess whether some treatment modalities are associated with a better qol score than others, and to assess the directions of the differences in distribution of the variables.

Note

More background, theoretical and mathematical information of crosstabs is given in Statistics applied to clinical studies 5th edition, Chap. 3, The analysis of safety data, pp. 41–59, Edited by Springer Heidelberg Germany, 2012, from the same authors.

Chapter 11
Predictions from Ordinal Clinical Data (450 Patients)

General Purpose

In Chap. 9 the typology of medical data was reviewed. Ordinal data are, like nominal data (Chap. 10), discrete data, however, with a stepping pattern, like severity scores, intelligence levels, physical strength scores. They are usually assessed with frequency tables and bar charts. Unlike scale data, that also have a stepping pattern, they do not necessarily have to have steps with equal intervals. Statistical testing is not of much interest. Statistical testing becomes, however, interesting, if we want to know whether two ordinal variables like levels of satisfaction with treatment and treatment outcome are differently distributed between one another. An interaction matrix of these two ordinal variables could then be used to test whether one treatment level performs better than the other. We should add that sometimes an ordinal variable can very well be analyzed as a nominal one (e.g., treatment outcome in the current Chapter and in Chap. 10).

Background

Nominal data
> Nominal data are discrete data without a stepping pattern, like genders, age classes, family names. They can be assessed with pie charts, frequency tables and bar charts.

Ordinal data

Electronic Supplementary Material The online version of this chapter (https://doi.org/10.1007/978-3-030-33970-8_11) contains supplementary material, which is available to authorized users.

Ordinal data are also discrete data, however, with a stepping pattern, like severity scores, intelligence levels, physical strength scores. They are usually assessed with frequency tables and bar charts.

Scale data

Scale data also have a stepping pattern, but, unlike ordinal data, they have steps with equal intervals. With small steps they are called continuous data. They are sometimes called quantitative data, while nominal and ordinal data are traditionally called qualitative data. The scale data are assessed with summary tables and histograms.

Having understanding of different data types, also called measurement scales, is a prerequisite for doing exploratory data analysis (EDA), since you can use certain statistical measurements only for specific data types. You also need to know which data type you are dealing with to choose the right visualization method. Think of data types as a way to categorize different types of variables. We will discuss the main types of variables and look at examples for the purpose.

The typology of the data values becomes particularly important, when it comes to statistical analyses. E.g.:

1. Means and standard deviations makes no sense with nominal data.
2. The problem with ordinal data is, that the steps are usually not equal, like with scale data. With ordinal data you will usually have a mix-up of larger and smaller steps.
3. This biases the outcome, if you use a scale data test for their analysis. The Chap. 37 of the current book, entitled "Ordinal scaling for clinical scores with inconsistent intervals", shows how this problem can mathematically be largely solved by complementary log-log transformations.

Primary Scientific Question

This chapter assesses the relationship between five levels of satisfaction with the treating doctor, and, as outcome, five levels of quality of life (qol). Can an interaction matrix, otherwise called contingency table or crosstab, be used to assess whether some "satisfaction-with-treating-doctor" levels are associated with a better qol score than others, and to assess the directions of the differences in distribution of the variables.

Example

In 450 patients with coronary artery disease the satisfaction level of patients with their doctor was assumed to be an important predictor of patient qol (quality of life).

Example   81

treatment	counseling	qol	sat doctor
3	1	4	4
4	0	2	1
2	1	5	4
3	0	4	4
2	1	2	1
2	0	1	4
4	0	4	1
3	0	4	1
4	1	4	4
2	1	3	4

Treatment	= treatment modality (1 = cardiac fitness, 2 = physiotherapy, 3 = wellness, 4 = hydrotherapy, 5 = nothing)
counseling	= counseling given (0 = no, 1 = yes)
qol	= quality of life score (1 = very low, 5 = vey high)
sat doctor	= satisfaction with doctor (1 = very low, 5 = very high).

The above table gives the first 10 patients of a 450 patients study of the effects of doctors' satisfaction level and qol. The data are also used in the Chap. 16. The entire data file is in extras.springer.com and is entitled "qol.sav".

SPSS is used for analysis.

Command

Analyze....Descriptive Statistics....Crosstabs....Rows: enter "sat doctor".... Columns: enter "qol score"....click Statistics....mark Gamma, Somer's d, Kendall's tau-b, Kendall's tau-c....click Continue....click OK.

sat with doctor * qol score Crosstabulation

Count

		qol score					Total
		very low	low	medium	high	very high	
sat with doctor	very low	11	12	12	11	4	50
	low	24	16	23	28	15	106
	medium	21	23	17	22	27	110
	high	18	16	15	32	36	117
	very high	12	6	4	16	29	67
Total		86	73	71	109	111	450

The above matrix of observed counts is shown in the output sheets. Very high qol was frequently observed in patients who were very satisfied with their doctor, while few patients with very high qol (only 4) had a very low satisfaction with their doctor. We wish to assess whether this association is chance or statistically significant.

"Ordinal x ordinal crosstabs" work differently from "nominal x nominal crosstabs" (Chap. 16). The latter compares the magnitude of the cells, the former compares the magnitude of the concordant and those of the discordant cells, whereby the concordant cells are, e.g., "very low versus very low", "low versus low", etc.

Directional Measures

			Value	Asymp. Std. Error[a]	Approx. T[b]	Approx. Sig.
Ordinal by Ordinal	Somers' d	Symmetric	,178	,037	4,817	,000
		sat with doctor Dependent	,177	,037	4,817	,000
		qol score Dependent	,179	,037	4,817	,000

a. Not assuming the null hypothesis.
b. Using the asymptotic standard error assuming the null hypothesis.

Symmetric Measures

		Value	Asymp. Std. Error[a]	Approx. T[b]	Approx. Sig.
Ordinal by Ordinal	Kendall's tau-b	,178	,037	4,817	,000
	Kendall's tau-c	,175	,036	4,817	,000
	Gamma	,225	,046	4,817	,000
N of Valid Cases		450			

a. Not assuming the null hypothesis.
b. Using the asymptotic standard error assuming the null hypothesis.

The above tables are also in the output. The gamma value equals probability$_{concordance}$ − probability$_{discordance}$, whereby the tied cells are excluded (the cells that have the same order of both variables). Somer's d measures the same but includes the ties. The measures demonstrate that the association of the two variables is closer than could happen by chance. A positive value means a positive correlation, the higher the order in one variable, the higher it will be in the other one. Tau b and c have similar meanings, but are more appropriate for data where numbers of categories between the two variables are different. Both directional and symmetry measures are statistically very significant. This means that high satisfaction levels with the treating doctors are strongly associated with high qol levels, and that low satisfaction levels are strongly associated with low qol levels.

Conclusion

We can conclude from this analysis that there is a statistically significant positive association between the qol score levels and the levels of satisfaction with the patients' doctors, can make predictions from the levels of satisfaction with the doctor about the expected quality of life in future patients, and could consider to recommend doctors to try and perform better to that aim. An interaction matrix, otherwise called contingency table or crosstab, can be used to assess whether treatment levels are associated with a better outcome score than others, and to assess the directions of the differences in distribution of the variables.

Note

More background, theoretical and mathematical information of crosstabs is given in Statistics applied to clinical studies 5th edition, Chap. 3, The analysis of safety data, pp. 41–59, Edited by Springer Heidelberg Germany, 2012, from the same authors.

Chapter 12
Assessing Relative Health Risks (3000 Subjects)

General Purpose

This chapter is to assess whether interaction matrices, otherwise called contingency tables or simply crosstabs, can be used to test the effect of personal characteristics like gender, age, married status etc. on a person's health risks.

Background

Absolute risk of a disease is your risk of developing the disease over a time period. We all have absolute risks of developing various diseases such as heart disease, cancer, stroke, etc. The same absolute risk can be expressed in different ways. For example, say you have a 1 in 10 risk of developing a certain disease in your life. This can also be said to be a 10% risk, or a 0.1 risk – depending on whether you use percentages or decimals.

Relative risk is used to compare the risk in two different groups of people. For example, the groups could be smokers and non-smokers. All sorts of groups are compared to others in medical research to see, if belonging to a group increases or decreases your risk of developing certain diseases. For example, research has shown, that smokers have a higher risk of developing heart disease compared to (relative to) non-smokers.

Electronic Supplementary Material The online version of this chapter (https://doi.org/10.1007/978-3-030-33970-8_12) contains supplementary material, which is available to authorized users.

T. J. Cleophas, A. H. Zwinderman, *Machine Learning in Medicine – A Complete Overview*, https://doi.org/10.1007/978-3-030-33970-8_12

Primary Scientific Question

Can marital status affect a person's health risks.

Example

In 3000 subjects the effect of married status on being healthy was assessed.

ageclass	married	healthy
4,00	1	0
3,00	0	0
2,00	1	0
1,00	1	0
4,00	1	0
3,00	0	0
2,00	1	0
1,00	0	0
4,00	1	0
3,00	1	0

ageclass 1 = 30-40, 2 = 40-50, 3 = 50-60, 4 = 60-70
married 0 = no, 1 = yes
healthy 0 = no, 1 = yes

In the above table the first 10 patients are given. The entire data file is entitled "healthrisk.sav" and is in extras.springer.com. We will start the analysis by opening the data file in SPSS.

Command

Analyze....Descriptive Statistics....Crosstabs....Row(s): enter married....Column(s): enter health....Statistics: mark Observed....mark Rows....click Continue....click OK.

married * healthy Crosstabulation

			healthy		Total
			no	yes	
married	no	Count	192	1104	1296
		% within married	14,8%	85,2%	100,0%
	yes	Count	167	1537	1704
		% within married	9,8%	90,2%	100,0%

Example   87

The crosstab is in the output sheets. It shows that 14.8% of the unmarried subjects were unhealthy, leaving 85,2% being healthy. In contrast, 9.8% of the married subjects were unhealthy, 90.2% being healthy. And so, the risk of being unhealthy in this population was 14.8% in the unmarried and 9.8% in the married subjects. The relative risk of being unhealthy in unmarried versus married subjects was, thus, 14.8/9.8 = 1.512. Similarly, the relative risk of being healthy in unmarried versus married subjects was 85.2/90.2 = 0.944.

Risk Estimate

	Value	95% Confidence Interval	
		Lower	Upper
Odds Ratio for married (no / yes)	1,601	1,283	1,997
For cohort healthy = no	1,512	1,245	1,836
For cohort healthy = yes	,944	,919	,971
N of Valid Cases	3000		

The odds of being unhealthy in unmarried subjects was 192/1104 = 0.1739.
The odds of being unhealthy in married subjects was 167/1537 = 0.1087.
The ratio of the two, the odds ratio was thus 0.1739/0.1087 = 1.601, as shown in the above table. It is easy to see that this odds ratio is equal to

$$= \frac{\text{the relative risk of being unhealthy in the unmarried versus married subjects}}{\text{the relative risk of being healthy in the unmarried versus married subjects}}$$
$$= 1.512/0.944 = 1.601.$$

In order to assess whether this finding is robust, we will add age classes as a layer variable, and test whether different age classes have similar odds ratios.

Command
Analyze....Descriptive Statistics....Crosstabs....Row(s): enter married....Column(s): enter health....Layer 1 of 1: enter ageclass....Statistics: mark Observed....mark Rows ....mark Cochran and Mantel Haenszel Statistics.... click Continue....click OK.

married * healthy * ageclass Crosstabulation

ageclass					healthy no	healthy yes	Total
30-40	married	no		Count	52	138	190
				% within married	27,4%	72,6%	100,0%
		yes		Count	53	327	380
				% within married	13,9%	86,1%	100,0%
	Total			Count	105	465	570
				% within married	18,4%	81,6%	100,0%
40-50	married	no		Count	69	352	421
				% within married	16,4%	83,6%	100,0%
		yes		Count	67	593	660
				% within married	10,2%	89,8%	100,0%
	Total			Count	136	945	1081
				% within married	12,6%	87,4%	100,0%
50-60	married	no		Count	28	201	229
				% within married	12,2%	87,8%	100,0%
		yes		Count	17	287	304
				% within married	5,6%	94,4%	100,0%
	Total			Count	45	488	533
				% within married	8,4%	91,6%	100,0%
60-70	married	no		Count	43	413	456
				% within married	9,4%	90,6%	100,0%
		yes		Count	30	330	360
				% within married	8,3%	91,7%	100,0%
	Total			Count	73	743	816
				% within married	8,9%	91,1%	100,0%

Example   89

Risk Estimate

ageclass		Value	95% Confidence Interval	
			Lower	Upper
30-40	Odds Ratio for married (no / yes)	2,325	1,511	3,578
	For cohort healthy = no	1,962	1,396	2,759
	For cohort healthy = yes	,844	,767	,929
	N of Valid Cases	570		
40-50	Odds Ratio for married (no / yes)	1,735	1,209	2,490
	For cohort healthy = no	1,614	1,180	2,208
	For cohort healthy = yes	,931	,886	,978
	N of Valid Cases	1081		
50-60	Odds Ratio for married (no / yes)	2,352	1,254	4,411
	For cohort healthy = no	2,186	1,227	3,896
	For cohort healthy = yes	,930	,879	,983
	N of Valid Cases	533		
60-70	Odds Ratio for married (no / yes)	1,145	,703	1,866
	For cohort healthy = no	1,132	,725	1,766
	For cohort healthy = yes	,988	,946	1,031
	N of Valid Cases	816		

In the output are the crosstabs the odds ratios of the 4 ageclasses. The odds ratios are pretty heterogeneous, between 1.145 and 2.352, but 95% confidence intervals were pretty wide. Yet, it is tested whether these odds ratios are significantly different from one another.

Tests of Homogeneity of the Odds Ratio

	Chi-Squared	df	Asymp. Sig. (2-sided)
Breslow-Day	5,428	3	,143
Tarone's	5,422	3	,143

The above Breslow and the Tarone's tests are the heterogeneity tests. They were insignificant. The differences could, thus, be ascribed to chance findings, rather than real effects. It seems appropriate, therefore, to say that an overall odds ratio of these data adjusted for age classes is meaningful. For that purpose a Mantel Haenszel (MH) odds ratio (OR) will be calculated.

		healthy	
		no	yes
unmarried	no	a	b
	yes	c	d

Having 4 odds ratios with the above structure, it is calculated as follows
(n = a + b + c + d):

$$\text{Odds Ratio}_{MH} = \frac{\Sigma \, ad/n}{\Sigma \, cd/n}$$

Tests of Conditional Independence

	Chi-Squared	df	Asymp. Sig. (2-sided)
Cochran's	26,125	1	,000
Mantel-Haenszel	25,500	1	,000

Under the conditional independence assumption,
Cochran's statistic is asymptotically distributed as a 1 df
chi-squared distribution, only if the number of strata is
fixed, while the Mantel-Haenszel statistic is always
asymptotically distributed as a 1 df chi-squared
distribution. Note that the continuity correction is removed
from the Mantel-Haenszel statistic when the sum of the
differences between the observed and the expected is 0.

Mantel-Haenszel Common Odds Ratio Estimate

Estimate			1,781
ln(Estimate)			,577
Std. Error of ln(Estimate)			,115
Asymp. Sig. (2-sided)			,000
Asymp. 95% Confidence Interval	Common Odds Ratio	Lower Bound	1,422
		Upper Bound	2,230
	ln(Common Odds Ratio)	Lower Bound	,352
		Upper Bound	,802

The Mantel-Haenszel common odds ratio estimate is asymptotically normally distributed
under the common odds ratio of 1,000 assumption. So is the natural log of the estimate.

The Cochran's and Mantel Haenszel tests assess whether married status remains
an independent predictor of health after adjustment for ageclasses. They are significantly larger than an odds ratio (OR) of 0 at p < 0.0001. The lower graph gives the
OR_{MH} is thus 1.781. This OR is adjusted, and, therefore, more adequate than the
unadjusted OR of page 1 of this chapter.

Conclusion

Interaction matrices, otherwise called contingency tables or simply crosstabs, can be used to test the effect of personal characteristics like gender, age, married status etc. on a person's health risks. Results can be adjusted for concomitant effects like the effect of age classes on the relationship between married status and health status. Prior to assessment the homogeneity of the concomitant factors have to be tested.

We should add a limitation of relative risks here. Currently, medical literature is snowed under with mortality trials, and invariably the relative rise in survival is over 10% and up to 30%. A relative rise in survival of 30% = an absolute risk reduction of 1%. Mortality is an insensitive variable for studies begun at middle-age due to comorbidity. A more sensitive endpoint of such studies would be morbidity. If, by some health measure, your risk of death goes from 3% to 2%, then your absolute difference will be only 1%, but your relative difference will be 33%. Relative risks tend to be overemphasized in the medical literature.

Note

More background, theoretical and mathematical information of relative risk assessments are in Statistics applied to clinical studies 5th edition, Chap. 3, The analysis of safety data, pp. 41–59, Edited by Springer Heidelberg Germany, 2012, from the same authors.

Chapter 13
Measuring Agreement (30 Patients)

General Purpose

Interaction matrices have myriad applications. In the Chap. 12 it can be observed that they perform well for assessing relative health risks, making predictions from nominal and ordinal clinical data (Chap. 9, 10 and 11), and statistical testing of outcome scores. In this chapter we will assess, if they also can be applied to measure agreement. Agreement, otherwise called reproducibility or reliability, of duplicate observations is the fundament of diagnostic procedures, and, therefore, also the fundament of much of scientific research.

Background

Jacob Cohen was a statistician at New York University who gave his name to Cohen's kappa (1960). It is commonly used for estimating reproducibility of qualitative diagnostic tests. An example is given.

Electronic Supplementary Material The online version of this chapter (https://doi.org/10.1007/978-3-030-33970-8_13) contains supplementary material, which is available to authorized users.

© Springer Nature Switzerland AG 2020

T. J. Cleophas, A. H. Zwinderman, *Machine Learning in Medicine – A Complete Overview*, https://doi.org/10.1007/978-3-030-33970-8_13

A lab-test of 30 patients is performed.

		1st time (positive test = yes)		
		yes	no	
2nd time	yes	10	5	15
	no	4	11	15
		14	16	30

If the test is not reproducible at all, then

	you should find	15 x twice the same,
	we do find	21 x twice the same.

$$\text{Kappa} = \frac{\text{observed - minimal}}{\text{maximal - minimal}} = \frac{21-15}{30-15} = 0.4 \quad \text{0 poor, 1 excellent}$$

Primary Scientific Question

Can a 2 × 2 interaction matrix also be used to demonstrate the level of agreement between duplicate observations of the effect of antihypertensive treatment.

Example

In 30 patients with hypertension the effect of an antihypertensive treatment was measured with normotension as outcome. Each patients was tested twice in order to assess the reproducibility of the procedure. The example was used before (Chap. 19, Reliability assessment of qualitative diagnostic tests, in: SPSS for starters part 1, pp. 69–70, Springer Heidelberg Germany, 2010, from the same authors as the current work).

Variables	
1	2
1,00	1,00
1,00	1,00
1,00	1,00
1,00	1,00
1,00	1,00
1,00	1,00
1,00	1,00
1,00	1,00
1,00	1,00
1,00	1,00
1,00	,00

Example 95

Variable 1 = responder after first test (0 = non responder, 1 = responder)
Variable 2 = responder after second test

The above table shows the results of first 11 patients. The entire data file is entitled "agreement", and is in extras.springer.com. We will start by opening the file in SPSS.

Command

Analyze....Descriptive Statistics....Crosstabs....Row(s): enter Variable 1....Column(s): enter Variable 2....click Statistics....Mark: kappa....click Continue....click Cells.....mark Observed....click continue....click OK.

VAR00001 * VAR00002 Crosstabulation

Count

		VAR00002		Total
		,00	1,00	
VAR00001	,00	11	4	15
	1,00	5	10	15
Total		16	14	30

In the output sheets a interaction matrix of the data is shown. If agreement is 100%, then the cells b and c would be empty, and the cells a and d would contain 30 patients.

		variable 2	
		0	1
variable 1	0	a	b
	1	c	d

However, the cells a and d contain only 21 patients.

If agreement would be 0%, then the cells a and d would contain 15 patients. However, 21 is more than 15, and so, this may indicate that agreement is better than 0%, although less than 100%. Cohen's Kappa is computed by SPSS to estimate the exact level of agreement.

Symmetric Measures

		Value	Asymp. Std. Error[a]	Approx. T[b]	Approx. Sig.
Measure of Agreement	Kappa	,400	,167	2,196	,028
N of Valid Cases		30			

a. Not assuming the null hypothesis.

b. Using the asymptotic standard error assuming the null hypothesis.

The above table shows that the kappa-value equals 0.400. A kappa-value of 0 means poor reproducibility or agreement, a kappa-value of 1 means excellent. This result of 0.400 is moderate. This result is significantly different from an agreement of 0 at $p = 0.028$.

Conclusion

In this chapter it is assessed if interaction matrices can be applied to measure agreement. Agreement, otherwise called reproducibility or reliability, of duplicate observations is the fundament of diagnostic procedures, and, therefore, also the fundament of much of scientific research.

A 2×2 interaction matrix can be used to demonstrate the level of agreement between duplicate observations of the effect of antihypertensive treatment. We should add that kappa-values can also be computed from larger interaction matrices, like 3×3, 4×4 contingency tables, etc.

Note

More background, theoretical and mathematical information of correct and incorrect methods for assessing reproducibility or agreement are given in Chap. 45, Testing reproducibility, pp. 499–508, in: Statistics applied to clinical studies 5th edition, Springer Heidelberg Germany, 2012, from the same authors.

Chapter 14
Column Proportions for Testing Differences between Outcome Scores (450 Patients)

General Purpose

In the Chap. 10 the relationships between treatment modality and quality of life (qol) score levels were assessed using a chi-square test of the interaction matrix. Many high qol scores were in the hydrotherapy and physiotherapy treatments, and in the subgroup that received counseling the overall differences from other treatments were statistically significant at $p < 0.0001$. In this chapter, using the same data, we will try and test what levels of qol scores were significantly different from one another, and, thus, provide more details about differences in effects.

Background

The "Column Proportion" test looks at the rows of a table, in an independent way, and it is used to compare pairs of columns, while testing, whether the proportions of respondents in one column is significantly different from the proportions in another column. The proportion is the count in the cell divided by the base for the column.

Electronic Supplementary Material The online version of this chapter (https://doi.org/10.1007/978-3-030-33970-8_14) contains supplementary material, which is available to authorized users.

T. J. Cleophas, A. H. Zwinderman, *Machine Learning in Medicine – A Complete Overview*, https://doi.org/10.1007/978-3-030-33970-8_14

Specific Scientific Question

Can the effects of different treatment modalities on outcome score levels previously assessed with a chi-square test of the interaction matrix, be assessed with better precision applying column proportion comparisons using Bonferroni-adjusted z-tests?

Example

A parallel group study of 450 patients assessed the effect of different complementary treatment modalities on qol score levels. The first 11 patients of the data file is underneath. The entire data file is entitled "qol.sav", and is in extras.springer.com.

treatment	counseling	qol	satdoctor
3	1	4	4
4	0	2	1
2	1	5	4
3	0	4	4
2	1	2	1
2	0	1	4
4	0	4	1
3	0	4	1
4	1	4	4
2	1	3	4
4	1	5	5

treatment	= treatment modality (1 = cardiac fitness, 2 = physiotherapy, 3 = wellness, 4 = hydrotherapy
counseling	= counseling given (0 = no, 1 = yes)
qol	= quality of life scores (1 = very low, 5 = very high)
satdoctor	= satisfaction with treating doctor (1 = very low, 5 = very high)

We will start by opening the data file in SPSS.

Command

Analyze....Descriptive Statistics....Crosstabs....Row(s): enter treatment.... Column(s): enter qol....click Cells....mark Observed....mark Columns....mark: Compare column properties....mark: Adjusted p-values (Bonferroni method) .... click Continue....click OK.

Example   99

treatment * qol score Crosstabulation

			qol score					Total
			very low	low	medium	high	very high	
treatment	cardiac fitness	Count	21$_a$	21$_a$	16$_a$	24$_a$	36$_a$	118
		% within qol score	24,4%	28,8%	22,5%	22,0%	32,4%	26,2%
	physiotherapy	Count	22$_a$	20$_a$	18$_a$	20$_a$	20$_a$	100
		% within qol score	25,6%	27,4%	25,4%	18,3%	18,0%	22,2%
	wellness	Count	23$_a$	14$_a$	12$_a$	30$_a$	25$_a$	104
		% within qol score	26,7%	19,2%	16,9%	27,5%	22,5%	23,1%
	hydrotherapy	Count	20$_a$	18$_a$	25$_a$	35$_a$	30$_a$	128
		% within qol score	23,3%	24,7%	35,2%	32,1%	27,0%	28,4%
Total		Count	86	73	71	109	111	450
		% within qol score	100,0%	100,0%	100,0%	100,0%	100,0%	100,0%

Each subscript letter denotes a subset of qol score categories whose column proportions do not differ significantly from each other at the ,05 level.

The above table is in the output sheets. All of the counts in the cells are given with the subscript letter a.

The interpretation of the subscript letters are pretty obvious (vs = versus):

> looking in a single row
> a vs a $p > 0.10$
> a vs a,b $0.05 < p < 0.10$
> a vs b $p < 0.05$
> a vs c $p < 0.01$
> a vs d $p < 0.001$
> b vs a,b $0.05 < p < 0.10$

This means, that, in the above table, none of the counts is significantly different from one another. This is consistent with the insignificant chi-square test of Chap. 16. We have clinical arguments that counseling may support the beneficial effects of treatments, and, therefore, perform an analysis with two layers, one in the patients with and one in those without counseling.

Command

Analyze....Descriptive Statistics....Crosstabs....Row(s): enter treatment.... Column(s): enter qol....Layer 1 of 1: enter counseling....click Cells....mark Observed....mark Columns....mark: Compare column properties....mark: Adjusted p-values (Bonferroni method)....click Continue....click OK.

treatment * qol score * counseling Crosstabulation

counseling				very low	low	medium	high	very high	Total
						qol score			
No	treatment	cardiac fitness	Count	19$_a$	16$_a$	8$_a$	8$_a$	14$_a$	65
			% within qol score	29,2%	34,8%	26,7%	20,0%	28,6%	28,3%
		physiotherapy	Count	8$_a$	8$_{a,b}$	7$_{a,b}$	7$_{a,b}$	15$_b$	45
			% within qol score	12,3%	17,4%	23,3%	17,5%	30,6%	19,6%
		wellness	Count	23$_a$	8$_b$	6$_{a,b}$	15$_a$	9$_b$	61
			% within qol score	35,4%	17,4%	20,0%	37,5%	18,4%	26,5%
		hydrotherapy	Count	15$_a$	14$_a$	9$_a$	10$_a$	11$_a$	59
			% within qol score	23,1%	30,4%	30,0%	25,0%	22,4%	25,7%
	Total		Count	65	46	30	40	49	230
			% within qol score	100,0%	100,0%	100,0%	100,0%	100,0%	100,0%
Yes	treatment	cardiac fitness	Count	2$_a$	5$_{a,b}$	8$_{a,b}$	16$_{a,b}$	22$_b$	53
			% within qol score	9,5%	18,5%	19,5%	23,2%	35,5%	24,1%
		physiotherapy	Count	14$_a$	12$_{a,b}$	11$_{b,c}$	13$_{c,d}$	5$_d$	55
			% within qol score	66,7%	44,4%	26,8%	18,8%	8,1%	25,0%
		wellness	Count	0$_a$	6$_b$	6$_{a,b}$	15$_b$	16$_b$	43
			% within qol score	,0%	22,2%	14,6%	21,7%	25,8%	19,5%
		hydrotherapy	Count	5$_{a,b}$	4$_b$	16$_a$	25$_a$	19$_{a,b}$	69
			% within qol score	23,8%	14,8%	39,0%	36,2%	30,6%	31,4%
	Total		Count	21	27	41	69	62	220
			% within qol score	100,0%	100,0%	100,0%	100,0%	100,0%	100,0%
Total	treatment	cardiac fitness	Count	21$_a$	21$_a$	16$_a$	24$_a$	36$_a$	118
			% within qol score	24,4%	28,8%	22,5%	22,0%	32,4%	26,2%
		physiotherapy	Count	22$_a$	20$_a$	18$_a$	20$_a$	20$_a$	100
			% within qol score	25,6%	27,4%	25,4%	18,3%	18,0%	22,2%
		wellness	Count	23$_a$	14$_a$	12$_a$	30$_a$	25$_a$	104
			% within qol score	26,7%	19,2%	16,9%	27,5%	22,5%	23,1%
		hydrotherapy	Count	20$_a$	18$_a$	25$_a$	35$_a$	30$_a$	128
			% within qol score	23,3%	24,7%	35,2%	32,1%	27,0%	28,4%
	Total		Count	86	73	71	109	111	450
			% within qol score	100,0%	100,0%	100,0%	100,0%	100,0%	100,0%

Each subscript letter denotes a subset of qol score categories whose column proportions do not differ significantly from each other at the ,05 level.

The above table is now shown. It gives the computations for the patients previously counseled separately. Now differences particularly in the patients counseled were larger.

In the cardiac fitness row the very low and very high qol cells the percentages of patients present are 9.5 and 23.2% (significantly different at $p < 0.05$ Bonferroni adjusted), and "very low" versus the three scores in between have a trend to significance $0.05 < p < 0.10$. The same is true with "very high" versus (vs) the three scores in between. In the physiotherapy row differences were even larger. In the physiotherapy row we have:

1. both 14 vs 11 and 11 vs 5 significantly different at $p < 0.05$
2. 14 vs 12, 12 vs 11, 11 vs 13, 13 vs 5 with a trend to significantly different at $0.05 < p < 0.10$.

Similarly, in the wellness and hydrotherapy rows significant differences and trends to significance were observed.

In the no-counseling patients differences were smaller, but some trends, and two significant differences at $p < 0.05$ (a vs b) were, nonetheless, observed.

In conclusion, only in the physiotherapy row the low qol fraction is large, in the other three the high qol fractions are large. And so, with respect to qol physiotherapy does not perform very well, and may better be skipped from the program.

Note: Bonferroni adjustment for multiple testing works as follows. In order for p-values to be significant, with two tests they need to be smaller than 0.025, with four tests smaller than 0.0125, with ten tests smaller than 0.005, etc.

Conclusion

When assessing the outcome effects of different treatments, column proportions comparisons of interaction matrices can be applied to precisely find what outcome scores are significantly different from one another. This may provide relevant information about some treatment modalities, and may give cause for some treatment modalities to be skipped.

Note

More background, theoretical and mathematical information of interaction matrices is given in Statistics applied to clinical studies 5th edition, Chap. 3, The analysis of safety data, pp. 41–59, Springer Heidelberg Germany, 2012, from the same authors, and in the Chaps. 10, 11, 12 and 13 of this work.

Chapter 15
Pivoting Trays and Tables for Improved Analysis of Multidimensional Data (450 Patients)

General Purpose

Pivot tables is for multilevel analyses with frequencies or percentages. It can visualize multiple variables data with the help of interactive displays of multiple dimensions. They have been in SPSS statistical software for a long time (from version 7.0), and, gradually, they take over in most modules. They are helpful for improving the analysis by visualizing interaction patterns you so far did not notice.

Background

Default tables, as produced by statistical software programs, may not display information as neatly or clearly, as it should. Pivot tables are interactive. You can transpose rows and columns ("flip" the table), adjust the order of data in a table, and modify the table in many other ways. For example, you can change a short, wide table into a long thin one by transposing rows and columns. Changing the layout of the table does not affect the results. Instead, it's a way of displaying your information into a different or more desirable manner. The interactive pivot tables are not only a way of showing the same as the default table in another perspective, but they are also more than that, because they help you better notice, what is going on at difference levels of the analysis, and, so, they, actually, can improve the analysis by visualizing data patterns, you did not notice before. Pivot tables are widely applied, not only in SPSS and most other larger statistical software programs, but also in spreadsheets programs, like Excel. In SPSS they are being applied with Anova (analysis of

Electronic Supplementary Material The online version of this chapter (https://doi.org/10.1007/978-3-030-33970-8_15) contains supplementary material, which is available to authorized users.

T. J. Cleophas, A. H. Zwinderman, *Machine Learning in Medicine – A Complete Overview*, https://doi.org/10.1007/978-3-030-33970-8_15

variance), Correlations, Crosstabs, Descriptives, Examine, Frequencies, General Linear Models, Nonparametric Tests, Regression, T-tests.

Primary Scientific Question

Are pivot tables able to visualize interaction pattern in your clinical data that so far were unnoticed?

Example

We will use as example the data also used in the Chaps. 10, 11, 12, 13 and 14. A parallel group study of 450 patients assessed the effect of different complementary treatment modalities on qol score levels. The first 11 patients of the data file is underneath. The entire data file is entitled "qol.sav", and is in extras.springer.com.

treatment	counseling	qol	satdoctor
3	1	4	4
4	0	2	1
2	1	5	4
3	0	4	4
2	1	2	1
2	0	1	4
4	0	4	1
3	0	4	1
4	1	4	4
2	1	3	4
4	1	5	5

treatment	= treatment modality (1 = cardiac fitness, 2 = physiotherapy, 3 = wellness, 4 = hydrotherapy
counseling	= counseling given (0 = no, 1 = yes)
qol	= quality of life scores (1 = very low, 5 = very high)
satdoctor	= satisfaction with treating doctor (1 = very low, 5 = very high)

We will start by opening the data file in your computer mounted with SPSS statistical software.

Command
Analyze....Descriptive Statistics....Crosstabs....Row(s): enter treatment.... Column(s): enter qol....click Cells....mark Observed....mark Columns....click Continue....click OK.

Example   105

The underneath table is shown in the output sheets.

treatment * qol score * counseling Crosstabulation

counseling				very low	low	medium	high	very high	Total
						qol score			
No	treatment	cardiac fitness	Count	19	16	8	8	14	65
			% within qol score	29,2%	34,8%	26,7%	20,0%	28,6%	28,3%
		physiotherapy	Count	8	8	7	7	15	45
			% within qol score	12,3%	17,4%	23,3%	17,5%	30,6%	19,6%
		wellness	Count	23	8	6	15	9	61
			% within qol score	35,4%	17,4%	20,0%	37,5%	18,4%	26,5%
		hydrotherapy	Count	15	14	9	10	11	59
			% within qol score	23,1%	30,4%	30,0%	25,0%	22,4%	25,7%
	Total		Count	65	46	30	40	49	230
			% within qol score	100,0%	100,0%	100,0%	100,0%	100,0%	100,0%
Yes	treatment	cardiac fitness	Count	2	5	8	16	22	53
			% within qol score	9,5%	18,5%	19,5%	23,2%	35,5%	24,1%
		physiotherapy	Count	14	12	11	13	5	55
			% within qol score	66,7%	44,4%	26,8%	18,8%	8,1%	25,0%
		wellness	Count	0	6	6	15	16	43
			% within qol score	,0%	22,2%	14,6%	21,7%	25,8%	19,5%
		hydrotherapy	Count	5	4	16	25	19	69
			% within qol score	23,8%	14,8%	39,0%	36,2%	30,6%	31,4%
	Total		Count	21	27	41	69	62	220
			% within qol score	100,0%	100,0%	100,0%	100,0%	100,0%	100,0%
Total	treatment	cardiac fitness	Count	21	21	16	24	36	118
			% within qol score	24,4%	28,8%	22,5%	22,0%	32,4%	26,2%
		physiotherapy	Count	22	20	18	20	20	100
			% within qol score	25,6%	27,4%	25,4%	18,3%	18,0%	22,2%
		wellness	Count	23	14	12	30	25	104
			% within qol score	26,7%	19,2%	16,9%	27,5%	22,5%	23,1%
		hydrotherapy	Count	20	18	25	35	30	128
			% within qol score	23,3%	24,7%	35,2%	32,1%	27,0%	28,4%
	Total		Count	86	73	71	109	111	450
			% within qol score	100,0%	100,0%	100,0%	100,0%	100,0%	100,0%

We will apply this table for pivoting the data, using the "user interface for pivot tables", otherwise called the pivoting tray.

Command
Double-click the above table....the term Pivot is added to the menu bar....click Pivot in the menu bar....the underneath Pivoting Tray consisting of all of the variables appears....qol score is a column variables....counseling, treatment, and statistics are row variables....left click the counseling icon and drag it to the column variables....similarly have statistics dragged to the layer dimension....close the Pivoting Tray.

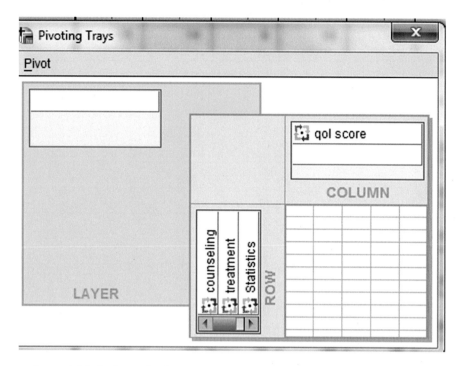

A new table is shown in the output.

Statistics: % within qol score

treatment * qol score * counseling Crosstabulation

| | | very low | | | low | | | medium | | | high | | | very high | | |
| | | counseling | | | counseling | | | counseling | | | counseling | | | counseling | | |
		No	Yes	Total	No	Yes	Total	No	Yes	Total	No	Yes	Total	No	Yes	Total
treatment	cardiac fitness	29,2%	9,5%	24,4%	34,8%	18,5%	28,8%	26,7%	19,5%	22,5%	20,0%	23,2%	22,0%	28,6%	35,5%	32,4%
	physiotherapy	12,3%	66,7%	25,6%	17,4%	44,4%	27,4%	23,3%	26,8%	25,4%	17,5%	18,8%	18,3%	30,6%	8,1%	18,0%
	wellness	35,4%	,0%	26,7%	17,4%	22,2%	19,2%	20,0%	14,6%	16,9%	37,5%	21,7%	27,5%	18,4%	25,8%	22,5%
	hydrotherapy	23,1%	23,8%	23,3%	30,4%	14,8%	24,7%	30,0%	39,0%	35,2%	25,0%	36,2%	32,1%	22,4%	30,6%	27,0%
Total		100,0%	100,0%	100,0%	100,0%	100,0%	100,0%	100,0%	100,0%	100,0%	100,0%	100,0%	100,0%	100,0%	100,0%	100,0%

In it click Statistics and click "% within qol score" in the drop box of the table next to Statistics. In the now upcoming table the cell counts have disappeared. They are not relevant, anyway, only the percentages are so. From the Chaps. 2 and 6 we already know, that there is an overall difference between the cells of the yes-counseling matrix, and that the 67% very low qol is significantly different from the 5% very high qol in the physical therapy treatment groups. What more can the above pivoted table teach us? It underscores the finding from the Chaps. 2 and 6 by showing next to each other the no-counseling and yes-counseling percentages; very low qol with physiotherapy is observed in respectively 12.3 and 66.7%, low qol in 17.4 and 44.4%, and, in contrast, very high qol in respectively 30.6 and 8.1%.

Example   107

Restarting with the Above Unpivoted Table Once More, Give the Commands
Double-click the table....the term Pivot is added to the menu bar....click Pivot in
the menu bar....the Pivoting Tray consisting of all of the variables appears....qol
score is a column variables....counseling, treatment, and statistics are row
variables....drag treatment to the layer dimension....similarly have statistics
dragged to the layer dimension....the Pivoting Tray now looks like shown
underneath....close it.

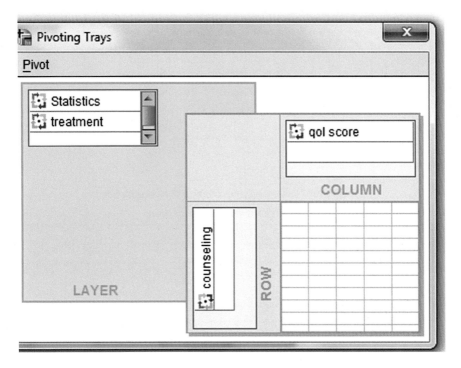

A new pivot table is given in the output. In the left upper angle of it, it has a
Statistics and a treatment drop box. Statistics: click Count and select "% within qol
score", treatment: select, subsequently, all of the four treatments given. The four
underneath tables are produced.

treatment * qol score * counseling Crosstabulation

Statistics: % within qol score,treatment: treatment cardiac fitness

counseling	qol score					Total
	very low	low	medium	high	very high	
No	29,2%	34,8%	26,7%	20,0%	28,6%	28,3%
Yes	9,5%	18,5%	19,5%	23,2%	35,5%	24,1%
Total	24,4%	28,8%	22,5%	22,0%	32,4%	26,2%

treatment * qol score * counseling Crosstabulation

Statistics: % within qol score,treatment: treatment physiotherapy

counseling	qol score					Total
	very low	low	medium	high	very high	
No	12,3%	17,4%	23,3%	17,5%	30,6%	19,6%
Yes	66,7%	44,4%	26,8%	18,8%	8,1%	25,0%
Total	25,6%	27,4%	25,4%	18,3%	18,0%	22,2%

treatment * qol score * counseling Crosstabulation

Statistics: % within qol score,treatment: treatment wellness

counseling	qol score					Total
	very low	low	medium	high	very high	
No	35,4%	17,4%	20,0%	37,5%	18,4%	26,5%
Yes	,0%	22,2%	14,6%	21,7%	25,8%	19,5%
Total	26,7%	19,2%	16,9%	27,5%	22,5%	23,1%

treatment * qol score * counseling Crosstabulation

Statistics: % within qol score,treatment: treatment hydrotherapy

counseling	qol score					Total
	very low	low	medium	high	very high	
No	23,1%	30,4%	30,0%	25,0%	22,4%	25,7%
Yes	23,8%	14,8%	39,0%	36,2%	30,6%	31,4%
Total	23,3%	24,7%	35,2%	32,1%	27,0%	28,4%

They visualize a big downward trend of percentages from very low to very high qol for the treatments cardiac fitness, wellness and hydrotherapy, and an upward trend for the treatment physiotherapy. Although this is in agreement with the findings from the Chaps. 2 and 6, the patterns are relevant, because they give you an additional idea about how patients experience their treatments.

Conclusion

The interactive pivot tables are not only a way of showing the same in another perspective, but they are also more than that, because they help you better notice what is going on at difference levels of the analysis, and, so, they, actually, can improve the analysis by visualizing data patterns you did not notice before.

Note

Pivot tables are applied not only in SPSS and most of the larger statistical software programs, but also in spreadsheets programs like Excel. In SPSS they are being applied with Anova (analysis of variance), Correlations, Crosstabs, Descriptives, Examine, Frequencies, General Linear Models, Nonparametric Tests, Regression, T-tests. In the current book pivot tables were applied in many more Chapters, e.g., the Chaps. 4, 16 and 29.

Chapter 16
Online Analytical Procedure Cubes, a More Rapid Approach to Analyzing Frequencies (450 Patients)

General Purpose

Traditional analyses of interaction matrices of frequencies are in the Chaps. 9, 10 and 11. The OLAP (online analytical procedures) cube is another approach with similar results, but it works more rapidly than the other methods. An *OLAP cube* is a multi-dimensional array of data. Online analytical processing (OLAP) is a computer-based technique of analyzing data to look for insights. OLAP is a category of software that allows users to analyze information from multiple database systems at the same time. It is a technology that enables analysts to extract and view business data from different points of view. OLAP stands for Online Analytical Processing. Analysts frequently need to group, aggregate and join data. These operations in relational databases are resource intensive. With OLAP data can be pre-calculated and pre-aggregated, making analysis faster. OLAP databases are divided into one or more cubes. The cubes are designed in such a way that creating and viewing reports become easy. This chapter will assess whether online analytical procedures can be applied on health outcomes instead of business outcomes.

Background

OLAP means "online analytical procedures". Cubes is a term used to indicate multidimensional datasets. OLAP cubes were first used in 1970, by "SQL (structure query language) Express", a software package for storing business data, like financial data, in an electronic warehouse, and, at the same time, turning raw data into meaningful information (business intelligence), and was initially called "layered

Electronic Supplementary Material The online version of this chapter (https://doi.org/10.1007/ 978-3-030-33970-8_16) contains supplementary material, which is available to authorized users.

reports". Generally, financial data or production data are being summarized, and from these summaries sub-summaries are computed like productions by time-periods, cities, and other subgroups. Instead of quantities of business data, quantities of health outcomes could, similarly, be analyzed. However, to date no such analyses have been performed. This chapter is to assess, whether online analytical procedures can also be applied on health outcomes instead of business outcomes.

Primary Scientific Question

Can online analytical processing (OLAP) using summaries and sub-summaries of clinical outcome data support traditional crosstab analyses?

Example

We will use as example the data also used in the Chaps. 10 and 11. A parallel group study of 450 patients assessed the effect of different complementary treatment modalities on qol score levels. The first 11 patients of the data file is underneath. The entire data file is entitled "qol.sav", and is in extras.springer.com.

treatment	counseling	qol	satdoctor
3	1	4	4
4	0	2	1
2	1	5	4
3	0	4	4
2	1	2	1
2	0	1	4
4	0	4	1
3	0	4	1
4	1	4	4
2	1	3	4
4	1	5	5

treatment	= treatment modality (1 = cardiac fitness, 2 = physiotherapy, 3 = wellness, 4 = hydrotherapy
counseling	= counseling given (0 = no, 1 = yes)
qol	= quality of life scores (1 = very low, 5 = very high)
satdoctor	= satisfaction with treating doctor (1 = very low, 5 = very high)

We will start by opening the data file in SPSS.

Command
Analyze....Reports....OLAP Cubes....Summary Variable(s): enter qol score....Grouping Variable(s): enter treatment, counseling....click OK.

Example   113

Case Processing Summary

	Cases					
	Included		Excluded		Total	
	N	Percent	N	Percent	N	Percent
qol score * treatment * counseling	450	100,0%	0	,0%	450	100,0%

OLAP Cubes

treatment:Total
counseling:Total

	Sum	N	Mean	Std. Deviation	% of Total Sum	% of Total N
qol score	1436	450	3,19	1,457	100,0%	100,0%

The above tables are in the output sheets. The add-up sum of all scores are given (1436), and the overall mean score of the 450 patients (3.19). Next we can slice these results into subgroups, and calculate mean scores by treatment modality. A pivoting tray is used for that purpose.

Command
Double-click the above table....the term Pivot is added to the menu bar....click Pivot in the menu bar....the underneath Pivoting Tray consisting of all of the variables appears....close the Pivoting Tray.

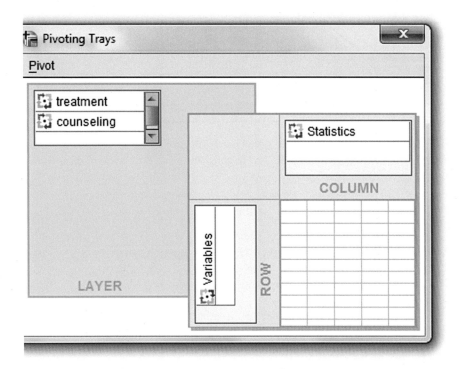

The above table now has in the upper right corner two drop boxes: treatment, and counseling. Treatment: click Total (in blue), and produce the underneath four tables with summary statistics of the four treatment modalities.

OLAP Cubes

treatment:cardiac fitness
counseling:Total

	Sum	N	Mean	Std. Deviation	% of Total Sum	% of Total N
qol score	387	118	3,28	1,501	26,9%	26,2%

OLAP Cubes

treatment:physiotherapy
counseling:Total

	Sum	N	Mean	Std. Deviation	% of Total Sum	% of Total N
qol score	296	100	2,96	1,449	20,6%	22,2%

OLAP Cubes

treatment:wellness
counseling:Total

	Sum	N	Mean	Std. Deviation	% of Total Sum	% of Total N
qol score	332	104	3,19	1,501	23,1%	23,1%

OLAP Cubes

treatment:hydrotherapy
counseling:Total

	Sum	N	Mean	Std. Deviation	% of Total Sum	% of Total N
qol score	421	128	3,29	1,381	29,3%	28,4%

It is easy to see, that the mean qol score of physiotherapy is significantly lower than that of hydrotherapy according to an unpaired t-test ($^$ = symbol of power):

mean   Std Deviation n   Std Error
2.96   1.449   100   0.145
3.29   1.381   128   0.122
$t = (3.29-2.96) / \sqrt{(0.145^2+0.122^2)} = 1.96$
with $(100+128-2) = 226$ degrees of freedom

This would indicate that these two mean qol scores are significantly different from one another at $p < 0.05$.

In addition to summary statistics of different treatments, we can also compute summary statistics of qol scores by counseling yes or no.

Command

click the treatment drop box....select Total....next click the counseling drop box...first select counseling no....then select counseling yes.

The underneath tables are given.

OLAP Cubes

treatment:Total
counseling:Total

	Sum	N	Mean	Std. Deviation	% of Total Sum	% of Total N
qol score	1436	450	3,19	1,457	100,0%	100,0%

OLAP Cubes

treatment:Total
counseling:No

	Sum	N	Mean	Std. Deviation	% of Total Sum	% of Total N
qol score	652	230	2,83	1,530	45,4%	51,1%

OLAP Cubes

treatment:Total
counseling:Yes

	Sum	N	Mean	Std. Deviation	% of Total Sum	% of Total N
qol score	784	220	3,56	1,279	54,6%	48,9%

It is again easy to test whether the mean qol score of no-counseling is significantly lower than that of yes-counseling according to an unpaired t-test:

$$\begin{array}{llll} \text{mean} & \text{Std Deviation n} & & \text{Std Error} \\ 2.83 & 1.530 & 230 & 0.101 \\ 3.56 & 1.279 & 220 & 0.086 \\ \end{array}$$

$t = (3.56-2.83) / \sqrt{(0.101^2+0.086^2)} = 5.49$

with $(230+220 -2) = 448$ degrees of freedom

This would indicate that the two means are significantly different from one another at $p < 0.0001$.

Conclusion

In the current example the individual qol levels were estimated as 5 scores on a 5-points linear scale. In the Chaps. 2, 6 and 7 analyses took place by comparing frequencies of different qol scores with one another. In the OLAP cubes analysis a different approach is applied. Instead of working with frequencies of different qol scores, it works with mean scores and standard deviations. Other summary measure is also possible like sums of qol scores, medians, ranges or variances etc. Unpaired t-test can be used to test the significance of difference between various sub-summaries.

Although we have to admit that the crosstab analyses and OLAP cube lead to essentially the same results, the OLAP cube procedure is faster, and few simple tables are enough to tell you what is going on. Also additional statistical testing with the t-test is simple.

Note

More background, theoretical and mathematical information about the analyses of interaction matrices of frequencies are in the Chaps. 9, 10 and 11. The OLAP cube is another approach with similar results, but it works more rapidly than the other methods.

Chapter 17
Restructure Data Wizard for Data Classified the Wrong Way (20 Patients)

General Purpose

Underneath the opening page of the Restructure Data Wizard in SPSS is given. In the current chapter this tool will be applied for restructuring multiple variables in a single case to multiple cases with a single variables.

Electronic Supplementary Material The online version of this chapter (https://doi.org/10.1007/978-3-030-33970-8_17) contains supplementary material, which is available to authorized users.

Welcome to the Restructure Data Wizard!

This wizard helps you to restructure your data from multiple variables (columns) in a single case to groups of related cases (rows) or vice versa, or you can choose to transpose your data.

 The wizard replaces the current data set with the restructured data. Note that data restructuring cannot be undone.

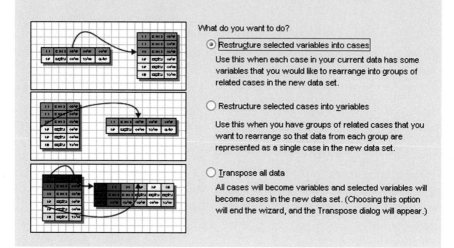

What do you want to do?

⦿ Restructure selected variables into cases

Use this when each case in your current data has some variables that you would like to rearrange into groups of related cases in the new data set.

◯ Restructure selected cases into variables

Use this when you have groups of related cases that you want to rearrange so that data from each group are represented as a single case in the new data set.

◯ Transpose all data

All cases will become variables and selected variables will become cases in the new data set. (Choosing this option will end the wizard, and the Transpose dialog will appear.)

Background

Suppose in a study the treatment outcome has been measured several times instead of once. In current clinical research repeated measures in a single subject are common. The problem with repeated measures is, that they are more close to one another than unrepeated measures. If this is not taken into account, then data analysis will lose power. The underneath table gives an example of a 2 group parallel-group study comparing two treatments for cholesterol reduction of 5 weeks. The example is taken from Chap. 6, Mixed linear models, pp. 65–77, in: Machine learning in medicine part one, Springer Heidelberg Germany, 2013, from the same authors.

It shows that 5 different variables present the 5 subsequent outcome measurements in each patient. In order to analyze these data appropriately, the table has to be restructured with each week given a separate row. This is a pretty laborious exercise, and it will get really annoying if you have 100 or more patients instead of 20. The restructure data wizard, however, should do the job within seconds.

Example   119

patientno	week 1	week 2	week 3	week 4	week 5	treatment modality
1	1,66	1,62	1,57	1,52	1,50	0,00
2	1,69	1,71	1,60	1,55	1,56	0,00
3	1,92	1,94	1,83	1,78	1,79	0,00
4	1,95	1,97	1,86	1,81	1,82	0,00
5	1,98	2,00	1,89	1,84	1,85	0,00
6	2,01	2,03	1,92	1,87	1,88	0,00
7	2,04	2,06	1,95	1,90	1,91	0,00
8	2,07	2,09	1,98	1,93	1,94	0,00
9	2,30	2,32	2,21	2,16	2,17	0,00
10	2,36	2,35	2,26	2,23	2,20	0,00
11	1,57	1,82	1,83	1,83	1,82	1,00
12	1,60	1,85	1,89	1,89	1,85	1,00
13	1,83	2,08	2,12	2,12	2,08	1,00
14	1,86	2,11	2,16	2,15	2,11	1,00
15	2,80	2,14	2,19	2,18	2,14	1,00
16	1,92	2,17	2,22	2,21	2,17	1,00
17	1,95	2,20	2,25	2,24	2,20	1,00
18	1,98	2,23	2,28	2,27	2,24	1,00
19	2,21	2,46	2,57	2,51	2,48	1,00
20	2,34	2,51	2,55	2,55	2,52	1,00

week 1 = hdl-cholesterol level after 1 week of trial
treatment modality = treatment modality (0 = treatment 0, 1 = treatment 1)

Primary Scientific Question

Can the restructure data wizard provide a table suitable for testing treatment efficacies adjusted for the repeated nature of the outcome data.

Example

The above data file is entitled "restructure.sav", and is in extras.springer.com. Start by opening the data file in SPSS statistical software.

Command
click Data....click Restructure....mark Restructure selected variables into cases.... click Next....mark One (for example, w1, w2, and w3)....click Next....Name: id (the patient id variable is already provided)....Target Variable: enter "firstweek, secondweek...... fifthweek"....Fixed Variable(s): enter treatment....click Next.... How many index variables do you want to create?.... mark One....click Next....click Next again....click Next again....click Finish.... Sets from the original data will still be in use...click OK.

Return to the main screen and observe that there are now 100 rows instead of 20 in the data file. The first 10 rows are given underneath.

id	treatment	Index1	Trans1
1	0,00	1	1,66
1	0,00	2	1,62
1	0,00	3	1,57
1	0,00	4	1,52
1	0,00	5	1,50
2	0,00	1	1,69
2	0,00	2	1,71
2	0,00	3	1,60
2	0,00	4	1,55
2	0,00	5	1,56

id = patient id
treatment = treatment modality
Index1 = week of treatment (1-5)
Trans1 = outcome values

We will now perform a mixed linear analysis of the data.

Command
Analyze....mixed models....linear....specify subjects and repeated....subject: enter id ....continue....linear mixed model....dependent: Trans1....factors: Index1, treatment....fixed....build nested term....treatment ....add.... Index1....add.... Index1 build term by* treatment....Index1 *treatment.... add....continue....OK (* = sign of multiplication).

The underneath table shows the main results from the above analysis. After adjustment for the repeated nature of the outcome data the treatment modality 0 performs much better than the treatment modality 1. The results from alternative analyses for these data were not only less appropriate but also less sensitive. The discussion of this is beyond the scope of the current chapter, but it can found in the Chap. 6, Mixed linear models, pp. 65–77, in: Machine learning in medicine part one, Springer Heidelberg Germany, 2013, from the same authors.

Type III Tests of Fixed Effects[a]

Source	Numerator df	Denominator df	F	Sig.
Intercept	1	76,570	6988,626	,000
week	4	31,149	,384	,818
treatment	1	76,570	20,030	,000
week * treatment	4	31,149	1,337	,278

a. Dependent Variable: outcome.

Conclusion

The restructure data wizard provides a table suitable for testing treatment efficacies adjusted for the repeated nature of the outcome data. It is particularly pleasant if your data file is big, and has many (repeated) observations. The Restructure function is not only a requirement with repeated outcome data, it is also often useful when dealing with data which is in long format and one needs the data in wide format, or vice versus. Long format refers to data in which each observation or participant has multiple rows. Wide format refers to data in which each observation or participant has only one row. Longitudinal research is an example of the type of research which often creates data files in long format.

Note

More background, theoretical and mathematical information of restructuring data files is in the Chap. 6, Mixed linear models, pp. 65–77, in: Machine learning in medicine part one, Springer Heidelberg Germany, 2013, from the same authors.

Chapter 18
Control Charts for Quality Control of Medicines (164 Tablet Desintegration Times)

General Purpose

The control chart is a graph used to study how a process changes over time. Data are plotted in time order. A control chart always has a central line for the average, an upper line for the upper control limit and a lower line for the lower control limit. These lines are determined from historical data. This chapter will use control charts for quality control of desintegration times of medicines.

Background

A consistent quality of a process or product, like the manufacturing of tablets is, traditionally, tested by 1 sample chi-square tests of their weights, diameters, desintegration times. E.g., tablets may only be approved, if the standard deviation of their diameters is less than 0.7 mm. E.g., a 50 tablet sample with a standard deviation of 0.9 mm is significantly different from 0.7 ($^$ = symbol of power term).

$$\text{Chi-square} = (50\text{-}1)\ 0.9^2 / 0.7^2 = 81$$
$$50\text{-}1 \text{ degrees of freedom}$$
$$p < 0.01 \text{ (one sided)}$$

The example is from the Chap. 44, entitled "Clinical data where variability is more important than averages", pp. 487–497, in: Statistics applied to clinical studies fifth edition, Springer Heidelberg Germany, 2012, from the same authors). Nowadays, we live in an era of machine learning, and ongoing quality control, instead of

Electronic Supplementary Material The online version of this chapter (https://doi.org/10.1007/978-3-030-33970-8_18) contains supplementary material, which is available to authorized users.

testing now and then, has become more easy, and, in addition, provides information of process variations over time and process performance. Control charts available in SPSS and other data mining software is helpful to that aim.

Primary Scientific Question

Control charts are currently routinely applied for the process control of larger factories, but they are, virtually, unused in the medical field. We will assess, whether they can be helpful to process control of pharmaceuticals.

Example

A important quality criterion of tablets is the desintegration time in water of 37 °C within 30 min or so. If it is considerably longer, the tablet will be too hard for consumption, if shorter it will be too soft for storage. 164 Tablets were tested over a period of 40 days.

day	desintegration (min)
1	33,2
1	31,0
1	32,7
1	30,8
1	32,2
1	31,3
2	30,1
2	31,5
2	33,6
2	32,2
4	32,9
4	32,2

The desintegration times of the first 11 tablets are above. The entire data file is in "qolcontrol.sav", and is in extras.springer.com. We will start the analysis by opening the data file in SPSS statistical software.

Command

Analyze....Quality Control....Control Charts....mark Cases are units....click Define....Process Measurement: enter "desintegration".....Subgroups Defined by: enter "days".....click Control Rules....mark: Above +3 sigma,

Example   125

Below -3 sigma,
2 out of last 3 above +2 sigma,
2 out of last 3 below -2 sigma,
4 out of 5 last above +1 sigma,
4 out of last 5 below -1 sigma

....click Continue....click Statistics....Specification Limits: Upper: type 36,0....Lower: type 30,0....Target: type 33,0....mark Actual % outside specification limits....Process Capability Indices....in Capacity Indices mark.

	CP
	CpL
	CpU
	k
	CpM....
....in Performance Indices mark	PP
	PpL
	PpU
	PpM....

Process capability and process performance indices are explained briefly.

Process capability indices:

CP	ratio of differences between the specification limits and the observed process variation, it should be >1, <1 indicates too much variation.
CpL and CpU	answer whether the process variations are symmetric, they should be close to CP.
K	measure of capability of the data, which should have their centers close to the specified target, a small K value is good (particularly if CP is >1).
CpM	same meaning as K, it should be close to CP.

Process performance indices:

	The values are similar to those of the process capability indices, but a bit smaller, because they overall instead of sample variability is taken into account. If a lot smaller, they indicate selection bias in the data.
PP	similar meaning as CP.
PpL and PpU	similar meaning as CpL and CpU.

The Above Commands Will be Completed Next

....click continue....click OK.

In the output sheets are two pivot figures and two pivot tables. Many details of the analyses can be called up after double-clicking them, then clicking the term pivot in the menu bar, and closing the upcoming pivoting tray. Drop boxes appear everywhere, and are convenient to visualize statistical details and textual explanations about what is going on (see the Chap. 15 for additional information on the use of pivoting figures and tables).

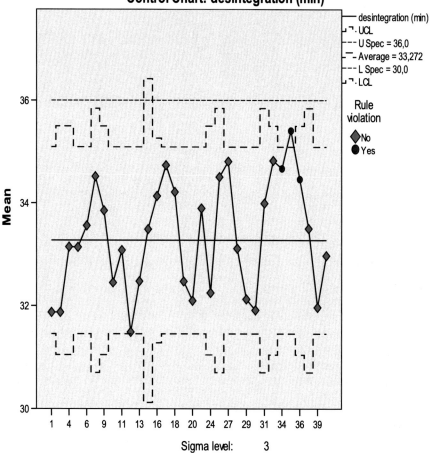

The above pivot figure shows a pattern of the mean desintegration times of the daily subsamples. The pattern is mostly within the 3 standard deviation limits. The straight interrupted lines give upper and lower specification limits (= overall mean ± 3 standard deviations, the lower one coincides with the x-axis, and is therefore not visible). The UCL (upper control limit) and LCL (lower control limit) curves describe sample ranges used to monitor spread in the daily subsamples. There are just three violations of the above set control rules of ±3 sigmas (= standard deviations) etc. The underneath table gives the details of the violations.

Example   127

Rule Violations for X-bar

day	Violations for Points
34	2 points out of the last 3 above +2 sigma
35	Greater than +3 sigma
35	2 points out of the last 3 above +2 sigma
36	4 points out of the last 5 above +1 sigma

3 points violate control rules.

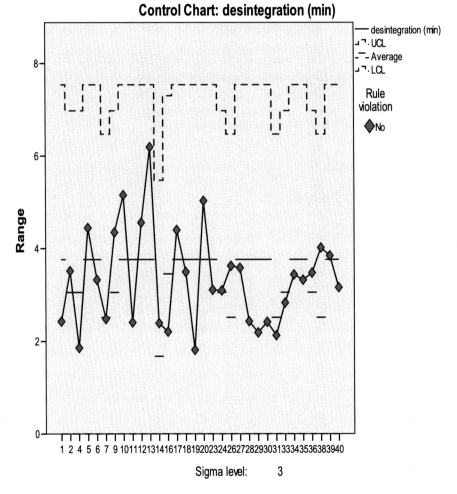

Control Chart: desintegration (min)

Sigma level: 3

The above table gives mean ranges of the daily subsamples. There are no violations of the control rules here.

The underneath table gives the process statistics.

Process Statistics

Act. % Outside SL		8,5%
Capability Indices	CP[a]	,674
	CpL[a]	,735
	CpU[a]	,613
	K	,091
	CpM[a,b]	,663
Performance Indices	PP	,602
	PpL	,657
	PpU	,548
	PpM[b]	,594

The normal distribution is assumed. LSL = 30,0 and USL = 36,0.

a. The estimated capability sigma is based on the mean of the sample group ranges.
b. The target value is 33,0.

The above table shows that the process stability is pretty bad with CP and PP values a lot < 1. K is small, which is good, because it indicates that the center of the data is close to the specified target.

Conclusion

The above analysis shows that control charts methodology may be helpful to process control of pharmaceuticals, and. The example data were largely in control, and the process mean was close to the specified target value of 33,0 min. Nonetheless, statistics of process stability were pretty weak, and precision of the data was pretty bad.

Note

More background, theoretical and mathematical information of the SPSS module Quality Control is in the Chap. 67. More information of process quality control is also in the Chap. 44, entitled "Clinical data where variability is more important than averages", pp. 487–497, in: Statistics applied to clinical studies fifth edition, Springer Heidelberg Germany 2012, from the same authors.

Part II
(Log) Linear Models

Chapter 19
Linear, Logistic, and Cox Regression for Outcome Prediction with Unpaired Data (20, 55, and 60 Patients)

General Purpose

To assess whether linear, logistic and Cox modeling can be used to train clinical data samples to make predictions about groups and individual patients.

Background

Outcome predictions from previous data analyses require a prediction file. Often an Extensible Markup Language (XML) file is applied for the purpose. It is really just a plain text file that uses custom tags to describe the structure and other features of the document. XML is a markup language created by the World Wide Web Consortium (W3C) to define a syntax for encoding documents that both humans and machines could read. It does this through the use of tags that define the structure of the document, as well as how the document should be stored and transported. It's probably easiest to compare it to another markup language with which you should be familiar—the Hypertext Markup Language (HTML) used to encode web pages. HTML uses a pre-defined set of markup symbols (short codes) that describe the format of content on a web page. For example, the following simple HTML code uses tags to make some words bold and some italic: The thing that differentiates XML, though, is that it's extensible. XML doesn't have a predefined markup language, like HTML does. Instead, XML allows users to create their own markup symbols to describe content, making an unlimited and self-defining symbol set.

This chapter was previously published in "Machine learning in medicine-cookbook 1" as Chap. 4, 2013.

Electronic Supplementary Material The online version of this chapter (https://doi.org/10.1007/978-3-030-33970-8_19) contains supplementary material, which is available to authorized users.

Essentially, HTML is a language that focuses on the presentation of content, while XML is a dedicated data-description language used to store data. XML is often used as the basis for other document formats – hundreds, in fact. However, here is a common feature you might recognize: an XML file doesn't necessarily tell you what app it's intended to use with. And typically, you won't need to worry about it, unless you're the one actually designing XML files. There are a few ways you can open an XML file directly. You can open and edit them with any text editor, view them with any web browser, or use a website that lets you view, edit, and even convert them to other formats. Since XML files are really just text files, you can open them in any text editor. The thing is, a lot of text editors – like Notepad – just aren't designed to show XML files with their proper structure. It might be okay for popping an XML file open and taking a quick look to help figure out what it is. But, there are much better tools for working with them. Right-click the XML file you want to open, point to "Open With" on the context menu, and then click the "Notepad" option.

Specific Scientific Question

How many hours will patients sleep, how large is the risk for patients to fall out of bed, how large is the hazard for patients to die.

Linear Regression, the Computer Teaches Itself to Make Predictions

Var 1	Var 2	Var 3	Var 4	Var 5
0,00	6,00	65,00	0,00	1,00
0,00	7,10	75,00	0,00	1,00
0,00	8,10	86,00	0,00	0,00
0,00	7,50	74,00	0,00	0,00
0,00	6,40	64,00	0,00	1,00
0,00	7,90	75,00	1,00	1,00
0,00	6,80	65,00	1,00	1,00
0,00	6,60	64,00	1,00	0,00
0,00	7,30	75,00	1,00	0,00
0,00	5,60	56,00	0,00	0,00
1,00	5,10	55,00	1,00	0,00
1,00	8,00	85,00	0,00	1,00
1,00	3,80	36,00	1,00	0,00
1,00	4,40	47,00	0,00	1,00
1,00	5,20	58,00	1,00	0,00
1,00	5,40	56,00	0,00	1,00

1,00	4,30	46,00	1,00	1,00
1,00	6,00	64,00	1,00	0,00
1,00	3,70	33,00	1,00	0,00
1,00	6,20	65,00	0,00	1,00

Var = variable
Var 1 = treatment 0 is placebo, treatment 1 is sleeping pill
Var 2 = hours of sleep
Var 3 = age
Var 4 = gender
Var 5 = comorbidity

SPSS 19.0 is used for analysis, with the help of an XML (eXtended Markup Language) file. The data file is entitled "linoutcomeprediction" and is in extras. springer.com. Start by opening the data file.

Command
Click Transform....click Random Number Generators....click Set Starting Point ....click Fixed Value (2000000)....click OK....click Analyze....Regression.... Linear....Dependent: enter hoursofsleep....Independent: enter treatment and age....click Save....Predicted Values: click Unstandardized....in XML Files click Export final model....click Browse....File name: enter "exportlin"....click Save....click Continue....click OK.

Coefficients[a]

Model		Unstandardized Coefficients		Standardized Coefficients		
		B	Std. Error	Beta	t	Sig.
1	(Constant)	,989	,366		2,702	,015
	treatment	-,411	,143	-,154	-2,878	,010
	age	,085	,005	,890	16,684	,000

a. Dependent Variable: hoursofsleep

The output sheets show in the coefficients table that both treatment and age are significant predictors at $p < 0.10$. Returning to the data file we will observe that SPSS has computed predicted values and gives them in a novel variable entitled PRE_1. The saved XML file will now be used to compute the predicted hours of sleep in 4 novel patients with the following characteristics. For convenience the XML file is given in extras.springer.com.

Var 1	Var 2	Var 3	Var 4	Var 5
,00	6,00	66,00	,00	1,00
,00	7,10	74,00	,00	1,00
,00	8,10	86,00	,00	,00

,00   7,50   74,00   ,00   ,00

Var 1 = treatment 0 is placebo, treatment 1 is sleeping pill
Var 2 = hours of sleep
Var 3 = age
Var 4 = gender
Var 5 = comorbidity

Enter the above data in a new SPSS data file.

Command
Utilities....click Scoring Wizard....click Browse....click Select....Folder: enter
the exportlin.xml file....click Select....in Scoring Wizard click Next....click Use
value substitution....click Next....click Finish.

The above data file now gives individually predicted hours of sleep as computed
by the linear model with the help of the XML file.

Var 1	Var 2	Var 3	Var 4	Var 5	Var 6
,00	6,00	66,00	,00	1,00	6,51
,00	7,10	74,00	,00	1,00	7,28
,00	8,10	86,00	,00	,00	8,30
,00	7,50	74,00	,00	,00	7,28

Var 1 = treatment 0 is placebo, treatment 1 is sleeping pill
Var 2 = hours of sleep
Var 3 = age
Var 4 = gender
Var 5 = comorbidity
Var 6 = predicted hours of sleep

Conclusion

The module linear regression can be readily trained to predict hours of sleep both in
groups and, with the help of an XML file, in individual future patients.

Note

More background, theoretical and mathematical information of linear regression is.
    available in Statistics applied to clinical studies, 5th edition, Chaps. 14 and 15,
entitled "Linear regression basic approach" and "Linear regression for assessing

precision, confounding, interaction", pp. 161–176 and 177–185, Springer Heidelberg Germany 2012, from the same authors.

Logistic Regression, the Computer Teaches Itself to Make Predictions

Var 1	Var 2	Var 3	Var 4	Var 5
,00	1,00	50,00	,00	1,00
,00	1,00	76,00	,00	1,00
,00	1,00	57,00	1,00	1,00
,00	1,00	65,00	,00	1,00
,00	1,00	46,00	1,00	1,00
,00	1,00	36,00	1,00	1,00
,00	1,00	98,00	,00	,00
,00	1,00	56,00	1,00	,00
,00	1,00	44,00	,00	,00
,00	1,00	76,00	1,00	1,00
,00	1,00	75,00	1,00	1,00
,00	1,00	74,00	1,00	1,00
,00	1,00	87,00	,00	,00

Var = variable
Var 1 department type
Var 2 falling out of bed (1 = yes)
Var 3 age
Var 4 gender
Var 5 letter of complaint (1 = yes)

Only the first 13 patients are given, the entire data file is entitled "logoutcomeprediction" and is in extras.springer.com.

SPSS 19.0 is used for analysis, with the help of an XML (eXtended Markup Language) file. Start by opening the data file.

Command
Click Transform....click Random Number Generators....click Set Starting Point ....click Fixed Value (2000000)....click OK....click Analyze....Regression .... Binary Logistic....Dependent: enter fallingoutofbed ....Covariates: enter departmenttype and letterofcomplaint....click Save....in Predicted Values click Probabilities....in Export model information to XML file click Browse.... File name: enter "exportlog"....click Save....click Continue....click OK.

Variables in the Equation

		B	S.E.	Wald	df	Sig.	Exp(B)
Step 1ª	departmenttype	1,349	,681	3,930	1	,047	3,854
	letterofcomplaint	2,039	,687	8,816	1	,003	7,681
	Constant	-1,007	,448	5,047	1	,025	,365

a. Variable(s) entered on step 1: departmenttype, letterofcomplaint.

In the above output table it is shown that both department type and letter of complaint are significant predictors of the risk of falling out of bed. Returning to the data file we will observe that SPSS has computed predicted values and gives them in a novel variable entitled PRE_1. The saved XML file will now be used to compute the predicted hours of sleep in 5 novel patients with the following characteristics. For convenience the XML file is given in extras.springer.com.

Var 1	Var 2	Var 3	Var 4	Var 5
,00	,00	67,00	,00	,00
1,00	1,00	54,00	1,00	,00
1,00	1,00	65,00	1,00	,00
1,00	1,00	74,00	1,00	1,00
1,00	1,00	73,00	,00	1,00

Var = variable
Var 1 department type
Var 2 falling out of bed (1 = yes)
Var 3 age
Var 4 gender
Var 5 letter of complaint (1 = yes)

Enter the above data in a new SPSS data file.

Command
Utilities....click Scoring Wizard....click Browse....click Select....Folder: enter the exportlog.xml file....click Select....in Scoring Wizard click Next....mark Probability of Predicted Category....click Next....click Finish.

The above data file now gives individually predicted probabilities of falling out of bed as computed by the logistic model with the help of the XML file.

Var 1	Var 2	Var 3	Var 4	Var 5	Var 6
,00	,00	67,00	,00	,00	,73
1,00	1,00	54,00	1,00	,00	,58
1,00	1,00	65,00	1,00	,00	,58
1,00	1,00	74,00	1,00	1,00	,92
1,00	1,00	73,00	,00	1,00	,92

Var 1 department type
Var 2 falling out of bed (1 = yes)
Var 3 age
Var 4 gender
Var 5 letter of complaint (1 = yes)
Var 6 Predicted Probability

Conclusion
The module binary logistic regression can be readily trained to predict probability of falling out of bed both in groups and, with the help of an XML file, in individual future patients.

Note
More background, theoretical and mathematical information of binary logistic regression is available in Statistics applied to clinical studies 5th edition, Chaps. 17, 19, and 65, entitled "Logistic and Cox regression, Markov models, Laplace transformations", "Post-hoc analyses in clinical trials", and "Odds ratios and multiple regression", pp. 199–218, 227–231, and 695–711, Springer Heidelberg Germany 2012, from the same authors.

Cox Regression, the Computer Teaches Itself to Make Predictions

Var 1	Var 2	Var 3	Var 4
1,00	1,00	,00	65,00
1,00	1,00	,00	66,00
2,00	1,00	,00	73,00
2,00	1,00	,00	91,00
2,00	1,00	,00	86,00
2,00	1,00	,00	87,00
2,00	1,00	,00	54,00
2,00	1,00	,00	66,00
2,00	1,00	,00	64,00
3,00	,00	,00	62,00
4,00	1,00	,00	57,00
5,00	1,00	,00	85,00
6,00	1,00	,00	85,00

Var = variable
Var 1 follow up in months
Var 2 event (1 = yes)
Var 3 treatment modality
Var 4 age

Only the first 13 patients are given, the entire data file is entitled "Coxoutcomeprediction" and is in extras.springer.com.

SPSS 19.0 is used for analysis, with the help of an XML (eXtended Markup Language) file. Start by opening the data file.

Command

Click Transform....click Random Number Generators....click Set Starting Point
....click Fixed Value (2000000)....click OK....click Analyze....Survival....Cox
Regression....Time: followupmonth....Status: event....Define event: enter 1....
Covariates: enter treatment and age....click Save....mark: Survival function.... In
Export Model information to XML file click Browse.... File name: enter
"exportCox"....click Save....click Continue....click OK.

Variables in the Equation

	B	SE	Wald	df	Sig.	Exp(B)
treatment	-,791	,332	5,686	1	,017	,454
age	,028	,012	5,449	1	,020	1,028

In the above output table it is shown that both treatment modality and age are
significant predictors of survival. Returning to the data file we will now observe that
SPSS has computed individual probabilities of survival and gave them in a novel
variable entitled SUR_1. The probabilities vary from 0.00 to 1.00. E.g., for the first
patient, based on follow up of 1 month, treatment modality 0, and age 65, the
computer has computed a mean survival chance at the time of observation of
0.95741 (= over 95%). Other patients had much less probability of survival. If
you would have limited sources for further treatment in this population, it would
make sense not to burden with continued treatment those with, e.g., less than 20%
survival probability. We should emphasize that the probability is based on the
information of the variables 1, 3, 4, and is assumed to be measured just prior to
the event, and the event is not taken into account here.

Var 1 Var 2 Var 3 Var 4 SUR_1
1,00   1,00   ,00   65,00 ,95,741

The saved XML file will now be used to compute the predicted probabilities of
survival in 5 novel patients with the following characteristics. For convenience the
XML file is given in extras.springer.com. We will skip the variable 2 for the above
reason.

Var 1 Var 2 Var 3 Var 4
30,00   1,00   88,00
29,00   1,00   67,00
29,00   1,00   56,00
29,00   1,00   54,00
28,00   1,00   57,00

Var = variable
Var 1 follow up in months

Var 2 event (1 = yes)
Var 3 treatment modality
Var 4 age

Enter the above data in a new SPSS data file.

Command
Utilities....click Scoring Wizard....click Browse....click Select....Folder: enter the exportCox.xml file....click Select....in Scoring Wizard click Next....mark Predicted Value....click Next....click Finish.

The above data file now gives individually predicted probabilities of survival as computed by the Cox regression model with the help of the XML file.

Var 1	Var 2	Var 3	Var 4	Var 5 PredictedValue
30,00		1,00	88,00	,18
29,00		1,00	67,00	,39
29,00		1,00	56,00	,50
29,00		1,00	54,00	,51
28,00		1,00	57,00	,54

Var = variable
Var 1 follow up in months
Var 2 event (1 = yes)
Var 3 treatment modality
Var 4 age
Var 5 predicted probability of survival (0.0–1.0)

Conclusion
The module Cox regression can be readily trained to predict probability of survival both in groups and, with the help of an XML file, in individual future patients. Like outcome prediction with linear and logistic regression models, Cox regression is an important method to determine with limited health care sources, who of the patients will be recommended expensive medications and other treatments.

Note
More background, theoretical and mathematical information of binary logistic regression is available in Statistics applied to clinical studies 5th edition, Chaps. 17 and 31, entitled "Logistic and Cox regression, Markov models, Laplace transformations", and "Time-dependent factor analysis", pp. 199–218, and pp. 353–364, Springer Heidelberg Germany 2012, from the same authors.

Chapter 20
Generalized Linear Models for Outcome Prediction with Paired Data (100 Patients and 139 Physicians)

General Purpose

With linear and logistic regression *unpaired* data can be used for outcome prediction. With generalized linear models *paired* data can be used for the purpose.

This chapter gives some examples.

Background

Generalized linear model (GLDM) is a flexible generalization of ordinary linear regression, that allows for response variables, that have error distribution models other than the normal distribution. In order to avoid misunderstandings about terminology, the term *general linear model* (GLM) is different and refers to conventional linear regression models for a continuous response variable given continuous and/or categorical predictors. It includes multiple linear regression, as well as ANOVA (analysis of variance) and ANCOVA (analysis of covariance). These models are fit by least squares and weighted least squares. The term *generalized linear model* (GLDM) refers to a larger class of models popularized by McCullagh and Nelder (1982, 2nd edition 1989). In these models, the response variable follows an exponential family distribution with mean, being some (often nonlinear) function. The generalized linear models (GLDMs) are a broad class of models that include linear regression, ANOVA, Poisson regression, log-linear models, gamma regression, Tweedie regression. In SPSS statistical software, GLDM also includes paired

This chapter was previously published in "Machine learning in medicine-cookbook 1" as Chap. 5, 2013.

Electronic Supplementary Material The online version of this chapter (https://doi.org/10.1007/978-3-030-33970-8_20) contains supplementary material, which is available to authorized users.

© Springer Nature Switzerland AG 2020

T. J. Cleophas, A. H. Zwinderman, *Machine Learning in Medicine – A Complete Overview*, https://doi.org/10.1007/978-3-030-33970-8_20

outcome data analysis, and event rate analysis. And a closely related module entitled generalized estimation equation models (GEE models) addresses paired binary outcomes. All of these analytical models will be assessed in various chapters of the current edition.

Traditional tests like paired t-tests and Wilcoxon signed rank tests require, just like multivariate data, two outcome variables, like the effects of two parallel treatments. Generalized Linear Models can simultaneously assess the difference between two outcomes, and, at the same time, the overall effect of additional predictors on the outcome data.

Specific Scientific Question

Can crossover studies (1) of sleeping pills and (2) of lifestyle treatments be used as training samples to predict hours of sleep and lifestyle treatment in groups and individuals.

Generalized Linear Modeling, the Computer Teaches Itself to Make Predictions

Var 1	Var 2	Var 3	Var 4
6,10	79,00	1,00	1,00
5,20	79,00	1,00	2,00
7,00	55,00	2,00	1,00
7,90	55,00	2,00	2,00
8,20	78,00	3,00	1,00
3,90	78,00	3,00	2,00
7,60	53,00	4,00	1,00
4,70	53,00	4,00	2,00
6,50	85,00	5,00	1,00
5,30	85,00	5,00	2,00
8,40	85,00	6,00	1,00
5,40	85,00	6,00	2,00

Var = variable
Var 1 = outcome (hours of sleep after sleeping pill or placebo)
Var 2 = age
Var 3 = patientnumber (patientid)
Var 4 = treatment modality (1 sleeping pill, 2 placebo)

Only the data from first 6 patients are given, the entire data file is entitled "generalizedlmpairedcontinuous" and is in extras.springer.com. SPSS 19.0 is used for analysis, with the help of an XML (eXtended Markup Language) file. Start by opening the data file.

Command

Click Transform....click Random Number Generators....click Set Starting Point ....click Fixed Value (2000000)....click OK....click Analyze....Generalized Linear Models....again click Generalized Linear models....click Type of Model.... click Linear....click Response....Dependent Variable: enter Outcome....Scale Weight Variable: enter patientid....click Predictors....Factors: enter treatment.... Covariates: enter age....click Model: Model: enter treatment and age....click Save: mark Predicted value of linear predictor....click Export....click Browse....File name: enter "exportpairedcontinuous"....click Save....click Continue.... click OK.

The output sheets show, that both treatment and age are significant predictors at p < 0.10.

Parameter Estimates

Parameter	B	Std. Error	95% Wald Confidence Interval		Hypothesis Test		
			Lower	Upper	Wald Chi-Square	df	Sig.
(Intercept)	6,178	,5171	5,165	7,191	142,763	1	,000
[treatment=1,00]	2,003	,2089	1,593	2,412	91,895	1	,000
[treatment=2,00]	0ª	.	.	.	.	.	.
age	-,014	,0075	-,029	,001	3,418	1	,064
(Scale)	27,825ᵇ	3,9351	21,089	36,713			

Dependent Variable: outcome
Model: (Intercept), treatment, age

a. Set to zero because this parameter is redundant.
b. Maximum likelihood estimate.

Returning to the data file we will observe, that SPSS has computed predicted values of hours of sleep, and has given them in a novel variable entitled XBPredicted (predicted values of linear predictor). The saved XML file entitled "exportpairedcontinuous") will now be used to compute the predicted hours of sleep in five novel patients with the following characteristics. For convenience the XML file is given in extras.springer.com.

Var 2	Var 3	Var 4
79,00	1,00	1,00
55,00	2,00	1,00
78,00	3,00	1,00
53,00	4,00	2,00
85,00	5,00	1,00

Var = variable

Var 2 = age
Var 3 = patientnumber (patientid)
Var 4 = treatment modality (1 sleeping pill, 2 placebo)

Enter the above data in a new SPSS data file.

Command

Utilities....click Scoring Wizard....click Browse....click Select....Folder: enter the exportpairedcontinuous.xml file....click Select....in Scoring Wizard click Next....click Use value substitution....click Next....click Finish.

The above data file now gives individually predicted hours of sleep as computed by the linear model with the help of the XML file.

Var 2	Var 3	Var 4	Var 5
79,00	1,00	1,00	7,09
55,00	2,00	1,00	7,42
78,00	3,00	1,00	7,10
53,00	4,00	2,00	5,44
85,00	5,00	1,00	7,00

Var = variable
Var 2 = age
Var 3 = patientnumber (patientid)
Var 4 = treatment modality (1 sleeping pill, 2 placebo)
Var 5 = predicted values of hours of sleep in individual patient

Conclusion

The SPSS module generalized linear models can be readily trained to predict hours of sleep in groups, and, with the help of an XML file, in individual future patients.

Generalized Estimation Equations, the Computer Teaches Itself to Make Predictions

Var 1	Var 2	Var 3	Var 4
,00	89,00	1,00	1,00
,00	89,00	1,00	2,00
,00	78,00	2,00	1,00
,00	78,00	2,00	2,00
,00	79,00	3,00	1,00

,00	79,00	3,00	2,00
,00	76,00	4,00	1,00
,00	76,00	4,00	2,00
,00	87,00	5,00	1,00
,00	87,00	5,00	2,00
,00	84,00	6,00	1,00
,00	84,00	6,00	2,00
,00	84,00	7,00	1,00
,00	84,00	7,00	2,00
,00	69,00	8,00	1,00
,00	69,00	8,00	2,00
,00	77,00	9,00	1,00
,00	77,00	9,00	2,00
,00	79,00	10,00	1,00
,00	79,00	10,00	2,00

Var = variable
Var 1 outcome (lifestyle advise given 0 = no, 1 = yes)
Var 2 physicians' age
Var 3 physicians' id
Var 4 prior postgraduate education regarding lifestyle advise (1 = no, 2 = yes)

Only the first 10 physicians are given, the entire data file is entitled "generalizedpairedbinary" and is in extras.springer.com. All physicians are assessed twice, once before lifestyle education and once after. The effect of lifestyle education on the willingness to provide lifestyle advise was the main objective of the study.

SPSS 19.0 is used for analysis, with the help of an XML (eXtended Markup Language) file. Start by opening the data file.

Command
Click Transform....click Random Number Generators....click Set Starting Point ....click Fixed Value (2000000)....click OK....click Analyze....Generalized Linear Models....Generalized Estimating Equations....click Repeated....in Subjects variables enter physicianid....in Within-subject variables enter lifestyle advise.... in Structure enter Unstructured....click Type of Model....mark Binary logistic.... click Response....in Dependent Variable enter outcome....click Reference Category....mark First....click Continue....click Predictors....in Factors enter lifestyleadvise....in Covariates enter age....click Model....in Model enter lifestyle and age....click Save....mark Predicted value of mean of response....click Export ....mark Export model in XML....click Browse.... In File name: enter "exportpairedbinary"....in Look in: enter the appropriate map in your computer for storage....click Save....click Continue....click OK.

Parameter Estimates

Parameter	B	Std. Error	95% Wald Confidence Interval		Hypothesis Test		
			Lower	Upper	Wald Chi-Square	df	Sig.
(Intercept)	2,469	,7936	,913	4,024	9,677	1	,002
[lifestyleadvise=1,00]	-,522	,2026	-,919	-,124	6,624	1	,010
[lifestyleadvise=2,00]	0ᵃ	.	.	.	.	.	.
age	-,042	,0130	-,068	-,017	10,563	1	,001
(Scale)	1						

Dependent Variable: outcome
Model: (Intercept), lifestyleadvise, age

a. Set to zero because this parameter is redundant.

The output sheets show that both prior lifestyle education and physicians' age are very significant predictors at p < 0.01. Returning to the data file we will observe that SPSS has computed predicted probabilities of lifestyle advise given or not by each physician in the data file, and a novel variable is added to the data file for the purpose. It is given the name MeanPredicted. The saved XML file entitled "exportpairedbinary" will now be used to compute the predicted probability of receiving lifestyle advise based on physicians' age and the physicians' prior lifestyle education in twelve novel physicians. For convenience the XML file is given in extras.springer.com.

Var 2	Var 3	Var 4
64,00	1,00	2,00
64,00	2,00	1,00
65,00	3,00	1,00
65,00	3,00	2,00
52,00	4,00	1,00
66,00	5,00	1,00
79,00	6,00	1,00
79,00	6,00	2,00
53,00	7,00	1,00
53,00	7,00	2,00
55,00	8,00	1,00
46,00	9,00	1,00

Var = variable
Var 2 age
Var 3 physicianid
Var 4 lifestyleadvise (prior postgraduate education regarding lifestyle advise (1 = no, 2 = yes))

Enter the above data in a new SPSS data file.

Command

Utilities....click Scoring Wizard....click Browse....click Select....Folder: enter
the exportpairedbinary.xml file....click Select....in Scoring Wizard click Next....
mark Probability of Predicted Category....click Next....click Finish.

The above data file now gives individually predicted probabilities of receiving
lifestyle advise as computed by the logistic model with the help of the XML file.

Var 2	Var 3	Var 4	Var 5
64,00	1,00	2,00	,56
64,00	2,00	1,00	,68
65,00	3,00	1,00	,69
65,00	3,00	2,00	,57
52,00	4,00	1,00	,56
66,00	5,00	1,00	,70
79,00	6,00	1,00	,80
79,00	6,00	2,00	,70
53,00	7,00	1,00	,57
53,00	7,00	2,00	,56
55,00	8,00	1,00	,59
46,00	9,00	1,00	,50

Var = variable
Var 2 age
Var 3 physicianid
Var 4 lifestyleadvise
Var 5 probability of predicted category (between 0.0 and 1.0)

Conclusion

The SPSS module generalized estimating equations can be readily trained to predict
with paired data the probability of physicians giving lifestyle advise as groups and,
with the help of an XML file, as individual physicians.

Note

More background, theoretical and mathematical information of paired analysis of
binary data is given in SPSS for starters part one, Chap. 13, entitled "Paired binary
(McNemar test)", pp. 47–49, Springer Heidelberg Germany, 2010, from the same
authors.

Chapter 21
Generalized Linear Models Event-Rates (50 Patients)

General Purpose

This chapter assesses, whether in a longitudinal study event rates, defined as numbers of events per person per period, can be analyzed with the generalized linear model module. This chapter gives some examples.

Background

Generalized linear model (GLDM) is a flexible generalization of ordinary linear regression that allows for response variables that have error distribution models other than the normal distribution. In order to avoid misunderstandings about terminology, the term *general linear model* (GLM) is different and refers to conventional linear regression models for a continuous response variable given continuous and/or categorical predictors. It includes multiple linear regression, as well as ANOVA (analysis of variance) and ANCOVA (analysis of covariance). These models are fit by least squares and weighted least squares. The term *generalized linear model* (GLDM) refers to a larger class of models popularized by McCullagh and Nelder (1982, 2nd edition 1989). In these models, the response variable follows an exponential family distribution with mean, being some (often nonlinear) function. The generalized linear models (GLDMs) are a broad class of models that include linear regression, ANOVA, Poisson regression, log-linear models, gamma regression, Tweedie regression. In SPSS statistical software GLDM also includes paired

This chapter was previously published in "Machine learning in medicine-cookbook 1" as Chap. 6, 2013.

Electronic Supplementary Material The online version of this chapter (https://doi.org/10.1007/978-3-030-33970-8_21) contains supplementary material, which is available to authorized users.

© Springer Nature Switzerland AG 2020
T. J. Cleophas, A. H. Zwinderman, *Machine Learning in Medicine – A Complete Overview*, https://doi.org/10.1007/978-3-030-33970-8_21

149

outcome data analysis, and event rate analysis. And a closely related module entitled generalized estimation equation models (GEE models) addresses paired binary outcomes. All of these analytical models will be assessed in various chapters of the current edition.

Traditional tests like paired t-tests and Wilcoxon signed rank tests require, just like multivariate data, two outcome variables, like the effects of two parallel treatments. Generalized Linear Models can simultaneously assess the difference between two outcomes, and the overall effect of additional predictors on the outcome data.

Specific Scientific Question

Can generalized linear modeling be trained to predict rates of episodes of paroxysmal atrial fibrillation both in groups and in individual future patients.

Example

Fifty patients were followed for numbers of episodes of paroxysmal atrial fibrillation (PAF), while on treated with two parallel treatment modalities. The data file is below.

Var 1	Var 2	Var 3	Var 4	Var 5
1	56,99	42,45	73	4
1	37,09	46,82	73	4
0	32,28	43,57	76	2
0	29,06	43,57	74	3
0	6,75	27,25	73	3
0	61,65	48,41	62	13
0	56,99	40,74	66	11
1	10,39	15,36	72	7
1	50,53	52,12	63	10
1	49,47	42,45	68	9
0	39,56	36,45	72	4
1	33,74	13,13	74	5

Var = variable
Var 1 = treatment modality
Var 2 = psychological score
Var 3 = social score
Var 4 = days of observation
Var 5 = number of episodes of paroxysmal atrial fibrillation (PAF)

The first 12 patients are shown only, the entire data file is entitled "generalizedlmeventrates" and is in extras.springer.com.

The Computer Teaches Itself to Make Predictions

SPSS 19.0 is used for training and outcome prediction. It uses XML (eXtended Markup Language) files to store data. We will perform the analysis with a linear regression analysis of variable 5 as outcome variable and the other 4 variables as predictors. Start by opening the data file.

Command
Analyze....Regression....Linear....Dependent Variable: episodes of paroxysmal atrial fibrillation....Independent: treatment modality, psychological score, social score, days of observation....click OK.

Coefficients^a

Model		Unstandardized Coefficients		Standardized Coefficients	t	Sig.
		B	Std. Error	Beta		
1	(Constant)	49,059	5,447		9,006	,000
	treat	-2,914	1,385	-,204	-2,105	,041
	psych	,014	,052	,036	,273	,786
	soc	-,073	,058	-,169	-1,266	,212
	days	-,557	,074	-,715	-7,535	,000

a. Dependent Variable: paf

The above table shows that treatment modality is weakly significant, and psychological and social scores are not. Furthermore, days of observation is very significant. However, it is not entirely appropriate to include this variable if your outcome is the numbers of events per person per time unit. Therefore, we will perform a linear regression, and adjust the outcome variable for the differences in days of observation using weighted least square regression.

Coefficients^{a,b}

Model		Unstandardized Coefficients		Standardized Coefficients	t	Sig.
		B	Std. Error	Beta		
1	(Constant)	10,033	2,862		3,506	,001
	treat	-3,502	1,867	-,269	-1,876	,067
	psych	,033	,069	,093	,472	,639
	soc	-,093	,078	-,237	-1,194	,238

a. Dependent Variable: paf

b. Weighted Least Squares Regression - Weighted by days

Command

Analyze....Regression....Linear....Dependent: episodes of paroxysmal atrial fibrillation....Independent: treatment modality, psychological score, social score ....WLS Weight: days of observation.... click OK.

The above table shows the results. A largely similar pattern is observed, but treatment modality is no more statistically significant. We will use the generalized linear modeling module to perform a Poisson regression which is more appropriate for rate data. The model applied will also be stored and reapplied for making predictions about event rates in individual future patients.

Command

Click Transform....click Random Number Generators....click Set Starting Point.... click Fixed Value (2000000)....click OK....click Generalized Linear Models ....click again Generalized Linear Models....mark: Custom....Distribution: Poisson.....Link function: Log....Response: Dependent variable: numbers of episodes of PAF....Scale Weight Variable: days of observation....Predictors: Main Effect: treatment modality....Covariates: psychological score, social score.... Model: main effects: treatment modality, psychological score, social score.... Estimation: mark Model-based Estimation ....click Save....mark Predicted value of mean of response....click Export....mark Export model in XML....click Browse.... in File name enter "exportrate"....in Look in: enter the appropriate map in your computer for storage....click Save....click OK.

Parameter Estimates

Parameter	B	Std. Error	95% Wald Confidence Interval		Hypothesis Test		
			Lower	Upper	Wald Chi-Square	df	Sig.
(Intercept)	1,868	,0206	1,828	1,909	8256,274	1	,000
[treat=0]	,667	,0153	,637	,697	1897,429	1	,000
[treat=1]	0[a]	.	.	.	.	.	.
psych	,006	,0006	,005	,008	120,966	1	,000
soc	-,019	,0006	-,020	-,017	830,264	1	,000
(Scale)	1[b]						

Dependent Variable: paf
Model: (Intercept), treat, psych, soc

a. Set to zero because this parameter is redundant.

b. Fixed at the displayed value.

The outcome sheets give the results. All of a sudden, all of the predictors including treatment modality, psychological and social score are very significant predictors of the PAF rate. When minimizing the output sheets the data file returns and now shows a novel variable entitled "PredictedValues" with the mean rates of PAF episodes per patient (per day). The saved XML file will now be used to compute the predicted PAF rate in 5 novel patients with the following characteristics. For convenience the XML file is given in extras.springer.com.

Var 1   Var 2   Var 3   Var 4   Var 5

1,00	56,99	42,45	73,00	4,00
1,00	30,09	46,82	34,00	4,00
,00	32,28	32,00	76,00	2,00
,00	29,06	40,00	36,00	3,00
,00	6,75	27,25	73,00	3,00

Var = variable
Var 1 = treatment modality
Var 2 = psychological score
Var 3 = social score
Var 4 = days of observation
Var 5 = number of episodes of paroxysmal atrial fibrillation (PAF)

Enter the above data in a new SPSS data file.

Command
Utilities....click Scoring Wizard....click Browse....click Select....Folder: enter
the exportrate.xml file....click Select....in Scoring Wizard click Next....click Use
value substitution....click Next....click Finish.

The above data file now gives individually predicted rates of PAF as computed by
the linear model with the help of the XML file. Enter the above data in a new SPSS
data file.

Var 1	Var 2	Var 3	Var 4	Var 5	Var 6
1,00	56,99	42,45	73,00	4,00	4,23
1,00	30,09	46,82	34,00	4,00	3,27
,00	32,28	32,00	76,00	2,00	8,54
,00	29,06	40,00	36,00	3,00	7,20
,00	6,75	27,25	73,00	3,00	7,92

Var = variable
Var 1 = treatment modality
Var 2 = psychological score
Var 3 = social score
Var 4 = days of observation
Var 5 = number of episodes of paroxysmal atrial fibrillation (PAF)
Var 6 = individually predicted mean rates of PAF (per day)

Conclusion

The module generalized linear models can be readily trained to predict event rate of PAF episodes both in groups, and, with the help of an XML file, in individual patients.

Note

More background, theoretical and mathematical information of generalized linear modeling is available in SPSS for Starters part two, Chap. 10, entitled "Poisson regression", pp. 43–48, Springer Heidelberg Germany 2012, from the same authors.

Chapter 22
Factor Analysis and Partial Least Squares (PLS) for Complex-Data Reduction (250 Patients)

General Purpose

A few unmeasured factors, otherwise called latent factors, are identified to explain a much larger number of measured factors, e.g., highly expressed chromosome-clustered genes. Unlike factor analysis, partial least squares (PLS) identifies not only exposure (x-value), but also outcome (y-value) variables. This chapter is to assess, whether factor analysis/PLS is better than traditional analysis for regression data with multiple exposure and outcome variables.

Background

The current chapter reviews, how to construct high quality latent variables, and how they can be successfully implemented in many modern methodologies for data analysis. Two of them will be reviewed.

First, factor analysis: it is an unsupervised learning methodology, i.e., it has no dependent variable.

Second, partial least squares: it is a supervised learrning methodology, where outcomes are separately included.

A third methodology is called discriminant analysis is pretty similar to the above two, but goes one step further. It includes a grouping predictor variable, e.g., treatment modality. It will be reviewed in the Chap. 24.

This chapter was previously published in "Machine learning in medicine-cookbook 1" as Chap. 7, 2013.

Electronic Supplementary Material The online version of this chapter (https://doi.org/10.1007/978-3-030-33970-8_22) contains supplementary material, which is available to authorized users.

All of the three methodologies are multivariate methods. Complex data reduction with the help of factor analysis is entirely different from complex samples methodologies as reviewed in the Chap. 56.

Many factors in life are complex and difficult to measure directly. Charles Spearman, a London UK psychometrician in the 40s, searched for a method to measure intelligence (Barthelemew, Br J Math Stat Psychol 1995; 48: 211). Intelligence has many aspects, that can be measured and modeled together. The simplest model is the use of add-up scores. However, add-up scores do not account for the relative importance of the separate aspects, their interactions and differences in units. All of this is accounted for by a technique called factor analysis: two or three unmeasured factors are identified to explain a much larger number of measured variables. Although factor analysis is a major research tool in behavioral sciences, social sciences, marketing, operational research, and other applied sciences, it is rarely applied in clinical research. When searching the internet we found, except for a few genetic studies (Meng J, www.cmsworldwide.com, 2011, Hochreiter et al. Bioinformatics 2006; 22: 943) no clinical studies applying factor analysis. This is a pity given the presence of large numbers of variables in this field, particularly, in diagnostic research.

In this chapter we will assess, whether the performance of a diagnostic battery for making clinical predictions can be improved by using factor analysis. We will also assess, whether factor analysis enables to make predictions about individuals. We hope, that this chapter will stimulate clinical investigators to start using this method. For factor analysis internal consistency between the original variables contributing to a factor is required. There should be a strong correlation between the answers given to questions within one factor: all of the questions should, approximately, predict one and the same thing. The level of correlation is expressed as Cronbach's alpha: 0 means poor, 1 perfect relationship. The test-retest reliability of the original variables should be assessed with one variable missing: all of the data files with one missing variable should produce at least for 80% the same result, as that of the non-missing data file (alphas > 80%).

Cronbach's alpha

$$\text{alpha} = \frac{k}{(k-1)} \cdot \left(1 - \sum \frac{s_i^2}{s_T^2}\right)$$

K = number of original variables
s_i^2 = variance of ith original variable
s_T^2 = variance of total score of the factor obtained by summing up all of the original variables

Also, there should not be a too strong correlation between different original variable values in a conventional linear regression. Correlation coefficient (R) > 0.80 means the presence of multicollinearity and, thus, of a flawed multiple regression analysis. R is the Pearson's correlation coefficient, and has the underneath mathematical equation with x and y, as the variables of the x- and y-axes of a linear regression.

$$R = \frac{\sum(x - \bar{x})(y - \bar{y})}{\sqrt{\sum(x - \bar{x})^2 \sum(y - \bar{y})^2}}$$

R is a measure for the strength of association between two variables. The stronger the association, the better one variable predicts the other. It varies between − 1 and + 1, zero means no correlation at all, −1 means 100% negative correlation, +1 100% positive correlation.

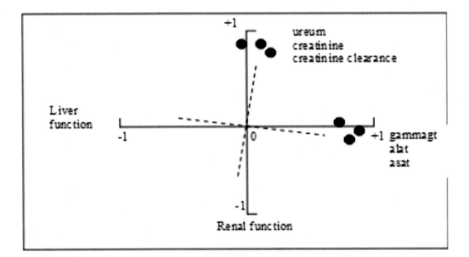

The factor analysis theory will be explained using the data of the above graph. ALAT (alanine aminotransferase), ASAT (aspartate aminotransferase) and gammaGT (gamma glutamyl tranferase) are a cluster of variables telling us something about a patient's liver function, while ureum, creatinine (creat) and creatininine clearance (c-clear) tell us something about the same patient's renal function. In order to make morbidity/mortality predictions from such variables, often, multiple regression is used. However, with multicollinearity, the variables cannot be used simultaneously in a regression model, and an alternative method has to be used. With factor analysis, all of the variables are replaced with a limited number of novel variables, that have the largest possible correlation coefficients with all of the original variables. As a multivariate technique, it is somewhat similar to Manova (multivariate analysis of variance), with the novel variables, otherwise called the factors, as outcomes, and the original variables, as predictors. However, it is less affected by multicollinearity, because the y- and x-axes are used to present the novel factors in an orthogonal way, and it can be shown, that with an orthogonal relationship between two variables the magnitude of their covariance is zero, and does not have to be taken into account. The magnitude of the latent factor values for individual patients are calculated as shown:

$$Factor_{liver\ function} = 0.87 \times ASAT + 0.90 \times ALAT + 0.85 \times GammaGT +$$
$$0.10 \times creatinine + 0.15 \times creatininine\ clearance$$
$$- 0.05 \times reum$$
$$Factor_{liver\ function} = -0.10 \times ASAT - 0.05 \times ALAT + 0.05 \times GammaGT +$$
$$0.91 \times creatinine + 0.88 \times creatininine\ clearance$$
$$+ 0.90 \times ureum$$

The term factor loadings is given to the linear correlation coefficients between the original variables and the estimated novel variable, the latent factor, adjusted for all of the manifest variables, and adjusted for eventual differences in units.

It can be demonstrated in a "2 factor" factor analysis, that, by slightly rotating both x and y-axes, the model can be fitted even better. When the y- and x-axes are rotated simultaneously, the two novel factors are assumed to be 100% independent of one another, and this rotation method is called varimax rotation. Independence needs not be true, and, if not true, the y-axis and x-axis can, alternatively, be rotated separately, in order to find the best fit model for the data given. Eigenvectors is a term often used with factor analysis. The R-values of the manifest variables versus latent factors are the eigenvalues of the original variables, their place in the above graph the eigenvectors (see Chap. 54). A scree plot is used to compare the relative importance of the latent factors with that of the manifest variables using eigenvector values.

Complex mathematical models are often laborious, so that even modern computers have difficulty to process them. Software packages currently make use of a technique called iterations: five or more calculations are estimated, and the one with the best fit is chosen.

The term components is often used to indicate the factors in a factor analysis, e.g., in rotated component matrix and in principal component analysis. The term latent factors is used to indicate the factors in a factor analysis. They are called latent, because they are not directly measured, but, rather, derived from the original variables. An y- and x-axis are used to represent them in a two factor model. If a third factor existed in your data model, it could be represented by a third axis, a z-axis creating a 3-d graph. Also additional factors can be added to the model, but they cannot be presented in a 2- or 3-d drawing anymore, but, just like with multiple regression modeling, the software programs have no problem with multidimensional computations similar to the above 2-d calculations.

Specific Scientific Question

As another example twelve highly expressed genes are used to predict drug efficacy. Is factor analysis/ PLS better than traditional analysis for regression data with multiple exposure and outcome variables.

G1	G2	G3	G4	G16	G17	G18	G19	G24	G25	G26	G27	O1	O2	O3	O4
8	8	9	5	7	10	5	6	9	9	6	6	6	7	6	7
9	9	10	9	8	8	7	8	8	9	8	8	8	7	8	7
9	8	8	8	8	9	7	8	9	8	9	9	9	8	8	8
8	9	8	9	6	7	6	4	6	6	5	5	7	7	7	6
10	10	8	10	9	10	10	8	8	9	9	9	8	8	8	7
7	8	8	8	8	7	6	5	7	8	8	7	7	6	6	7
5	5	5	5	5	6	4	5	5	6	6	5	6	5	6	4
9	9	9	9	8	8	8	8	9	8	3	8	8	8	8	8
9	8	9	8	9	8	7	7	7	7	5	8	8	7	6	6
10	10	10	10	10	10	10	10	10	8	8	10	10	10	9	10
2	2	8	5	7	8	8	8	9	3	9	8	7	7	7	6
7	8	8	7	8	6	6	7	8	8	8	7	8	7	8	8
8	9	9	8	10	8	8	7	8	8	9	9	7	7	8	8

Var G1–27 highly expressed genes estimated from their arrays' normalized ratios
Var O1–4 drug efficacy scores (the variables 20–23 from the initial data file)

The data from the first 13 patients are shown only (see extras.springer.com for the entire 250 patient data file entitled "optscalingfactorplscanonical").

Factor Analysis

First the reliability of the model was assessed by assessing the test-retest reliability of the original predictor variables using the correlation coefficients after deletion of one variable: all of the data files should produce at least by 80% the same result as that of the non-deleted data file (alphas >80%). SPSS 19.0 is used. Start by opening the data file.

Command

Analyze....Scale....Reliability Analysis....transfer original variables to Variables box....click Statistics....mark Scale if item deleted....mark Correlations ....
Continue....click OK.

Item-Total Statistics

	Scale Mean if Item Deleted	Scale Variance if Item Deleted	Corrected Item-Total Correlation	Squared Multiple Correlation	Cronbach's Alpha if Item Deleted
geneone	80,8680	276,195	,540	,485	,902
genetwo	80,8680	263,882	,700	,695	,895
genethree	80,7600	264,569	,720	,679	,895
genefour	80,7960	282,002	,495	,404	,904
genesixteen	81,6200	258,004	,679	,611	,896
geneseventeen	80,9800	266,196	,680	,585	,896
geneeighteen	81,5560	263,260	,606	,487	,899
genenineteen	82,2040	255,079	,696	,546	,895
genetwentyfour	81,5280	243,126	,735	,632	,893
genetwentyfive	81,2680	269,305	,538	,359	,902
genetwentysix	81,8720	242,859	,719	,629	,894
genetwentyseven	81,0720	264,501	,540	,419	,903

None of the original variables after deletion reduce the test-retest reliability. The data are reliable. We will now perform the principal components analysis with three components, otherwise called latent variables.

Command

Analyze....Dimension Reduction....Factor....enter variables into Variables box....click Extraction....Method: click Principle Components....mark Correlation Matrix, Unrotated factor solution....Fixed number of factors: enter 3....Maximal Iterations plot Convergence: enter 25....Continue....click Rotation....
Method: click Varimax....mark Rotated solution....mark Loading Plots....Maximal Iterations: enter 25....Continue....click Scores.... mark Display factor score coefficient matrix ....click OK.

Rotated Component Matrix[a]

	Component		
	1	2	3
geneone	,211	,810	,143
genetwo	,548	,683	,072
genethree	,624	,614	,064
genefour	,033	,757	,367
genesixteen	,857	,161	,090
geneseventeen	,650	,216	,338
geneeighteen	,526	,297	,318
genenineteen	,750	,266	,170
genetwentyfour	,657	,100	,539
genetwentyfive	,219	,231	,696
genetwentysix	,687	,077	,489
genetwentyseven	,188	,159	,825

Extraction Method: Principal Component Analysis.
Rotation Method: Varimax with Kaiser Normalization.

a. Rotation converged in 8 iterations.

The best fit coefficients of the original variables constituting 3 new factors (unmeasured, otherwise called latent, factors) are given. The latent factor 1 has a very strong correlation with the genes 16–19, the latent factor 2 with the genes 1–4, and the latent factor 3 with the genes 24–27.

When returning to the data file, we now observe, that, for each patient, the software program has produced the individual values of these novel predictors.

In order to fit these novel predictors with the outcome variables, the drug efficacy scores (variables O1-4), multivariate analysis of variance (MANOVA) should be appropriate. However, the large number of columns in the design matrix caused integer overflow, and the command was not executed. Instead we will perform a univariate multiple linear regression with the add-up scores of the outcome variables (using the Transform and Compute Variable command) as novel outcome variable.

Command

Transform. . . .Compute Variable. . . .transfer outcomeone to Numeric Expression box. . . .click +. . . .outcometwo idem. . . .click+. . . .outcomethree idem. . . .click +. . . . outcomefour idem. . . .Target Variable: enter "summaryoutcome". . . . click OK.

In the data file the summaryoutcome values are displayed as a novel variable.

Command

Analyze. . . .Regression. . . .Dependent: enter summaryoutcome. . . .Independent: enter Fac 1, Fac 2, and Fac 3. . . .click OK.

Coefficients[a]

Model		Unstandardized Coefficients		Standardized Coefficients	t	Sig.
		B	Std. Error	Beta		
1	(Constant)	27,332	,231		118,379	,000
	REGR factor score 1 for analysis 1	5,289	,231	,775	22,863	,000
	REGR factor score 2 for analysis 1	1,749	,231	,256	7,562	,000
	REGR factor score 3 for analysis 1	1,529	,231	,224	6,611	,000

a. Dependent Variable: summaryoutcome

All of the 3 latent predictors were, obviously, very significant predictors of the summary outcome variable.

Partial Least Squares Analysis (PLS)

Because PLS is not available in the basic and regression modules of SPSS, the software program R Partial Least Squares, a free statistics and forecasting software available on the internet as a free online software calculator was used (www.wessa. net/rwasp). The data file is imported directly from the SPSS file entitled "optscalingfactorplscanonical" (cut/past commands).

Command

List the selected clusters of variables: latent variable 2 (here G16-19), latent variable 1 (here G24-27), latent variable 4 (here G1-4), and latent outcome variable 3 (here O 1-4).

A square boolean matrix is constructed with "0 or 1" values if fitted correlation coefficients to be included in the model were "no or yes" according to the underneath table.

Latent variable	1	2	3	4
Latent variable 1	0	0	0	0
2	0	0	0	0
3	1	1	0	0
4	0	0	1	0

Click "compute". After 15 s of computing the program produces the results. First, the data were validated using the GoF (goodness of fit) criteria. GoF = √ [mean of r-square values of comparisons in model * r-square overall model], where * is the sign of multiplication. A GoF value varies from 0 to 1 and values larger than 0.8 indicate that the data are adequately reliable for modeling.

GoF value	
Overall	0.9459
Outer model (including manifest variables)	0.9986
Inner model (including latent variables)	0.9466.

The data are, thus, adequately reliable. The calculated best fit r-values (correlation coefficients) are estimated from the model, and their standard errors would be available from second derivatives. However, the problem with the second derivatives is that they require very large data files in order to be accurate. Instead, distribution free standard errors are calculated using bootstrap resampling.

Latent Variables	Original r-value	Bootstrap r-value	Standard error	t-value
1 versus 3	0.57654	0.57729	0.08466	6.8189
2 versus 3	0.67322	0.67490	0.04152	16.2548
4 versus 3	0.18322	0.18896	0.05373	3.5168

All of the three correlation coefficients (r-values) are very significant predictors of the latent outcome variable.

Traditional Linear Regression

When using the summary scores of the main components of the 3 latent variables instead of the above modeled latent variables (using the above Transform and Compute Variable commands), the effects remained statistically significant, however, at lower levels of significance.

Command

Analyze....Regression....Linear....Dependent: enter summaryoutcome.... Independent: enter the three summary factors 1–3....click OK.

Coefficients[a]

Model		Unstandardized Coefficients		Standardized Coefficients	t	Sig.
		B	Std. Error	Beta		
1	(Constant)	1,177	1,407		,837	,404
	summaryfac1	,136	,059	,113	2,316	,021
	summaryfac2	,620	,054	,618	11,413	,000
	summaryfac3	,150	,044	,170	3,389	,001

a. Dependent Variable: summaryoutcome

   The partial least squares method produces smaller t-values than did factor analysis (t = 3.5–16.3 versus 6.6–22.9), but it is less biased, because it is a multivariate analysis adjusting relationships between the outcome variables. Both methods provided better t-values than did the above traditional regression analysis of summary variables (t = 2.3–11.4).

Conclusion

Factor analysis and PLS can handle many more variables than the standard methods, and account the relative importance of the separate variables, their interactions and differences in units. Partial least squares method is parsimonious to principal components analysis, because it can separately include outcome variables in the model.

Note

More background, theoretical and mathematical information of the three methods is given in Machine learning in medicine part one, Chaps. 14 and 16, Factor analysis pp. 167–181, and Partial least squares, pp. 197–212, Springer Heidelberg Germany 2013, from the same authors.

Chapter 23
Optimal Scaling of High-sensitivity Analysis of Health Predictors (250 Patients)

General Purpose

In linear models of health predictors (x-values) and health outcomes (y-values), better power of testing can sometimes be obtained, if continuous predictor variables are converted into the best fit discretized ones. Examples are given.

Background

Optimal scaling is an umbrella term for a host of different test methods. For instance, one form of optimal scaling is applicable in the context of multiple regression. Another form is applicable in the context of principal components analysis. Optimal scaling makes use of processes like discretization (converting continuous variables into discretized values), and regularization (correcting discretized variables for overfitting, otherwise called overdispersion).

Regularization has to take place for the purpose of correcting overdispersed models. Generally, the standard error is increased. Various methods for adjustment are possible. Hojsgaard and Halekoh, 2005, Danish Institute of Agriculture, recommended to use the [chi-square/degrees of freedom] ratio for adjustment. But shrinking the b-value is also adequate. Ridge regression is an important approach. The regression coefficient b is minimized by a shrinking factor λ such that $b_{ridge} = b/(1 + \lambda)$, and that, with $\lambda = 0$, $b_{ridge} = b$, and, with $\lambda = \infty$, $b_{ridge} = 0$. Calculations are based on likelihood statistics adjusted for degrees of freedom, and it seems true that

This chapter was previously published in "Machine learning in medicine-cookbook 1" as Chap. 8, 2013.

Electronic Supplementary Material The online version of this chapter (https://doi.org/10.1007/978-3-030-33970-8_23) contains supplementary material, which is available to authorized users.

© Springer Nature Switzerland AG 2020
T. J. Cleophas, A. H. Zwinderman, *Machine Learning in Medicine – A Complete Overview*, https://doi.org/10.1007/978-3-030-33970-8_23

there always exists a value for λ such that it provides a better scale model than did the traditional linear model. Knowing this, one elegant method is the Monte Carlo approach, i.e. perform multiple tests in order to find the best fit scale. For the purpose cross-validation splitting the data into a k-fold scale and comparing it with a k-1 fold scale is a common way. In addition to ridge regression, SPSS statistical software offers lasso regression and elastic net regression. Lasso, although it uses similarly sized factors to reduce the size of b-values, shrinks the smallest b-values in your data to 0, thereby eliminating some variables. This will improve the prediction accuracy, particularly if you are looking for a model with a limited number of strong predictors. In contrast, if you are looking for a complex model with a large number of predictors albeit weak ones, then ridge regression will perform better. Elastic net regression is like lasso, but performs better, if the number of predictors is larger than the number of observations.

Specific Scientific Question

Highly expressed genes were used to predict drug efficacy. The example from Chap. 22 was used once more. The gene expression levels were scored on a scale of 0–10, but some scores were rarely observed. Can the strength of prediction be improved by optimal scaling.

G1	G2	G3	G4	G16	G17	G18	G19	G24	G25	G26	G27	O1	O2	O3	O4
8	8	9	5	7	10	5	6	9	9	6	6	6	7	6	7
9	9	10	9	8	8	7	8	8	9	8	8	8	7	8	7
9	8	8	8	8	9	7	8	9	8	9	9	9	8	8	8
8	9	8	9	6	7	6	4	6	6	5	5	7	7	7	6
10	10	8	10	9	10	10	8	8	9	9	9	8	8	8	7
7	8	8	8	8	7	6	5	7	8	8	7	7	6	6	7
5	5	5	5	5	6	4	5	5	6	6	5	6	5	6	4
9	9	9	9	8	8	8	8	9	8	3	8	8	8	8	8
9	8	9	8	9	8	7	7	7	7	5	8	8	7	6	6
10	10	10	10	10	10	10	10	10	8	8	10	10	10	9	10
2	2	8	5	7	8	8	8	9	3	9	8	7	7	7	6
7	8	8	7	8	6	6	7	8	8	8	7	8	7	8	8
8	9	9	8	10	8	8	7	8	8	9	9	7	7	8	8

Var = variable

Var G1-27   highly expressed genes estimated from their arrays' normalized ratios

Var O1-4   drug efficacy scores (sum of the scores is used as outcome)

Only the data from the first 13 patients are shown. The entire data file entitled "optscalingfactorplscanonical" can be downloaded from extra.springer.com.

Traditional Multiple Linear Regression

SPSS 19.0 is used for data analysis. Open the data file and command.

Command
Analyze....Regression....Linear....Dependent: enter the 12 highly expressed genes....Independent: enter the summary scores of the 4 outcome variables (use Transform and Compute Variable command)....click OK.

Coefficients^a

Model		Unstandardized Coefficients		Standardized Coefficients	t	Sig.
		B	Std. Error	Beta		
1	(Constant)	3,293	1,475		2,232	,027
	geneone	-,122	,189	-,030	-,646	,519
	genetwo	,287	,225	,078	1,276	,203
	genethree	,370	,228	,097	1,625	,105
	genefour	,063	,196	,014	,321	,748
	genesixteen	,764	,172	,241	4,450	,000
	geneseventeen	,835	,198	,221	4,220	,000
	geneeighteen	,088	,151	,027	,580	,563
	genenineteen	,576	,154	,188	3,751	,000
	genetwentyfour	,403	,146	,154	2,760	,006
	genetwentyfive	,028	,141	,008	,198	,843
	genetwentysix	,320	,142	,125	2,250	,025
	genetwentyseven	-,275	,133	-,092	-2,067	,040

a. Dependent Variable: summaryoutcome

The number of statistically significant p-values (indicated here with Sig.), (< 0.10) was 6 out of 12. In order to improve this result the Optimal Scaling program of SPSS is used. Continuous predictor variables are converted into best fit discretized ones.

Optimal Scaling Without Regularization

Command
Analyze....Regression....Optimal Scaling....Dependent Variable: Var 28 (Define Scale: mark spline ordinal 2.2)....Independent Variables: Var 1, 2, 3, 4, 16, 17, 18, 19, 24, 25, 26, 27 (all of them Define Scale: mark spline ordinal 2.2).... Discretize: Method Grouping)....OK.

Coefficients

	Standardized Coefficients				
	Beta	Bootstrap (1000) Estimate of Std. Error	df	F	Sig.
geneone	-,109	,110	2	,988	,374
genetwo	,193	,107	3	3,250	,023
genethree	-,092	,119	2	,591	,555
genefour	,113	,074	3	2,318	,077
genesixteen	,263	,087	4	9,065	,000
geneseventeen	,301	,114	2	6,935	,001
geneeighteen	,113	,136	1	,687	,408
genenineteen	,145	,067	1	4,727	,031
genetwentyfour	,220	,097	2	5,166	,007
genetwentyfive	-,039	,094	1	,170	,681
genetwentysix	,058	,107	2	,293	,746
genetwentyseven	-,127	,104	2	1,490	,228

Dependent Variable: summaryoutcome

There is no intercept anymore and the t-tests have been replaced with F-tests. The optimally scaled model without regularization shows similarly sized effects.

The number of p-values <0.10 is 6 out of 12. In order to fully benefit from optimal scaling a regularization procedure for the purpose of correcting overdispersion (more spread in the data than compatible with Gaussian data) is desirable. Ridge regression minimizes the b-values such that $b_{ridge} = b /(1 + shrinking\ factor)$. With shrinking factor $= 0$, $b_{ridge} = b$, with ∞, $b_{ridge} = 0$.

Optimal Scaling with Ridge Regression

Command
Analyze....Regression....Optimal Scaling....Dependent Variable: Var 28 (Define Scale: mark spline ordinal 2.2)....Independent Variables: Var 1, 2, 3, 4, 16, 17, 18, 19, 24, 25, 26, 27 (all of them Define Scale: mark spline ordinal 2.2).... Discretize: Method Grouping, Number categories 7)....click Regularization.... mark Ridge.... click OK.

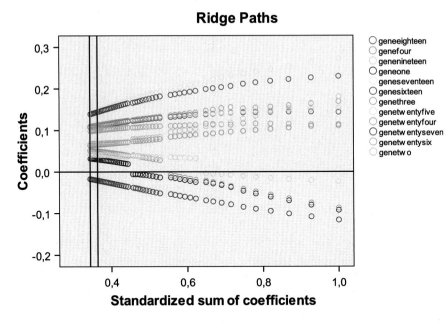

Ridge Paths

X-axis reference lines at optimal model and at most parsimonious model within 1 Std. Error.

The above figure is now in the output. The optimal scaled model with ridge regression shows the adjusted b-values of the best fit scale model (left vertical line). The b-values are also in the table included. The figure shows how the b-values of the different predictors gradually increase as the factor λ decreases. The right vertical line is the situation where the spread in the data has increased by one standard error above the best model (left line), and where the model has, thus, deteriorated correspondingly. The sensitivity of this model is much better than the traditional regression with 8 p-values <0.01, while the traditional and unregularized optimal scaling only produced 3 and 2 p-values <0.01.

Coefficients

| | Standardized Coefficients | | | | |
	Beta	Bootstrap (1000) Estimate of Std. Error	df	F	Sig.
geneone	,032	,033	2	,946	,390
genetwo	,068	,021	3	10,842	,000
genethree	,051	,030	1	2,963	,087
genefour	,064	,020	3	10,098	,000
genesixteen	,139	,024	4	34,114	,000
geneseventeen	,142	,025	2	31,468	,000
geneeighteen	,108	,040	2	7,236	,001
genenineteen	,109	,020	2	30,181	,000
genetwentyfour	,109	,021	2	27,855	,000
genetwentyfive	,041	,038	3	1,178	,319
genetwentysix	,098	,023	2	17,515	,000
genetwentyseven	-,017	,047	1	,132	,716

Dependent Variable: 20-23

The sensitivity of this model is better than the above two methods with 7 p-values <0.0001, and 9 p-values <0.10, while the traditional and unregularized Optimal Scaling only produced 6 and 6 p-values <0.10. Also the Lasso regularization model is possible (Var = variable). It shrinks the small b values to 0.

Optimal Scaling with Lasso Regression

Command
Analyze....Regression....Optimal Scaling....Dependent Variable: Var 28 (Define Scale: mark spline ordinal 2.2)....Independent Variables: Var 1, 2, 3, 4, 16, 17, 18, 19, 24, 25, 26, 27 (all of them Define Scale: mark spline ordinal 2.2)....Discretize: Method Grouping, Number categories 7)....click Regularization.... mark Lasso.... click OK.

Lasso Paths

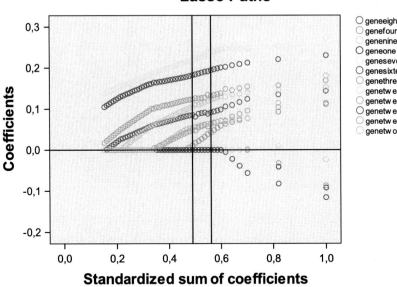

X-axis reference lines at optimal model and at most parsimonious model within 1 Std. Error.

The above figure of Lasso regression is in the output. The graph shows the adjusted b-values of the best fit scale model (left vertical line), the b-values are also in the underneath table. The graph shows how the b-value of different predictors gradually increase as the shrinking factor λ decreases (from the left to right end of the graph). The right vertical line is the situation where the spread in the data has increased by one standard error above the best model (left line), and this model has thus deteriorated correspondingly.

Coefficients

	Standardized Coefficients				
	Beta	Bootstrap (1000) Estimate of Std. Error	df	F	Sig.
geneone	,000	,020	0	,000	.
genetwo	,054	,046	3	1,390	,247
genethree	,000	,026	0	,000	.
genefour	,011	,036	3	,099	,960
genesixteen	,182	,084	4	4,684	,001
geneseventeen	,219	,095	3	5,334	,001
geneeighteen	,086	,079	2	1,159	,316
genenineteen	,105	,063	2	2,803	,063
genetwentyfour	,124	,078	2	2,532	,082
genetwentyfive	,000	,023	0	,000	.
genetwentysix	,048	,060	2	,647	,525
genetwentyseven	,000	,022	0	,000	.

Dependent Variable: 20-23

The b-values of the genes 1, 3, 25 and 27 are now shrunk to zero, and eliminated from the analysis. Lasso is particularly suitable if you are looking for a limited number of predictors and improves prediction accuracy by leaving out weak predictors. Finally, the elastic net method is applied. Like lasso it shrinks the small b-values to 0, but it performs better with many predictor variables.

Optimal Scaling with Elastic Net Regression

Command
Analyze. . . .Regression. . . .Optimal Scaling. . . .Dependent Variable: Var 28 (Define Scale: mark spline ordinal 2.2). . . .Independent Variables: Var 1, 2, 3, 4, 16, 17, 18, 19, 24, 25, 26, 27 (all of them Define Scale: mark spline ordinal 2.2). . . . Discretize: Method Grouping, Number categories 7). . . .click Regularization. . . . mark Elastic Net. . . .click OK.

Coefficients

| | Standardized Coefficients | | | | |
	Beta	Bootstrap (1000) Estimate of Std. Error	df	F	Sig.
geneone	,000	,016	0	,000	.
genetwo	,029	,039	3	,553	,647
genethree	,000	,032	3	,000	1,000
genefour	,000	,015	0	,000	.
genesixteen	,167	,048	4	12,265	,000
geneseventeen	,174	,051	3	11,429	,000
geneeighteen	,105	,055	2	3,598	,029
genenineteen	,089	,048	3	3,420	,018
genetwentyfour	,113	,053	2	4,630	,011
genetwentyfive	,000	,012	0	,000	.
genetwentysix	,062	,046	2	1,786	,170
genetwentyseven	,000	,018	0	,000	.

Dependent Variable: 20-23

The results are pretty much the same, as they are with lasso. Elastic net does not provide additional benefit in this example, but works better than lasso if the number of predictors is larger than the number of observations.

Conclusion

Optimal scaling of linear regression data provides little benefit due to overdispersion. Regularized optimal scaling using ridge regression provides excellent results. Lasso optimal scaling is suitable if you are looking for a limited number of strong predictors. Elastic net optimal scaling works better than lasso if the number of predictors is large.

Note

More background, theoretical and mathematical information of optimal scaling with or without regularization is available in Machine learning in medicine part one, Chaps. 3 and 4, entitled "Optimal scaling: discretization", and "Optimal scaling: regularization including ridge, lasso, and elastic net regression", pp. 25–37, and pp. 39–53, Springer Heidelberg Germany, 2013, from the same authors.

Chapter 24
Discriminant Analysis for Making a Diagnosis from Multiple Outcomes (45 Patients)

General Purpose

To assess whether discriminant analysis can be used to make a diagnosis from multiple outcomes both in groups and in individual patients.

Background

The current chapter reviews, how to construct high quality latent variables, and how they can be successfully implemented in many modern methodologies for data analysis. Two of them, factor analysis and partial least squares, have already been reviewed in the Chap. 22. A third one, called discriminant analysis is pretty similar to the above two, but goes one step further. It includes a grouping predictor variable, e.g., treatment modality. It will be reviewed in the current chapter.

All of the three methodologies are multivariate methods. We should add, that complex data reduction with the help of factor analysis is entirely different from complex samples methodologies as reviewed in the Chap. 56.

Many factors in life are complex and difficult to measure directly. Charles Spearman, a London UK psychometrician in the 40s, searched for a method to measure intelligence (Barthelemew, Br J Math Stat Psychol 1995; 48: 211). Intelligence has many aspects, that can be measured and modeled together. The simplest model is the use of add-up scores. However, add-up scores do not account for the relative importance of the separate aspects, their interactions and differences in units.

This chapter was previously published in "Machine learning in medicine-cookbook 1" as Chap. 9, 2013.

Electronic Supplementary Material The online version of this chapter (https://doi.org/10.1007/978-3-030-33970-8_24) contains supplementary material, which is available to authorized users.

The discriminant analysis module can adjust for all of these interactions and differences, and, at the same time, it can be be trained to provide from the data values of individual patients the best fit odds of having been in a particular diagnosis group. In this way discriminant analysis can support the hard work of physicians trying to make a diagnosis.

Specific Scientific Question

Laboratory screenings were performed in patients with different types of sepsis (urosepsis, bile duct sepsis, and airway sepsis). Can discriminant analysis of laboratory screenings improve reliability of diagnostic processes.

Var 1	Var 2	Var 3	Var 4	Var 5	Var 6	Var 7	Var 8	Var 9	Var10	Var 11
8,00	5,00	28,00	4,00	2,50	79,00	108,00	19,00	18,00	16,00	2,00
11,00	10,00	29,00	7,00	2,10	94,00	89,00	18,00	15,00	15,00	2,00
7,00	8,00	30,00	7,00	2,20	79,00	96,00	20,00	16,00	14,00	2,00
4,00	6,00	16,00	6,00	2,60	80,00	120,00	17,00	17,00	19,00	2,00
1,00	6,00	15,00	6,00	2,20	84,00	108,00	21,00	18,00	20,00	2,00
23,00	5,00	14,00	6,00	2,10	78,00	120,00	18,00	17,00	21,00	3,00
12,00	10,00	17,00	5,00	3,20	85,00	100,00	17,00	20,00	18,00	3,00
31,00	8,00	27,00	5,00	,20	68,00	113,00	19,00	15,00	18,00	3,00
22,00	7,00	26,00	5,00	1,20	74,00	98,00	16,00	16,00	17,00	3,00
30,00	6,00	25,00	4,00	2,40	69,00	90,00	20,00	18,00	16,00	3,00
2,00	12,00	21,00	4,00	2,80	75,00	112,00	11,00	14,00	19,00	1,00
10,00	21,00	20,00	4,00	2,90	70,00	100,00	12,00	15,00	20,00	1,00

Var = variable
Var 1 gammagt
Var 2 asat
Var 3 alat
Var 4 bilirubine
Var 5 ureum
Var 6 creatinine
Var 7 creatinine clearance
Var 8 erythrocyte sedimentation rate

Var 9 c-reactive protein
Var 10 leucocyte count
Var 11 type of sepsis (1–3 as described above)

The first 12 patients are shown only, the entire data file is entitled "discriminantanalysis" and is in extras.springer.com.

The Computer Teaches Itself to Make Predictions

SPSS 19.0 is used for training and outcome prediction. It uses XML (eXtended Markup Language) files to store data. Start by opening the data file.

Command
Click Transform....click Random Number Generators....click Set Starting Point.... click Fixed Value (2000000)....click OK....click Analyze.... Classify.... Discriminant Analysis....Grouping Variable: enter diagnosisgroup....Define Range: Minimum enter 1...Maximum enter 3....click Continue....Independents: enter all of the 10 laboratory variables....click Statistics....mark Unstandardized ....mark Separate-groups covariance....click Continue....click Classify....mark All groups equal....mark Summary table.... mark Within-groups....mark Combined groups....click Continue....click Save....mark Predicted group memberships....in Export model information to XML file enter: exportdiscriminant....click Browse and save the XML file in your computer....click Continue....click OK.

The scientific question "is the diagnosis group a significant predictor of the outcome estimated with 10 lab values" is hard to assess with traditional multivariate methods due to interaction between the outcome variables. It is, therefore, assessed with the question "is the clinical outcome a significant predictor of the odds of having had a particular prior diagnosis. This reasoning may seem incorrect, using an outcome for making predictions, but, mathematically, it is no problem. It is just a matter of linear cause-effect relationships, but just the other way around, and it works very conveniently with "messy" outcome variables like in the example given. However, first, the numbers of outcome variables have to be reduced. SPSS accomplishes this by orthogonal modeling of the outcome variables, which produces novel composite outcome variables. They are the y-values of linear equations. The x-values of these linear equations are the original outcome variables, and their regression coefficients are given in the underneath table.

Structure Matrix

	Function	
	1	2
asat	,574*	,184
gammagt	,460*	,203
c-reactive protein	-,034	,761*
leucos	,193	,537*
ureum	,461	,533*
creatinine	,462	,520*
alat	,411	,487*
bili	,356	,487*
esr	,360	,487*
creatinine clearance	-,083	-,374*

Pooled within-groups correlations between discriminating variables and standardized canonical discriminant functions
Variables ordered by absolute size of correlation within function.

*. Largest absolute correlation between each variable and any discriminant function

Wilks' Lambda

Test of Function(s)	Wilks' Lambda	Chi-square	df	Sig.
1 through 2	,420	32,500	20	,038
2	,859	5,681	9	,771

The two novel outcome variables significantly predict the odds of having had a prior diagnosis with $p = 0.038$ as shown above. When minimizing the output sheets we will return to the data file and observe that the novel outcome variables have been added (the variables entitled Dis1_1 and Dis1_2), as well as the predicted diagnosis group predicted from the discriminant model (the variable entitled Dis_1). For convenience the XML file entitled "exportdiscriminant" is stored in extras. springer.com.

The saved XML file can now be used to predict the odds of having been in a particular diagnosis group in five novel patients whose lab values are known but whose diagnoses are not yet obvious.

Var 1	Var 2	Var 3	Var 4	Var 5	Var 6	Var 7	Var 8	Var 9	Var 10
1049,00	466,00	301,00	268,00	59,80	213,00	−2,00	109,00	121,00	42,00
383,00	230,00	154,00	120,00	31,80	261,00	13,00	80,00	58,00	30,00
9,00	9,00	31,00	204,00	34,80	222,00	10,00	60,00	57,00	34,00
438,00	391,00	479,00	127,00	31,80	372,00	9,00	69,00	56,00	33,00
481,00	348,00	478,00	139,00	21,80	329,00	15,00	49,00	47,00	32,00

Var 1 gammagt
Var 2 asat
Var 3 alat
Var 4 bilirubine
Var 5 ureum
Var 6 creatinine
Var 7 creatinine clearance
Var 8 erythrocyte sedimentation rate
Var 9 c-reactive protein
Var 10 leucocyte count

Enter the above data in a new SPSS data file.

Command

Utilities....click Scoring Wizard....click Browse....click Select....Folder: enter the exportdiscriminant.xml file....click Select....in Scoring Wizard click Next.... click Use value substitution....click Next....click Finish.

The above data file now gives predicted odds of having been in a particular diagnosis group computed by the discriminant analysis module with the help of the xml file.

Var 1	Var 2	Var 3	Var 4	Var 5	Var 6	Var 7	Var 8	Var 9	Var 10	Var 11
1049,00	466,00	301,00	268,00	59,80	213,00	−2,00	109,00	121,00	42,00	2,00
383,00	230,00	154,00	120,00	31,80	261,00	13,00	80,00	58,00	30,00	2,00
9,00	9,00	31,00	204,00	34,80	222,00	10,00	60,00	57,00	34,00	1,00
438,00	391,00	479,00	127,00	31,80	372,00	9,00	69,00	56,00	33,00	1,00
481,00	348,00	478,00	139,00	21,80	329,00	15,00	49,00	47,00	32,00	2,00

Var 1 gammagt
Var 2 asat
Var 3 alat
Var 4 bilirubine
Var 5 ureum
Var 6 creatinine
Var 7 creatinine clearance
Var 8 erythrocyte sedimentation rate
Var 9 c-reactive protein
Var 10 leucocyte count

Var 11 predicted odds of having been in a particular diagnosis group

Conclusion

The discriminant analysis module can be readily trained to provide from the laboratory values of individual patients the best fit odds of having been in a particular diagnosis group. In this way discriminant analysis can support the hard work of physicians trying to make a diagnosis.

Note

More background, theoretical and mathematical information of discriminant analysis is available in Machine learning part one, Chap. 17, entitled "Discriminant analysis for supervised data ", pp. 215–224, Springer Heidelberg Germany, 2013, from the same authors.

Chapter 25
Weighted Least Squares for Adjusting Efficacy Data with Inconsistent Spread (78 Patients)

General Purpose

Linear regression assumes that the spread of the outcome-values is homoscedastic: it is the same for each predictor value. This assumption is, however, not warranted in many real life situations. This chapter is to assess the advantages of *weighted* least squares (WLS) instead of *ordinary* least squares (OLS) linear regression analysis.

Background

Knaub, statistician at the US Energy Information Department Washington DC developed weighted least squares (WLS) in 2007. WLS, also known as weighted linear regression, is a generalization of ordinary least squares and linear regression in which the errors covariance matrix is allowed to be different from an identity matrix. Socrates once said that all horses are animals, but not all animals are horses. Analogously, all ordinary least squares (OLS) regressions are weighted least squares (WLS) regressions, but not all WLS regressions are OLS. That is, OLS regression is a special case of WLS regression. Many of us may use OLS as a default, and in some applications that might be good enough, but just because we do not know the weights, it does not mean that we should avoid assigning weights by using WLS, while claiming that the weights are inequal.

This chapter was previously published in "Machine learning in medicine-cookbook 1" as Chap. 10, 2013.

Electronic Supplementary Material The online version of this chapter (https://doi.org/10.1007/978-3-030-33970-8_25) contains supplementary material, which is available to authorized users.

T. J. Cleophas, A. H. Zwinderman, *Machine Learning in Medicine – A Complete Overview*, https://doi.org/10.1007/978-3-030-33970-8_25

Specific Scientific Question

The effect of prednisone on peak expiratory flow was assumed to be more variable with increasing dosages. Can it, therefore, be measured with more precision if linear regression is replaced with weighted least squares procedure.

Var 1	Var 2	Var 3	Var 4
1	29	1,40	174
2	15	2,00	113
3	38	0,00	281
4	26	1,00	127
5	47	1,00	267
6	28	0,20	172
7	20	2,00	118
8	47	0,40	383
9	39	0,40	97
10	43	1,60	304
11	16	0,40	85
12	35	1,80	182
13	47	2,00	140
14	35	2,00	64
15	38	0,20	153
16	40	0,40	216

Var = variable
Var 1 Patient no
Var 2 prednisone (mg/24 h)
Var 3 peak flow (ml/min)
Var 4 beta agonist (mg/24 h)

Only the first 16 patients are given, the entire data file is entitled "weightedleastsquares" and is in extras.springer.com. SPSS 19.0 is used for data analysis. We will first make a graph of prednisone dosages and peak expiratory flows. Start with opening the data file.

Weighted Least Squares

Command
click Graphs....Legacy Dialogs....Scatter/Dot....click Simple Scatter....click Define....Y Axis enter peakflow....X Axis enter prednisone....click OK.

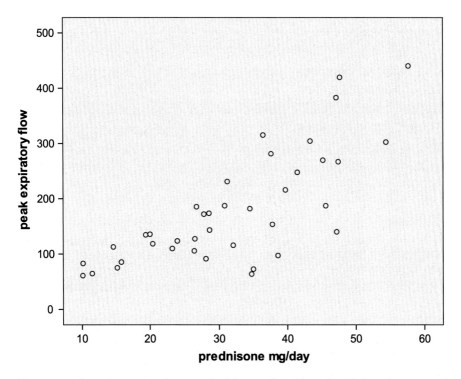

The output sheet shows that the spread of the y-values is small with low dosages and gradually increases. We will, therefore, perform both a traditional and a weighted least squares analysis of these data.

Command

Analyze....Regression....Linear....Dependent: enter peakflow....
   Independent: enter prednisone, betaagonist....click OK.

Model Summary[b]

Model	R	R Square	Adjusted R Square	Std. Error of the Estimate
1	,763[a]	,582	,571	65,304

a. Predictors: (Constant), beta agonist mg/24h, prednisone mg/day

b. Dependent Variable: peak expiratory flow

Coefficients[a]

Model		Unstandardized Coefficients		Standardized Coefficients	t	Sig.
		B	Std. Error	Beta		
1	(Constant)	-22,534	22,235		-1,013	,314
	prednisone mg/day	6,174	,604	,763	10,217	,000
	beta agonist mg/24h	6,744	11,299	,045	,597	,552

a. Dependent Variable: peak expiratory flow

In the output sheets an R value of 0.763 is observed, and the linear effects of prednisone dosages are a statistically significant predictor of the peak expiratory flow, but, surprisingly, the beta agonists dosages are not.

We will, subsequently, perform a WLS analysis.

Command

Analyze....Regression....Weight Estimation.... select: Dependent: enter peakflow .... Independent(s): enter prednisone, betaagonist....select prednisone also as Weight variable....Power

range: enter 0 through 5 by 0.5....click Options....select Save best weights as new variable....click Continue....click OK.

In the output sheets it is observed that the software has calculated likelihoods for different powers, and the best likelihood value is chosen for further analysis. When returning to the data file again a novel variable is added, the WGT_1 variable (the weights for the WLS analysis). The next step is to perform again a linear regression, but now with the weight variable included.

Command

Analyze....Regression....Linear.... select: Dependent: enter peakflow.... Independent(s): enter prednisone,

betaagonist....select the weights for the wls analysis (the GGT_1) variable as WLS Weight....click Save....select Unstandardized in Predicted Values....deselect Standardized in Residuals....click Continue....click OK.

Model Summary[b,c]

Model	R	R Square	Adjusted R Square	Std. Error of the Estimate
1	,846[a]	,716	,709	,125

a. Predictors: (Constant), beta agonist mg/24h, prednisone mg/day

b. Dependent Variable: peak expiratory flow

c. Weighted Least Squares Regression - Weighted by Weight for peakflow from WLS, MOD_6 PREDNISONE** -3,500

Coefficients[a,b]

Model		Unstandardized Coefficients		Standardized Coefficients	t	Sig.
		B	Std. Error	Beta		
1	(Constant)	5,029	7,544		,667	,507
	prednisone mg/day	5,064	,369	,880	13,740	,000
	beta agonist mg/24h	10,838	3,414	,203	3,174	,002

a. Dependent Variable: peak expiratory flow

b. Weighted Least Squares Regression - Weighted by Weight for peakflow from WLS, MOD_6 PREDNISONE** -3,500

The output table now shows an R value of 0.846. It has risen from 0.763, and provides thus more statistical power. The above lower table shows the effects of the two medicine dosages on the peak expiratory flows. The t-values of the medicine predictors have increased from approximately 10 and 0.5 to 14 and 3.2. The p-values correspondingly fell from 0.000 and 0.552 to respectively 0.000 and 0.002. Larger prednisone dosages and larger beta agonist dosages significantly and independently increased peak expiratory flows. After adjustment for heteroscedasticity, the beta agonist became a significant independent determinant of peak flow.

Conclusion

The current paper shows that, even with a sample of only 78 patients, WLS is able to demonstrate statistically significant linear effects that had been, previously, obscured by heteroscedasticity of the y-value.

Note

More background, theoretical and mathematical information of weighted least squares modeling is given in Machine learning in medicine part three, Chap. 10, Weighted least squares, pp. 107–116, Springer Heidelberg Germany, 2013, from the same authors.

Chapter 26
Partial Correlations for Removing Interaction Effects from Efficacy Data (64 Patients)

General Purpose

The outcome of cardiovascular research is generally affected by many more factors than a single one, and multiple regression assumes that these factors act independently of one another, but why should they not affect one another. This chapter is to assess whether partial correlation can be used to remove interaction effects from linear data.

Background

Partial correlations has a long history. Already in 1924 it was described by Fisher, otherwise famous from the F-test, in the article "Distribution of the partial correlation coefficient" in the journal *Metron* 1924: 3: 329. In probability theory and statistics, partial correlation measures the degree of association between two random variables, with the effect of a set of controlling random variables removed. Partial correlation is also used as expression in analyses of co-variance (ANCOVA) applied to questions of prediction and relationship.

This chapter was previously published in "Machine learning in medicine-cookbook 1" as Chap. 11, 2013.

Electronic Supplementary Material The online version of this chapter (https://doi.org/10.1007/978-3-030-33970-8_26) contains supplementary material, which is available to authorized users.

Specific Scientific Question

Both calorie intake and exercise are significant independent predictors of weight loss. However, exercise makes you hungry and patients on weight training are inclined to reduce (or increase) their calorie intake. Can partial correlations methods adjust the interaction between the two predictors.

Var 1	Var 2	Var 3	Var 4	Var 5
1,00	0,00	1000,00	0,00	45,00
29,00	0,00	1000,00	0,00	53,00
2,00	0,00	3000,00	0,00	64,00
1,00	0,00	3000,00	0,00	64,00
28,00	6,00	3000,00	18,000,00	34,00
27,00	6,00	3000,00	18,000,00	25,00
30,00	6,00	3000,00	18,000,00	34,00
27,00	6,00	1000,00	6000,00	45,00
29,00	0,00	2000,00	0,00	52,00
31,00	3,00	2000,00	6000,00	59,00
30,00	3,00	1000,00	3000,00	58,00
29,00	3,00	1000,00	3000,00	47,00
27,00	0,00	1000,00	0,00	45,00
28,00	0,00	1000,00	0,00	66,00
27,00	0,00	1000,00	0,00	67,00

Var = variable
Var 1 weight loss (kg)
Var 2 exercise (times per week)
Var 3 calorie intake (cal)
Var 4 interaction
Var 5 age (years)

Only the first fifteen patients are given, the entire file is entitled "partialcorrelations" and is in extras.springer.com.

Partial Correlations

We will first perform a linear regression of these data. SPSS 19.0 is used for the purpose. Start by opening the data file.

Command

Analyze....Regression....Linear....Dependent variable: enter weightloss....
Independent variables: enter exercise and calorieintake....click OK.

Coefficients[a]

Model		Unstandardized Coefficients		Standardized Coefficients	t	Sig.
		B	Std. Error	Beta		
1	(Constant)	29,089	2,241		12,978	,000
	exercise	2,548	,439	,617	5,802	,000
	calorieintake	-,006	,001	-,544	-5,116	,000

a. Dependent Variable: weightloss

The output sheets show that both calorie intake and exercise are significant independent predictors of weight loss. However, interaction between exercise and calorie intake is not accounted. In order to check, an interaction variable (x_3 = calorie intake $*$ exercise, with $*$ symbol of multiplication) is added to the model.

Command

Transform data....Compute Variable....in Target Variable enter the term "interaction"....to Numeric Expression: transfer from Type & Label "exercise" ....click $*$ ....transfer from Type & Label calorieintake....click OK.

The interaction variable is added by SPSS to the data file and is entitled "interaction". After the addition of the interaction variable to the regression model as third independent variable, the analysis is repeated.

Coefficients[a]

Model		Unstandardized Coefficients		Standardized Coefficients	t	Sig.
		B	Std. Error	Beta		
1	(Constant)	34,279	2,651		12,930	,000
	interaction	,001	,000	,868	3,183	,002
	exercise	-,238	,966	-,058	-,246	,807
	calorieintake	-,009	,002	-,813	-6,240	,000

a. Dependent Variable: weightloss

The output sheet now shows that exercise is no longer significant and interaction on the outcome is significant at p = 0.002. There is, obviously, interaction in the study, and the overall analysis of the data is, thus, no longer relevant. The best method to find the true effect of exercise would be to repeat the study with calorie intake held constant. Instead of this laborious exercise, a partial correlation analysis with calorie intake held artificially constant can be adequately performed, and would provide virtually the same result. Partial correlation analysis is performed using the SPSS module Correlations.

Command

Analyze....Correlate....Partial....Variables: enter weight loss and calorie intake ....Controlling for: enter exercise....OK.

Correlations

Control Variables			weightloss	calorieintake
exercise	weightloss	Correlation	1,000	-,548
		Significance (2-tailed)	.	,000
		df	0	61
	calorieintake	Correlation	-,548	1,000
		Significance (2-tailed)	,000	.
		df	61	0

Correlations

Control Variables			weightloss	exercise
calorieintake	weightloss	Correlation	1,000	,596
		Significance (2-tailed)	.	,000
		df	0	61
	exercise	Correlation	,596	1,000
		Significance (2-tailed)	,000	.
		df	61	0

The upper table shows, that, with exercise held constant, calorie intake is a significant negative predictor of weight loss with a correlation coefficient of -0.548 and a p-value of 0.0001. Also partial correlation with exercise as independent and calorie intake as controlling factor can be performed.

Command

Analyze....Correlate....Partial....Variables: enter weight loss and exercise ....
Controlling for: enter calorie intake....click OK.

The lower table shows that, with calorie intake held constant, exercise is a significant positive predictor of weight loss with a correlation coefficient of 0.596 and a p-value of 0.0001.

Why do we no longer have to account interaction with partial correlations. This is simply because, if you hold a predictor fixed, this fixed predictor can no longer change and interact in a multiple regression model.

Also higher order partial correlation analyses are possible. E.g., age may affect all of the three variables already in the model. The effect of exercise on weight loss with calorie intake and age fixed can be assessed.

Command

Analyze....Correlate....Partial....Variables: enter weight loss and exercise....
Controlling for: enter calorie intake and age....click OK.

Correlations

Control Variables			weightloss	exercise
age & calorieintake	weightloss	Correlation	1,000	,541
		Significance (2-tailed)	.	,000
		df	0	60
	exercise	Correlation	,541	1,000
		Significance (2-tailed)	,000	.
		df	60	0

In the above output sheet it can be observed that the correlation coefficient is still very significant.

Conclusion

Without the partial correlation approach the conclusion from this study would have been: no definitive conclusion about the effects of exercise and calorie intake is possible, because of a significant interaction between exercise and calorie intake. The partial correlation analysis allows to conclude that both exercise and calorie intake have a very significant linear relationship with weight loss effect. We should add that partial correlation methodology is also helpful for the identification and analysis of dependent adverse effects in clinical trials (Analysis of safety data of drug trials, Springer Heidelberg Germany, 2019, from the same authors).

Note

More background, theoretical and mathematical information of partial correlations methods is given in Machine learning in medicine part one, Chap. 5, Partial correlations, pp. 55–64, Springer Heidelberg Germany, 2013, from the same authors.

Chapter 27
Canonical Regression for Overall Statistics from Multivariate Data (250 Patients)

General Purpose

MANOVA (multivariate analysis of variance) tests the effects of separate predictors including both covariates (continuous) and fixed factors (categories), on.

1. all of the outcome combinations in a multivariate dataset,
2. the outcomes separately.

For statistics OLS (ordinary least squares) is used.

The general purpose of this chapter is, to assess in datasets with multiple predictor and outcome variables, whether canonical analysis, unlike traditional multivariate analysis of variance (MANOVA), can not only provide overall statistics of combined effects, but also account the relative importance of separate variables.

Background

Like MANOVA, canonical analysis is based on multiple linear regression, used to find the best fit correlation coefficients for your data. However, because it works with Wilks' statistic and beta distributions rather than Pillai's statistic and normal distributions, it is able to more easily calculate overall correlation coefficients between sets of variables. Yet, it also assesses, how a set of variables, as a whole is related to separate variables. Along this way, an overall canonical model can be further improved by removing unimportant variables. Canonical analysis may be

This chapter was previously published in "Machine learning in medicine-cookbook 1" as Chap. 12, 2013.

Electronic Supplementary Material The online version of this chapter (https://doi.org/10.1007/978-3-030-33970-8_27) contains supplementary material, which is available to authorized users.

arithmetically equivalent to factor-analysis/partial least squares analysis, but, conceptionally, it is very different. Unlike the latter, the former method does not produce new (latent) variables, but rather makes use of two sets of manifest variables. Also, unlike the latter, it complies with all of the requirements of traditional linear regression, and is, therefore, scientifically rigorous. A canonical analysis should start with a correlation matrix. Variables with large correlation coefficients must be removed from the model. If in canonical models the clusters of predictor and outcome variables have a significant relationship, then this finding can, just like with linear regression, be used for making predictions about individual patients. We will again use SPSS statistical software. The Menu does not offer canonical analysis, but the Syntax program does. Canonical analysis should start with a collinearity matrix. This is because the uncertainty of the canonical weights, being the main outcome of a canonical regression, are severely overestimated in case of collinearity. Variable versus variable correlation coefficients larger than 0.80 means that the models is collinear and that the collinear variables should be removed from the model.

Specific Scientific Question

The example of the Chaps. 22 and 23 is used once again. Twelve highly expressed genes are used to predict four measures of drug efficacy. We are more interested in the combined effect of the predictor variables on the outcome variables than we are in the separate effects of the different variables.

G1	G2	G3	G4	G16	G17	G18	G19	G24	G25	G26	G27	O1	O2	O3	O4
8	8	9	5	7	10	5	6	9	9	6	6	6	7	6	7
9	9	10	9	8	8	7	8	8	9	8	8	8	7	8	7
9	8	8	8	8	9	7	8	9	8	9	9	9	8	8	8
8	9	8	9	6	7	6	4	6	6	5	5	7	7	7	6
10	10	8	10	9	10	10	8	8	9	9	9	8	8	8	7
7	8	8	8	8	7	6	5	7	8	8	7	7	6	6	7
5	5	5	5	5	6	4	5	5	6	6	5	6	5	6	4
9	9	9	9	8	8	8	8	9	8	3	8	8	8	8	8
9	8	9	8	9	8	7	7	7	7	5	8	8	7	6	6
10	10	10	10	10	10	10	10	10	8	8	10	10	10	9	10
2	2	8	5	7	8	8	8	9	3	9	8	7	7	7	6
7	8	8	7	8	6	6	7	8	8	8	7	8	7	8	8
8	9	9	8	10	8	8	7	8	8	9	9	7	7	8	8

Var G1–27 highly expressed genes estimated from their arrays' normalized ratios
Var O1–4 drug efficacy scores (the variables 20–23 from the initial data file)

The data from the first 13 patients are shown only (see extra.springer.com for the entire data file entitled "optscalingfactorplscanonical"). First, MANOVA (multivariate analysis of variance) was performed with the four drug efficacy scores as outcome variables and the twelve gene expression levels as covariates. We can now use SPSS 19.0. Start by opening the data file.

Canonical Regression

Command
click Analyze....click General Linear Model....click Multivariate....Dependent Variables: enter the four drug efficacy scores....Covariates: enter the 12 genes.... OK.

	Effect value	F	Hypothesis df	Error df	p-value
Intercept	0.043	2.657	4.0	234.0	0.034
Gene 1	0.006	0.362	4.0	234.0	0.835
Gene 2	0.27	1.595	4.0	234.0	0.176
Gene 3	0.042	2.584	4.0	234.0	0.038
Gene 4	0.013	0.744	4.0	234.0	0.563
Gene 16	0.109	7.192	4.0	234.0	0.0001
Gene 17	0.080	5.118	4.0	234.0	0.001
Gene 18	0.23	1.393	4.0	234.0	0.237
Gene 19	0.092	5.938	4.0	234.0	0.0001
Gene 24	0.045	2.745	4.0	234.0	0.029
Gene 25	0.017	1.037	4.0	234.0	0.389
Gene 26	0.027	1.602	4.0	234.0	0.174
Gene 27	0.045	2.751	4.0	234.0	0.029

The MANOVA table is given (F = F-value, df = degrees of freedom). It shows that MANOVA can be considered as another regression model with intercepts and regression coefficients. We can conclude that the genes 3, 16, 17, 19, 24, and 27 are significant predictors of all four drug efficacy outcome scores. Unlike ANOVA, MANOVA does not give overall p-values, but rather separate p-values for separate covariates. However, we are, particularly, interested in the combined effect of the set of predictors, otherwise called covariates, on the set of outcomes, rather than we are in modeling the separate variables. In order to asses the overall effect of the cluster of genes on the cluster of drug efficacy scores canonical regression is performed.

Command
click File....click New....click Syntax....the Syntax Editor dialog box is displayed....enter the following text: "manova" and subsequently enter all of the outcome variables....enter the text "WITH"....then enter all of the gene-names.... then enter the following text: /discrim all alpha(1)/print = sig(eigen dim).... click Run.

Numbers variables (covariates v outcome variables).

	Canon cor	Sq cor	Wilks L	F	Hypoth df	Error df	p
12 v 4	0.87252	0.7613	0.19968	9.7773	48.0	903.4	0.0001
7 v 4	0.87054	0.7578	0.21776	16.227	28.0	863.2	0.0001
7 v 3	0.87009	0.7571	0.22043	22.767	21.0	689.0	0.0001

The above table is given (cor = correlation coefficient, sq. = squared, L = lambda, hypoth = hypothesis, df = degree of freedom, p = p-value, v = versus). The upper row, shows the result of the statistical analysis. The correlation coefficient between the 12 predictor and 4 outcome variables equals 0.87252. A squared correlation coefficient of 0.7613 means that 76% of the variability in the outcome variables is explained by the 12 covariates. The cluster of predictors is a very significant predictor of the cluster of outcomes, and can be used for making predictions about individual patients with similar gene profiles. Repeated testing after the removal of separate variables gives an idea about relatively unimportant contributors as estimated by their coefficients, which are kind of canonical b-values (regression coefficients). The larger they are, the more important they are.

Canonical Correlations

Model	12 v 4	7 v 4	7 v 3
Raw			
Outcome 1	-0.24620	-0.24603	0.25007
Outcome 2	-0.20355	-0.19683	0.20679
Outcome 3	-0.02113	-0.02532	
Outcome 4	-0.07993	-0.08448	0.09037
Gene 1	0.01177		
Gene 2	-0.01727		
Gene 3	-0.05964	-0.08344	0.08489
Gene 4	-0.02865		
Gene 16	-0.14094	-0.13883	0.13755
Gene 17	-0.12897	-0.14950	0.14845
Gene 18	-0.03276		
Gene 19	-0.10626	-0.11342	0.11296
Gene 24	-0.07148	-0.07024	0.07145
Gene 25	-0.00164		
Gene 26	-0.05443	-0.05326	0.05354
Gene 27	0.05589	0.04506	-0.04527
Standardized			
Outcome 1	-0.49754	-0.49720	0.50535
Outcome 2	-0.40093	-0.38771	0.40731
Outcome 3	-0.03970	-0.04758	
Outcome 4	-0.15649	-0.16539	0.17693
Gene 1	0.02003		
Gene 2	-0.03211		
Gene 3	-0.10663	-0.14919	0.15179
Gene 4	-0.04363		
Gene 16	-0.30371	-0.29918	0.29642
Gene 17	-0.23337	-0.27053	0.26862
Gene 18	-0.06872		
Gene 19	-0.23696	-0.25294	0.25189
Gene 24	-0.18627	-0.18302	0.18618
Gene 25	-0.00335		
Gene 26	-0.14503	-0.14191	0.14267
Gene 27	0.12711	0.10248	-0.10229

The above table left column gives an overview of raw and standardized (z transformed) canonical coefficients, otherwise called canonical weights (the multiple b-values of canonical regression), (Canon Cor = canonical correlation coefficient, v = versus, Model = analysis model after removal of one or more variables). The outcome 3, and the genes 2, 4, 18 and 25 contributed little to the overall result. When restricting the model by removing the variables with canonical coefficients smaller than 0.05 or larger than −0.05 (the middle and right columns of the table), the results were largely unchanged. And so were the results of the overall tests (the second and third rows). Seven versus three variables produced virtually the same correlation coefficient but with much more power (lambda increased from 0.1997 to 0.2204, the F value from 9.7773 to 22.767, in spite of a considerable fall in the degrees of freedom. It, therefore, does make sense to try and remove the weaker variables from the model ultimately to be used. The weakest contributing covariates of the MANOVA were virtually identical to the weakest canonical predictors, suggesting that the two methods are closely related and one method confirms the results of the other.

Conclusion

Canonical analysis is wonderful, because it can handle many more variables than MANOVA, accounts for the relative importance of the separate variables and their interactions, provides overall statistics. Unlike other methods for combining the effects of multiple variables like factor analysis /partial least squares (Chap. 22), canonical analysis is scientifically entirely rigorous. This is so, because canonical regression just like Manova, and unlike latent variables methods, leaves little room for subjective decisions. It was invented by Harold Hotelling, a professor of statistics in the early seventies at Chapel Hill University North Carolina, who used the term canonical, stemming from Hebrew and meaning being an important part or element of something, just like a canunic in the Catholic church. It works with canonical weights, rather than subjectively gathered latent variables. Canonical weights are like regression coefficients in linear regression. In its simplest version they are the best fit a and b values in the underneath regression eqs. (CV = canonical variable) in the underneath mathematical model to provide a maximal correlation between two orthogonal canonical variates (CVs)

$$CVx = a_1x_1 + a_2x_2 + a_3x_3 + a_4x_4 \ldots \ldots$$
$$CVy = b_1y_1 + b_2y_2 + b_3y_3 + b_4y_4 \ldots \ldots$$

This means, that they provide the best fit a and b values of the dependent and independent variables in the data model. Canonical correlations is increasingly important in big data statistics and, it will, therefore, be addressed again in the

Chaps. 83 and 84, covering respectively "omics research" and "sparse penalized canonical correlations".

Note

More background, theoretical and mathematical information of canonical regression is given in Machine learning in medicine part one, Chap. 18, Canonical regression, pp. 225–240, Springer Heidelberg Germany, 2013, from the same authors.

Chapter 28
Multinomial Regression for Outcome Categories (55 Patients)

General Purpose

This chapter will assess, whether multinomial regression can be trained to make predictions about.

(1) patients being in a category and
(2) the probability of it.

Examples are given.

Background

Multinomial logistic regression is used, when the dependent variable in question is nominal (equivalently categorical, meaning that it falls into any one of a set of categories that cannot be ordered in any meaningful way) and for which there are more than two categories. In clinical research it is not uncommon that outcome variables are categorical, e.g., the choice of food, treatment modality, type of doctor etc. If such outcome variables are binary, then binary logistic regression is appropriate. If, however, we have three or more alternatives, then multinomial logistic regression must be used. It works, essentially, similarly to the recoding procedure commonly used on categorical predictor variables. Multinomial logistic regression should not be confounded with ordered logistic regression, which is used in case the

---

This chapter was previously published in "Machine learning in medicine-cookbook 2" as Chap. 4, 2014.

Electronic Supplementary Material The online version of this chapter (https://doi.org/10.1007/978-3-030-33970-8_28) contains supplementary material, which is available to authorized users.

T. J. Cleophas, A. H. Zwinderman, *Machine Learning in Medicine – A Complete Overview*, https://doi.org/10.1007/978-3-030-33970-8_28

outcome variable consists of categories, that can be ordered in a meaningful way, e.g., anginal class or quality of life class.

Specific Scientific Question

Patients from different hospital departments and ages are assessed for falling out of bed (0 = no, 1 = yes without injury, 2 = yes with injury). The falloutofbed categories are the outcome, the department and ages are the predictors. Can a data file of such patients be trained to make predictions in future patients about their best fit category and probability of being in it.

department	falloutofbed	age(years)
,00	1	56,00
,00	1	58,00
,00	1	87,00
,00	1	64,00
,00	1	65,00
,00	1	53,00
,00	1	87,00
,00	1	77,00
,00	1	78,00
,00	1	89,00

Only the first 10 patients are given, the entire data file is entitled. categoriesasoutcome" and is in extras.springer.com.

The Computer Teaches Itself to Make Predictions

SPSS versions 18 and up can be used. SPSS will produce an XML (eXtended Markup Language) file of the prediction model from the above data. We will start. by opening the above data file.

Command
click Transform....click Random Number Generators....click Set Starting Point....click Fixed Value (2000000)....click OK....click Analyze.... Regression ....Multinomial Logistic Regression....Dependent: falloutofbed....

Factor: department....Covariate: age....click Save....mark: Estimated response probability, Predicted category, Predicted category probability, Actual category probability....click Browse....various folders in your personal computer come up....in "File name" of the appropriate folder enter "exportcategoriesasoutcome". ....click Save....click Continue....click OK.

Parameter Estimates

fall with/out injury[a]		B	Std. Error	Wald	df	Sig.	Exp(B)	95% Confidence Interval for Exp (B)	
								Lower Bound	Upper Bound
0	Intercept	5,337	2,298	5,393	1	,020			
	age	-,059	,029	4,013	1	,045	,943	,890	,999
	[department= ,00]	-1,139	,949	1,440	1	,230	,320	,050	2,057
	[department= 1,00]	0[b]	.	.	0	.	.	.	.
1	Intercept	3,493	2,333	2,241	1	,134			
	age	-,022	,029	,560	1	,454	,978	,924	1,036
	[department= ,00]	-1,945	,894	4,735	1	,030	,143	,025	,824
	[department= 1,00]	0[b]	.	.	0	.	.	.	.

a. The reference category is: 2.
b. This parameter is set to zero because it is redundant.

The above table is in the output. The independent predictors of falloutofbed are given. Per year of age there are 0,943 less "no falloutofbeds" versus "falloutofbeds with injury". The department 0,00 has 0,143 less falloutofbeds with versus without injury. The respective p-values are 0,045 and 0,030. When returning to the main data view, we will observe that SPSS has provided 6 novel variables for each patient.

1. EST1_1 estimated response probability (probability of the category 0 for each patient)
2. EST2_1 idem for category 1
3. EST3_1 idem for category 2
4. PRE_1 predicted category (category with highest probability score)
5. PCP_1 predicted category probability (the highest probability score predicted by model)
6. ACP_1 actual category probability (the highest probability computed from data)

With the Scoring Wizard and the exported XML file entitled "exportcategoriesasoutcome" we can now try and predict from the department and age of future patients (1) the most probable category they are in, and (2) the very probability of it. The department and age of 12 novel patients are as follow.

department	age
,00	73,00
,00	38,00
1,00	89,00
,00	75,00
,00	84,00
,00	74,00
1,00	90,00
1,00	72,00
1,00	62,00
1,00	34,00
1,00	85,00
1,00	43,00

Enter the Above Data in a Novel Data File and Command

Utilities. . . .click Scoring Wizard. . . .click Browse. . . .Open the appropriate folder. with the XML file entitled "exportcategoriesasoutcome". . . .click on the latter and click Select. . . .in Scoring Wizard double-click Next. . . .mark Predicted category and Probability of it. . . .click Finish.

department	age	probability of being in predicted category	predicted category
,00	73,00	,48	1,00
,00	38,00	,48	1,00
1,00	89,00	,36	2,00
,00	75,00	,47	1,00
,00	84,00	,48	2,00
,00	74,00	,48	1,00
1,00	90,00	,37	2,00
1,00	72,00	,55	,00
1,00	62,00	,65	,00
1,00	34,00	,84	,00
1,00	85,00	,39	,00
1,00	43,00	,79	,00

0 = no falloutofbed
1 = falloutofbed without injury
2 = falloutofbed with injury

In the data file SPSS has provided two novel variables as requested. The first patient from department 0,00 and 73 years of age has a 48% chance of being in the "falloutofbed without injury". His/her chance of being in the other two categories is smaller than 48%.

Conclusion

Multinomial, otherwise called polytomous logistic regression can be readily trained to make predictions in future patients about their best fit category and the probability of being in it.

Note

More background theoretical and mathematical information of analyses using categories as outcome is available in Machine learning in medicine part two, Chap. 10, Anomaly detection, pp. 93–103, Springer Heidelberg Germany, 2013, from the same authors.

Chapter 29
Various Methods for Analyzing Predictor Categories (60 and 30 Patients)

General Purpose

Categories unlike continuous data need not have stepping functions. In order to apply regression analysis for their analysis we need to recode them into multiple binary (dummy) variables. Particularly, if Gaussian distributions in the outcome are uncertain, automatic non-parametric testing is an adequate and very convenient modern alternative. Examples are given.

Background

A major objective of clinical research is to improve the effectiveness of individual therapies by studying treatment effects and health effects in subgroups of patients, for example age-groups, races, genders etc. Sometimes, the use of continuous or binary variables are possible for the purpose. However, races, numbers of co-medications, co-morbidities and many more variables in clinical research may or may not have stepping functions with a limited number of values, e.g., *four* races, *zero to eight* co-medications etc. If such stepping functions are analyzed using continuous variables in a linear or logistic regression model, we assume that the outcome variable will rise linearly, but this needs not necessarily be so. This assumption raises the risk of underestimating the effects. In the given situation, it may be more safe to recode the stepping variables into the form of categorical variables. Until the late nineties the proper handling of categories received little

This chapter was previously published in "Machine learning in medicine-cookbook 2" as Chap. 5, 2014.

Electronic Supplementary Material The online version of this chapter (https://doi.org/10.1007/978-3-030-33970-8_29) contains supplementary material, which is available to authorized users.

attention from the scientific community. In 1996 Nichols polled statistical software users, and found out that the proper use of categorical variables was of major concern (in: Using categorical variables in regression, SPSS Keywords: 1996; 1–4). In the past few years adequate methods for coding categorical predictor variables have been published. Unfortunately, statistical software programs, to date, do not routinely allow for recoding stepping variables into categorical ones. For example, with linear regression analysis in SPSS statistical software, categorical variables have to be created. In contrast, logistic regression in SPSS provides a special dialog box for the purpose. In this chapter we will demonstrate from examples how recoding works. The examples show, that the stepping functions, if used as continuous variables, do not produce significant effects, whereas they produce very significant effects after recoding. We hope this explanatory chapter will be helpful to researchers assessing categories. We should add, that, particularly, if the Gaussian distributions in the outcome are uncertain, automatic non-parametric testing with the help of Kruskal Wallis tests will be an adequate and very convenient alternative.

Specific Scientific Questions

1. Does race have an effect on physical strength (the variable race has a categorical rather than linear pattern).
2. Are the hours of sleep/levels of side effects different in categories treated with different sleeping pills.

Example 1

The effects on physical strength (scores 0–100) assessed in 60 subjects of different races (hispanics (1), blacks (2), asians (3), and whites (4), and ages (years), are in the left three columns of the data file entitled "categoriesaspredictor".

patient number	physical strength	race	age
1	70,00	1,00	35,00
2	77,00	1,00	55,00
3	66,00	1,00	70,00
4	59,00	1,00	55,00
5	71,00	1,00	45,00
6	72,00	1,00	47,00
7	45,00	1,00	75,00
8	85,00	1,00	83,00
9	70,00	1,00	35,00
10	77,00	1,00	49,00

Example 1   209

Only the first 10 patients are displayed above. The entire data file in www. springer.com. For the analysis we will use multiple linear regression.

Command
Analyze....Regression....Linear....Dependent: physical strength score.... Independent: race, age, ...OK.

Coefficients[a]

Model		Unstandardized Coefficients		Standardized Coefficients	t	Sig.
		B	Std. Error	Beta		
1	(Constant)	92,920	7,640		12,162	,000
	race	-,330	1,505	-,027	-,219	,827
	age	-,356	,116	-,383	-3,071	,003

a. Dependent Variable: strengthscore

The above table shows that age is a significant predictor but race is not. However, the analysis is not adequate, because the variable race is analyzed as a stepwise function from 1 to 4, and the linear regression model assumes that the outcome variable will rise (or fall) linearly, but, in the data given, this needs not be necessarily so. It may, therefore, be more safe to recode the stepping variable into the form of a categorical variable. The underneath data overview shows in the right 4 columns how it is manually done.

patient number	physical strength	race	age	race 1 hispanics	race 2 blacks	race 3 asians	race 4 whites
1	70,00	1,00	35,00	1,00	0,00	0,00	0,00
2	77,00	1,00	55,00	1,00	0,00	0,00	0,00
3	66,00	1,00	70,00	1,00	0,00	0,00	0,00
4	59,00	1,00	55,00	1,00	0,00	0,00	0,00
5	71,00	1,00	45,00	1,00	0,00	0,00	0,00
6	72,00	1,00	47,00	1,00	0,00	0,00	0,00
7	45,00	1,00	75,00	1,00	0,00	0,00	0,00
8	85,00	1,00	83,00	1,00	0,00	0,00	0,00
9	70,00	1,00	35,00	1,00	0,00	0,00	0,00
10	77,00	1,00	49,00	1,00	0,00	0,00	0,00

We, subsequently, will use again linear regression, but now for categorical analysis of race.

Command
click Transform....click Random Number Generators....click Set Starting Point....click Fixed Value (2000000)....click OK....click Analyze....Regression ....Linear....Dependent: physical strength score....Independent: race 1, race

3, race 4, age....click Save....mark Unstandardized....in Export model information   to   XML   (eXtended   Markup   Language)   file: type
"exportcategoriesaspredictor"....click   Browse....File   name: enter
"exportcategoriesaspredictor"....click Continue....click OK.

Coefficients[a]

Model		Unstandardized Coefficients		Standardized Coefficients	t	Sig.
		B	Std. Error	Beta		
1	(Constant)	97,270	4,509		21,572	,000
	age	-,200	,081	-,215	-2,457	,017
	race1	-17,483	3,211	-,560	-5,445	,000
	race3	-25,670	3,224	-,823	-7,962	,000
	race4	-8,811	3,198	-,282	-2,755	,008

a. Dependent Variable: strengthscore

The above table is in the output. It shows that race 1, 3, 4 are significant predictors
of physical strength compared to race 2. The results can be interpreted as follows.
The underneath regression equation is used:

$$y = a + b_1\, x_1\ + b_2\, x_2 + b_3\, x_3 + b_4\, x_4$$

$$a\ = \text{intercept}$$
$$b_1 = \text{regression coefficient for} \quad \text{age}$$
$$b_2 = \qquad\qquad\qquad\qquad\qquad\quad \text{hispanics}$$
$$b_3 = \qquad\qquad\qquad\qquad\qquad\quad \text{asians}$$
$$b_4 = \qquad\qquad\qquad\qquad\qquad\quad \text{white}$$

If an individual is black (race 2), then x_2, x_3, and x_4 will turn into 0, and the
regression equation becomes.

$$y = a + b_1 x_1$$

If hispanic, $y = a + b_1 x_1 + b_2 x_2$

If asian, $y = a + b_1 x_1 + b_3 x_3$

If white, $y = a + b_1 x_1 + b_4 x_4.$

So, e.g., the best predicted physical strength score of a white male of 25 years of
age would equal

$$y = 97.270 + 0.20 * 25 - 8.811 * 1 = 93.459,$$

($*$ = sign of multiplication).

Example 1   211

Obviously, all of the races are negative predictors of physical strength, but the blacks scored highest and the asians lowest. All of these results are adjusted for age.

If we return to the data file page, we will observe that SPSS has added a new variable entitled "PRE_1". It represents the individual strengthscores as predicted by the recoded linear model. They are pretty similar to the measured values.

We can now with the help of the Scoring Wizard and the exported XML (eXtended Markup Language) file entitled "exportcategoriesaspredictor" try and predict strength scores of future patients with known race and age.

race	age
1,00	40,00
2,00	70,00
3,00	54,00
4,00	45,00
1,00	36,00
2,00	46,00
3,00	50,00
4,00	36,00

First, recode the stepping variable race into 4 categorical variables.

race	age	race1	race3	race4
1,00	40,00	1,00	,00	,00
2,00	70,00	,00	,00	,00
3,00	54,00	,00	1,00	,00
4,00	45,00	,00	,00	1,00
1,00	36,00	1,00	,00	,00
2,00	46,00	,00	,00	,00
3,00	50,00	,00	1,00	,00
4,00	36,00	,00	,00	1,00

Then Command

click Utilities....click Scoring Wizard....click Browse....click Select....Folder: enter the exportcategoriesaspredictor.xml file....click Select....in Scoring Wizard click Next....click Finish.

race	age	race1	race3	race4	predicted strength score
1,00	40,00	1,00	,00	,00	71,81
2,00	70,00	,00	,00	,00	83,30
3,00	54,00	,00	1,00	,00	60,83
4,00	45,00	,00	,00	1,00	79,48
1,00	36,00	1,00	,00	,00	72,60
2,00	46,00	,00	,00	,00	88,09
3,00	50,00	,00	1,00	,00	61,62
4,00	36,00	,00	,00	1,00	81,28

The above data file now gives predicted strength scores of the 8 future patients as computed with help of the XML file.

Also with a binary outcome variable categorical analysis of covariates is possible. Using logistic regression in SPSS is convenient for the purpose, we need not *manually* transform the quantitative estimator into a categorical one. For the analysis we have to apply the usual commands.

Command

Analyze ....Regression....Binary logistic....Dependent variable.... Independent variables....then, open dialog box labeled Categorical Variables.... select the categorical variable and transfer it to the box Categorical Variables....then click Continue....OK.

Example 2

Particularly, if Gaussian distributions in the outcome are uncertain, automatic non-parametric testing is an adequate and very convenient modern alternative. Three parallel-groups were treated with different sleeping pills. Both hours of sleep and side effect score were assessed.

Group	efficacy	gender	comorbidity	side effect score
0	6,00	,00	1,00	45,00
0	7,10	,00	1,00	35,00
0	8,10	,00	,00	34,00
0	7,50	,00	,00	29,00
0	6,40	,00	1,00	48,00
0	7,90	1,00	1,00	23,00
0	6,80	1,00	1,00	56,00
0	6,60	1,00	,00	54,00
0	7,30	1,00	,00	33,00
0	5,60	,00	,00	75,00

Only the first ten patients are shown. The entire data file is in extras.springer.com and is entitled "categoriesaspredictor2". Automatic nonparametric tests is available in SPSS 18 and up. Start by opening the above data file.

Example 2   213

Command

Analyze....Nonparametric Tests....Independent Samples....click Objective.... mark Automatically compare distributions across groups....click Fields....in Test fields: enter "hours of sleep" and "side effect score"....in Groups: enter "group".... click Settings....Choose Tests....mark "Automatically choose the tests based on the data"....click Run.

In the interactive output sheets the underneath table is given. Both the distribution of hours of sleep and side effect score are significantly different across the three categories of treatment. The traditional assessment of these data would have been a multivariate analysis of variance (MANOVA) with treatment-category as predictor and both hours of sleep and side effect score as outcome. However, normal distributions are uncertain in this example, and the correlation between the two outcome measures may not be zero, reducing the sensitivity of MANOVA. A nice thing about the automatic nonparametric tests is that, like discriminant analysis (Machine learning in medicine part one, Chap. 17, Discriminant analysis for supervised data, pp. 215–224, Springer Heidelberg Germany, 2013, from the same authors), they assume orthogonality of the two outcomes, which means that the correlation level between the two does not have to be taken into account. By double-clicking the table you will obtain an interactive set of views of various details of the analysis, entitled the Model Viewer.

Hypothesis Test Summary

	Null Hypothesis	Test	Sig.	Decision
1	The distribution of hours of sleep is the same across categories of group.	Independent-Samples Kruskal-Wallis Test	,001	Reject the null hypothesis.
2	The distribution of side effect score is the same across categories of group.	Independent-Samples Kruskal-Wallis Test	,036	Reject the null hypothesis.

Asymptotic significances are displayed. The significance level is ,05.

One view provides the box and whiskers graphs (medians, quartiles, and ranges) of hours of sleep of the three treatment groups. Group 0 seems to perform better than the other two, but we don't know where the significant differences are.

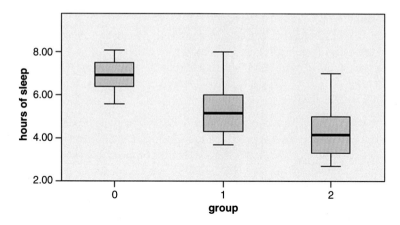

Also the box and whiskers graph of side effect scores is given. Some groups again seem to perform better than the other. However, we cannot see whether 0 versus (vs) 1, 1 vs 2, and/or 0 vs 2 are significantly different.

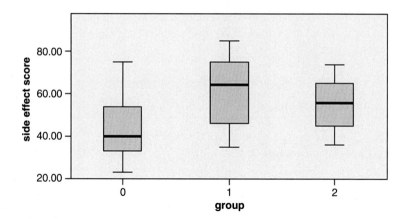

In the view space at the bottom of the auxiliary view (right half of the Model Viewer) several additional options are given. When clicking Pairwise Comparisons, a distance network is displayed with yellow lines corresponding to statistically significant differences, and black ones to insignificant ones. Obviously, the differences in hours of sleep of group 1 vs (versus) 0 and group 2 vs 0 are statistically significant, and 1 vs 2 is not. Group 0 had significantly more hours of sleep than the other two groups with p = 0.044 and 0.0001.

Example 2   215

Pairwise Comparisons of group

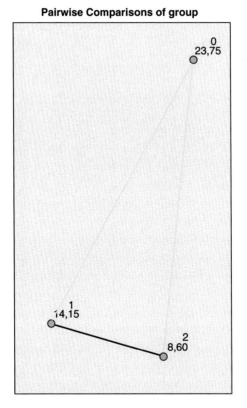

Each node shows the sample average rank of group.

Sample1-Sample2	Test Statistic	Std. Error	Std. Test Statistic	Sig.	Adj. Sig.
2- 1	5,550	3,936	1,410	,158	,475
2- 0	15,150	3,936	3,849	,000	,000
1- 0	9,600	3,936	2,439	,015	,044

Each row tests the null hypothesis that the Sample 1 and Sample 2 distributions are the same.
Asymptotic significances (2-sided tests) are displayed. The significance level is ,05.

As shown below, the difference in side effect score of group 1 vs 0 is also statistically significant, and 1 vs 0, and 1 vs 2 are not. Group 0 has a significantly better side effect score than the 1 with p = 0.035, but group 0 vs 2 and 1 vs 2 are not significantly different.

Pairwise Comparisons of group

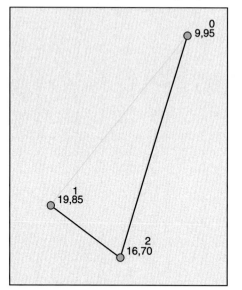

Each node shows the sample average rank of group.

Sample1-Sample2	Test Statistic	Std. Error	Std. Test Statistic	Sig.	Adj. Sig.
0- 2	−6,750	3,931	−1,717	,086	,258
0- 1	−9,900	3,931	−2,518	,012	,035
2- 1	3,150	3,931	,801	,423	1,000

Each row tests the null hypothesis that the Sample 1 and Sample 2
distributions are the same.
Asymptotic significances (2-sided tests) are displayed. The significance level
is ,05.

Conclusion

Predictor variables with a categorical rather than linear character should be recoded
for the purpose into categorical variables before analysis in a regression model. An
example is given. Particularly if the Gaussian distributions in the outcome are
uncertain, automatic non-parametric testing is an adequate and very convenient
alternative.

Note

More background theoretical and mathematical information of categories as predictor is given in SPSS for starters part two, Chap. 5, Categorical data, pp. 21–24, and Statistics applied to clinical studies 5th edition, Chap. 21, Races as a categorical variable, pp. 244–252, both of them from the same authors and edited by Springer Heidelberg Germany 2012.

Chapter 30
Random Intercept Models for Both Outcome and Predictor Categories (55 Patients)

General Purpose

Generalized linear mixed models are suitable for analyzing data with multiple categorical variables, both outcome and exposure variables. Do random intercept versions of these models provide better sensitivity of testing than fixed intercept models.

Background

Categories are very common in medical research. Examples include age classes, income classes, education levels, drug dosages, diagnosis groups, disease severities, etc. Statistics has generally difficulty to assess categories, and traditional models require either binary or continuous variables. If as outcome variables, categories can be assessed with multinomial regression (see the above Chap. 28), if as predictors, they can be assessed with automatic nonparametric tests (see the above Chap. 29). However, with multiple categories or with categories both in the outcome and as predictors, random intercept models may provide better sensitivity of testing. The latter models assume that for each predictor category or combination of categories x_1, x_2, slightly different a-values can be computed with a better fit for the outcome category y than a single a-value.

This chapter was previously published in "Machine learning in medicine-cookbook 2" as Chap. 6, 2014.

Electronic Supplementary Material The online version of this chapter (https://doi.org/10.1007/978-3-030-33970-8_30) contains supplementary material, which is available to authorized users.

T. J. Cleophas, A. H. Zwinderman, *Machine Learning in Medicine – A Complete Overview*, https://doi.org/10.1007/978-3-030-33970-8_30

$$y = a + b_1 \, x_1 + b_2 \, x_2 + \ldots.$$

We should add that, instead of the above linear equation, even better results may be obtained with log-linear equations (log = natural logarithm).

$$\log \, y = a + b_1 \, x_1 + b_2 \, x_2 + \ldots.$$

A random intercept model is a model in which intercepts are allowed to vary, and therefore, the scores on the dependent variable for each individual observation are predicted by the intercept that varies across groups. For example, the rat growth data, will fit the *random intercept model* if it fits the growth for the same two explanatory variables, a time and a group variable. Fitting a random intercept model allows the linear regression fit for each rat to differ in *intercept* from that of other rats. Generalized linear mixed-effects models as applied in R software, SAS software, SPSS statistical software, is appropriate for analysis. In the examples given in this chapter we will use the latter.

Specific Scientific Question

In a study three hospital departments (no surgery, little surgery, lot of surgery), and three patient age classes (young, middle, old) were the predictors of the risk class of falling out of bed (fall out of bed no, yes but no injury, yes and injury). Are the predictor categories significant determinants of the risk of falling out of bed with or without injury. Does a random intercept provide better statistics.

Example

department	falloutofbed	agecat	patient_id
0	1	1,00	1,00
0	1	1,00	2,00
0	1	2,00	3,00
0	1	1,00	4,00
0	1	1,00	5,00
0	1	,00	6,00
1	1	2,00	7,00
0	1	2,00	8,00
1	1	2,00	9,00
0	1	,00	10,00

Example   221

Variable 1:   department = department class (0 = no surgery, 1 = little surgery, 2 = lot of surgery)
Variable 2:   falloutofbed = risk of falling out of bed (0 = fall out of bed no, 1 = yes but no injury, 2 = yes and injury)
Variable 3:   agecat = patient age classes (young, middle, old)
Variable 4:   patient_id = patient identification

Only the first 10 patients of the 55 patient file is shown above. The entire data file is in extras.springer.com and is entitled "randomintercept.sav". SPSS version 20 and up can be used for analysis. First, we will perform a fixed intercept log-linear analysis.

Command
click Analyze....Mixed Models....Generalized Linear Mixed Models....click Data Structure....click "patient_id" and drag to Subjects on the Canvas....click Fields and Effects....click Target....Target: select "fall with/out injury"....click Fixed Effects....click "agecat"and "department" and drag to Effect Builder:.... mark Include intercept....click Run.

The underneath results show that both the various regression coefficients as well as the overall correlation coefficients between the predictors and the outcome are, generally, statistically significant.

Source	F	df1	df2	Sig.
Corrected Model ▼	9,398	4	10	,002
agecat	6,853	2	10	,013
department	9,839	2	10	,004

Probability distribution:Multinomial
Link function:Cumulative logit

Model Term		Coefficient ▶	Sig.
Threshold for falloutofbed=	0	2,140	,028
	1	7,229	,000
agecat=0		5,236	,005
agecat=1		-0,002	,998
agecat=2		0,000[a]	
department=0		3,660	,008
department=1		4,269	,002
department=2		0,000[a]	

Probability distribution: Multinomial
Link function: Cumulative logit

[a]This coefficient is set to zero because it is redundant.

Subsequently, a random intercept analysis is performed.

Command

Analyze....Mixed Models....Generalized Linear Mixed Models....click Data Structure....click "patient_id" and drag to Subjects on the Canvas....click Fields and Effects....click Target....Target: select "fall with/out injury"....click Fixed Effects....click "agecat"and "department" and drag to Effect Builder:....mark Include intercept....click Random Effects....click Add Block...mark Include intercept....Subject combination: select patient_id....click OK....click Model Options....click   Save   Fields...mark   PredictedValue....mark PredictedProbability....click Save....click Run.

The underneath results show the test statistics of the random intercept model. The random intercept model shows better statistics:

Example   223

	p = 0.007 and 0.013	overall for age,
	p = 0.001 and 0.004	overall for department,
	p = 0.003 and 0.005	regression coefficients for age class 0 versus 2,
	p = 0.900 and 0.998	for age class 1 versus 2,
	p = 0.004 and 0.008	for department 0 versus 2, and
	p = 0.001 and 0.0002	for department 1 versus 2.

Source	F	df1	df2	Sig.
Corrected Model ▼	7,935	4	49	,000
agecat	5,513	2	49	,007
department	7,602	2	49	,001

Probability distribution: Multinomial
Link function: Cumulative logit

Model Term		Coefficient ▶	Sig.
Threshold for falloutofbed=	0	2,082	,015
	1	5,464	,000
agecat=0		3,869	,003
agecat=1		0,096	,900
agecat=2		0,000ᵃ	
department=0		3,228	,004
department=1		3,566	,000
department=2		0,000ᵃ	

Probability distribution:Multinomial
Link function:Cumulative logit

ᵃThis coefficient is set to zero because it is redundant.

In the random intercept model we have also commanded predicted values (variable 7) and predicted probabilities of having the predicted values as computed by the software (variables 5 and 6).

1	2	3	4	5	6	7 (variables)
0	1	1,00	1,00	,224	,895	1
0	1	1,00	2,00	,224	,895	1
0	1	2,00	3,00	,241	,903	1
0	1	1,00	4,00	,224	,895	1
0	1	1,00	5,00	,224	,895	1
0	1	,00	6,00	,007	,163	2
1	1	2,00	7,00	,185	,870	1
0	1	2,00	8,00	,241	,903	1
1	1	2,00	9,00	,185	,870	1
0	1	,00	10,00	,007	,163	2

Variable 1:   department
Variable 2:   falloutofbed
Variable 3:   agecat
Variable 4:   patient_id
Variable 5:   predicted probability of predicted value of target accounting the department score only
Variable 6:   predicted probability of predicted value of target accounting both department and agecat scores
Variable 7:   predicted value of target

Like automatic linear regression (see Chap. 31) and other generalized mixed linear models (see Chap. 33) random intercept models include the possibility to make XML files from the analysis, that can subsequently be used for making predictions about the chance of falling out of bed in future patients. However, SPSS uses here slightly different software called winRAR ZIP files that are "shareware". This means that you pay a small fee and be registered if you wish to use it. Note that winRAR ZIP files have an archive file format consistent of compressed data used by Microsoft since 2006 for the purpose of filing XML (eXtended Markup Language) files. They are only employable for a limited period of time like e.g. 40 days.

Conclusion

Generalized linear mixed models are suitable for analyzing data with multiple categorical variables, both outcome and exposure variables. Random intercept versions of these models provide better sensitivity of testing than fixed intercept models.

Note

More information on statistical methods for analyzing data with categories is in the Chaps. 28 and 29 of this edition.

Chapter 31
Automatic Regression for Maximizing Linear Relationships (55 Patients)

General Purpose

This chapter is to assess whether automatic regression for maximizing linear relationships is helpful to obtain an improved precision of analysis of clinical trials. Examples are given.

Background

Automatic linear regression is in the Statistics Base add-on module SPSS statistical software version 19 and up. X-variables are automatically transformed in order to provide an improved data fit, and SPSS statistical software uses rescaling of time and other measurement values, outlier trimming, category merging and other methods. The computer teaches itself to make predictions. By the software modeled regression coefficients are used to make predictions about future data using the Scoring Wizard and an XML (eXtended Markup Language) file (winRAR ZIP file) of the data file. Like random intercept models (see Chap. 30), and other generalized mixed linear models, automatic linear regression includes the possibility to make XML files from the analysis, that can, subsequently, be used for making outcome predictions about future patients. SPSS uses here software called winRAR ZIP files that are "shareware". This means, that you pay a small fee, and be registered, if you wish to use it. Note that winRAR ZIP files have an archive file format consistent of compressed data used by Microsoft since 2006 for the purpose of filing XML files.

This chapter was previously published in "Machine learning in medicine-cookbook 2" as Chap. 7, 2014.

Electronic Supplementary Material The online version of this chapter (https://doi.org/10.1007/978-3-030-33970-8_31) contains supplementary material, which is available to authorized users.

Specific Scientific Question

In a clinical crossover trial an old laxative is tested against a new one. Numbers of stools per month is the outcome. The old laxative and the patients' age are the predictor variables. Does automatic linear regression provide better statistics of these data than traditional multiple linear regression does.

Data Example

Patno	newtreat	oldtreat	age categories
1,00	24,00	8,00	2,00
2,00	30,00	13,00	2,00
3,00	25,00	15,00	2,00
4,00	35,00	10,00	3,00
5,00	39,00	9,00	3,00
6,00	30,00	10,00	3,00
7,00	27,00	8,00	1,00
8,00	14,00	5,00	1,00
9,00	39,00	13,00	1,00
10,00	42,00	15,00	1,00

patno = patient number
newtreat = frequency of stools on a novel laxative
oldtreat = frequency of stools on an old laxative
agecategories = patients' age categories (1 = young, 2 = middle-age, 3 = old)

Only the first 10 patients of the 55 patients are shown above. The entire file is in extras.springer.com and is entitled "automaticlinreg". We will first perform a standard multiple linear regression.

Command

Analyze....Regression....Linear....Dependent: enter newtreat....Independent: enter oldtreat and agecategories....click OK.

Model Summary

Model	R	R Square	Adjusted R Square	Std. Error of the Estimate
1	,429[a]	,184	,133	9,28255

a. Predictors: (Constant), oldtreat, agecategories

ANOVA[a]

Model		Sum of Squares	df	Mean Square	F	Sig.
1	Regression	622,869	2	311,435	3,614	,038[b]
	Residual	2757,302	32	86,166		
	Total	3380,171	34			

a. Dependent Variable: newtreat

b. Predictors: (Constant), oldtreat, agecategories

Coefficients[a]

Model		Unstandardized Coefficients		Standardized Coefficients	t	Sig.
		B	Std. Error	Beta		
1	(Constant)	20,513	5,137		3,993	,000
	agecategories	3,908	2,329	,268	1,678	,103
	oldtreat	,135	,065	,331	2,070	,047

a. Dependent Variable: newtreat

Automatic Data Preparation

Target: newtreat

Field	Role	Actions Taken
(agecategories_transformed)	Predictor	Merge categories to maximize association with target
(oldtreat_transformed)	Predictor	Trim outliers

If the original field name is X, then the transformed field is displayed as (X_transformed). The original field is excluded from the analysis and the transformed field is included instead.

An interactive graph shows the predictors as lines with thicknesses corresponding to their predictive power and the outcome in the form of a histogram with its best fit Gaussian pattern. Both of the predictors are now statistically very significant with a correlation coefficient at $p < 0.0001$, and regression coefficients at p-values of respectively 0.001 and 0.007.

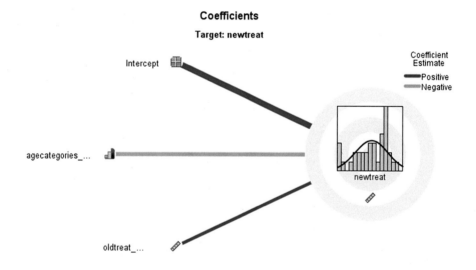

Coefficients

Target: newtreat

Model Term	Coefficient ▶	Sig.	Importance
Intercept	35,926	,000	
agecategories_transformed=0	-11,187	,001	0,609
agecategories_transformed=1	0,000ᵃ		0,609
oldtreat_transformed	0,209	,007	0,391

ᵃThis coefficient is set to zero because it is redundant.

Effects

Target: newtreat

Source	Sum of Squares	df	Mean Square	F	Sig.
Corrected Model ▶	1.289,960	2	644,980	9,874	,000
Residual	2.090,212	32	65,319		
Corrected Total	3.380,171	34			

Returning to the data view of the original data file, we now observe that SPSS has provided a novel variables with values for the new treatment as predicted from statistical model employed. They are pretty close to the real outcome values.

Patno	newtreat	oldtreat	age categories	Predicted Values
1,00	24,00	8,00	2,00	26,41
2,00	30,00	13,00	2,00	27,46
3,00	25,00	15,00	2,00	27,87
4,00	35,00	10,00	3,00	38,02
5,00	39,00	9,00	3,00	37,81
6,00	30,00	10,00	3,00	38,02
7,00	27,00	8,00	1,00	26,41
8,00	14,00	5,00	1,00	25,78
9,00	39,00	13,00	1,00	27,46
10,00	42,00	15,00	1,00	27,87

patno = patient number
newtreat = frequency of stools on a novel laxative
oldtreat = frequency of stools on an old laxative
agecategories = patients' age categories (1 = young, 2 = middle-age, 3 = old)

The Computer Teaches Itself to Make Predictions

The modeled regression coefficients are used to make predictions about future data using the Scoring Wizard and an XML (eXtended Markup Language) file (winRAR ZIP file) of the data file. Like random intercept models (see Chap. 6) and other generalized mixed linear models (see Chap. 9) automatic linear regression includes the possibility to make XML files from the analysis, that can subsequently be used for making outcome predictions in future patients. SPSS uses here software called winRAR ZIP files that are "shareware". This means that you pay a small fee and be registered if you wish to use it. Note that winRAR ZIP files have a archive file format consistent of compressed data used by Microsoft since 2006 for the purpose of filing XML files. They are only employable for a limited period of time like e.g. 40 days. Below the data of 9 future patients are given.

Newtreat	oldtreat	agecategory
	4,00	1,00
	13,00	1,00
	15,00	1,00
	15,00	1,00
	11,00	2,00
	80,00	2,00
	10,00	3,00
	18,00	2,00
	13,00	2,00

Enter the Above Data in a Novel Data File and Command
Utilities. . . .click Scoring Wizard. . . .click Browse. . . .Open the appropriate folder
with the XML file entitled "exportautomaticlinreg". . . .click on the latter and click
Select. . . .in Scoring Wizard double-click Next. . . .mark Predicted Value. . . .click
Finish.

Newtreat	oldtreat	agecategory	predictednewtreat
	4,00	1,00	25,58
	13,00	1,00	27,46
	15,00	1,00	27,87
	15,00	1,00	27,87
	11,00	2,00	27,04
	80,00	2,00	41,46
	10,00	3,00	38,02
	18,00	2,00	28,50
	13,00	2,00	27,46

In the data file SPSS has provided the novel variable as requested. The first patient
with only 4 stools per month on the old laxative and young of age will have over
25 stools on the new laxative.

Conclusion

SPSS' automatic linear regression can be helpful to obtain an improved precision of
analysis of clinical trials and provided in the example given better statistics than
traditional multiple linear regression did.

Note

More background theoretical and mathematical information of linear regression is available in Statistics applied to clinical studies 5th edition, Chap. 14, entitled Linear regression basic approach, and Chap. 15, Linear regression for assessing precision confounding interaction, Chap. 18, Regression modeling for improved precision, pp. 161–176, 177–185, 219–225, Springer Heidelberg Germany, 2012, from the same authors.

Chapter 32
Simulation Models for Varying Predictors (9000 Patients)

General Purpose

In medicine predictors are often varying, like, e.g., the numbers of complications and the days in hospital in patients with various conditions. This chapter is to assess, whether Monte Carlo simulation of the varying predictors can improve the outcome predictions.

Background

What is a Monte Carlo simulation? Monte Carlo simulations are used to model the probability of different outcomes in a process that cannot easily be predicted due to the intervention of random variables. It is a technique used to understand the impact of risk and uncertainty in prediction and forecasting models. Monte Carlo simulation can be used to assess questions in virtually every field including finance, engineering, supply chain, and science. Monte Carlo simulation is also named multiple probability simulation.

This chapter was previously published in "Machine learning in medicine-cookbook 2" as Chap. 8, 2014.

Electronic Supplementary Material The online version of this chapter (https://doi.org/10.1007/978-3-030-33970-8_32) contains supplementary material, which is available to authorized users.

When faced with significant uncertainty in the process of making a forecast or estimation, rather than just replacing the uncertain variable with a single average number, the Monte Carlo Simulation might prove to be a better solution. Since business and finance are plagued by random variables, Monte Carlo simulations have a vast array of potential applications in these fields. They are used to estimate the probability of cost overruns in large projects and the likelihood that an asset price will move in a certain way. Telecoms use them to assess network performance in different scenarios, helping them to optimize the network. Analysts use them to assess the risk that an entity will default and to analyze derivatives such as options. Insurers and oil well drillers also use them. Monte Carlo simulations have countless applications outside of business and finance, such as in meteorology, astronomy and particle physics.

Monte Carlo simulations are named after the gambling hot spot in Monaco, since chance and random outcomes are central to the modeling technique, much as they are to games like roulette, dice, and slot machines. The technique was first developed by Stanislaw Ulam, a mathematician who worked on the Manhattan Project. After world war II, while recovering from brain surgery, Ulam entertained himself by playing countless games of solitaire. He became interested in plotting the outcome of each of these games in order to observe their distribution and determine the probability of winning. After he shared his idea with John Von Neumann, the two collaborated to develop the Monte Carlo simulation.

Specific Scientific Question

The hospital costs for patients with heart infarction are supposed to be dependent on factors like patients' age, intensive care hours (ichours), numbers of complications. What percentage of patients will cost the hospital over 20,000 Euros, what percentage over 10,000. How will costs develop if the numbers of complications are reduced by 2 and the numbers of ichours by 20.

Instead of Traditional Means and Standard Deviations, Monte Carlo Simulations of the Input and Outcome Variables Are Used to Model the Data. This Enhances Precision, Particularly, with Non-normal Data

Age Years	complication number	ic hours	costs Euros
48	7	36	5488
66	7	57	8346
75	7	67	6976
72	6	45	5691
60	6	58	3637
84	9	54	16369
74	8	54	11349
42	9	26	10213
71	7	49	6474
73	10	35	30018
53	8	37	7632
79	6	46	6538
50	10	39	13797

Only the first 13 patients of this 9000 patient hypothesized data file is shown. The entire data file is in extras.springer.com and is entitled "simulation1.sav". SPSS 21 or 22 can be used. Start by opening the data file. We will first perform a traditional linear regression with the first three variables as input and the fourth variable as outcome.

Command:
click Transform....click Random Number Generators....click Set Starting Point ....click Fixed Value (2000000)....click OK....click Analyze ....Regression.... Linear....Dependent: costs...Independent: age, complication, ichours....click Save....click Browse....Select the desired folder in your computer....File name: enter "exportsimulation"....click Save....click Continue....click OK.

In the output sheets it is observed that all of the predictors are statistically very significant. Also a PMML (predictive model markup language) document, otherwise called XML (eXtended Markup Language) document has been produced and filed in your computer entitled "exportsimulation".

Coefficients[a]

Model	Unstandardized Coefficients		Standardized Coefficients	t	Sig.
	B	Std. Error	Beta		
(Constant)	-28570,977	254,044		-112,465	,000
age(years)	202,403	2,767	,318	73,136	,000
complications(n)	4022,405	21,661	,807	185,696	,000
ichours(hours)	-111,241	2,124	-,227	-52,374	,000

a. Dependent Variable: cost(Euros)

We will now perform the Monte Carlo simulation.

Command:
Analyze. . . .Simulation. . . .click Select SPSS Model File. . . .click Continue. . . .in
Look in: select folder with "exportsimulation.xml" file. . . .click Open. . . .click Simulation Fields. . . .click Fit All. . . .click Save. . . .mark Save the plan file for this
simulation. . . .click Browse. . . .in Look in: select the appropriate folder for storage
of a simulation plan document and entitle it, e.g., "splan". . . .click Save. . . .
click Run.

In the output the underneath interactive probability density graph is exhibited.
After double-clicking the vertical lines can be moved and corresponding areas under
the curve percentages are shown.

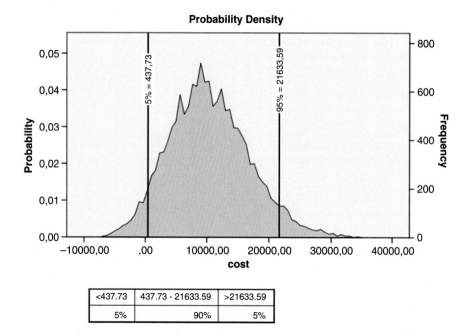

<437.73	437.73 - 21633.59	>21633.59
5%	90%	5%

Overall 90 % of the heart attacks patients will cost the hospital between 440 and
21.630 Euros. In the graph click Chart Options. . . .in View click Histogram. . . .click
Continue.

The histogram below is displayed. Again the vertical lines can be moved as
desired. It can, e.g., be observed that, around, 7.5 % of the heart attack patients will
cost the hospital over 20.000 Euros, around 50% of them will cost over 10.000
Euros.

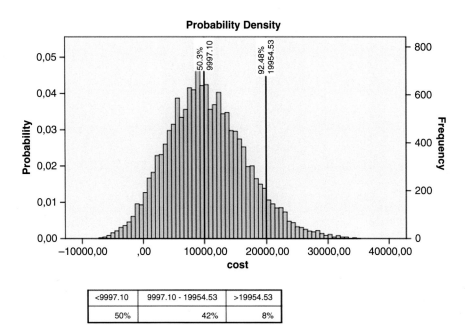

<9997.10	9997.10 - 19954.53	>19954.53
50%	42%	8%

Monte Carlo can also be used to answer questions like " What will happen to costs, if the numbers of complications are reduced by two or the ic hours are reduced by 20". For that purpose we will use the original data file entitled "chap8simulation1.sav" again. Also the document entitled "splan" which contains software syntax for performing a simulation is required.

Open "simulation1.sav" and Command:
Transform....Compute Variable....in Numeric Expression enter "complications" from the panel below Numeric Expressions enter "-" and "2"....in Target Variable type complications....click OK....in Change existing variable click OK.

In the data file all of the values of the variable "complications" have now been reduced by 2. This transformed data file is saved in the desired folder and entitled e.g. "simulation2.sav". We will now perform a Monte Carlo simulation of this transformed data file using the simulation plan "splan".

In "simulation2.sav" command: Analyze....Simulation....click Open an Existing Simulation Plan....click Continue....in Look in: find the appropriate folder in your computer....click "splan.splan"....click Open....click Simulation....click Fit All....click Run.

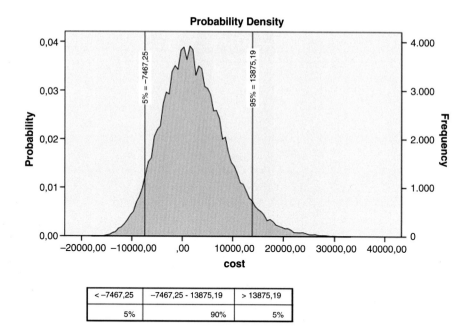

< -7467,25	-7467,25 - 13875,19	> 13875,19
5%	90%	5%

The above graph shows that fewer complications reduces the costs, e.g., 5% of the patients cost over 13.875 Euros, while the same class costed over 21.633 Euros before.

What about the effect of the hours in the ic unit. For that purpose, in "simulation1. sav" perform the same commands as shown directly above, and transform the ic hours variable by −20 h. The transformed document can be named "simulation3. sav" and saved. The subsequent simulation procedure in this data file using again "splan.splan" produces the underneath output.

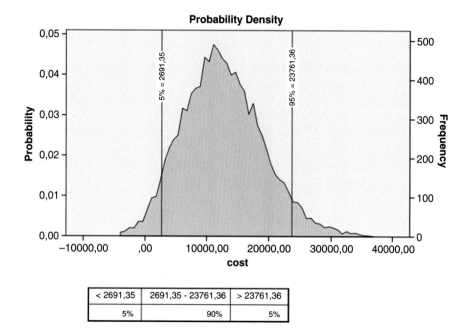

< 2691,35	2691,35 - 23761,36	> 23761,36
5%	90%	5%

It is observed that the costs are now not reduced, but rather somewhat increased with 5% of the patients costing over 23.761 Euros instead of 21.633. This would make sense, nonetheless, because it is sometimes assumed by hospital managers that the reduction of stay-days in hospital is accompanied with more demanding type of care (Statistics Applied to Clinical Studies 5th edition, Chap. 44, Clinical data where variability is more important than averages, pp 487–498, Springer Heidelberg Germany, 2012).

Conclusion

Monte Carlo simulations of inputs where variability is more important than means can model outcome distributions with increased precision. This is, particularly, so with non-normal data. Also questions, like "how will hospital costs develop, if the numbers of complications are reduced by 2 or numbers of hours in the intensive care unit reduced by 20", can be answered.

Note

More background, theoretical and mathematical information of Monte Carlo simulation is provided in Statistics applied to clinical studies 5th edition, Chap. 44, Clinical data where variability is more important than averages, pp 487–498, Springer Heidelberg Germany, 2012, from the same authors as the current publication.

Chapter 33
Generalized Linear Mixed Models for Outcome Prediction from Mixed Data (20 Patients)

General Purpose

To assess, whether generalized linear mixed models can be used to train clinical samples with both fixed and random effects about individual future patients. Examples are given.

Background

In statistics terminologies are often rather inconsistent. As an example, a mixed data file is a term sometimes used for naming data files in which a group of individuals is described both by quantitative and qualitative variables. However, traditionally, mixed research models is a name used for advanced analysis-of-variance models (see Statistics applied to clinical studies 5th edition, Chap. 56, Springer Heidelberg Germany, 2012, from the same authors). These research models are assumed to include variables with fixed rather than random effects.

It means, that the patients selected for a specific treatment are assumed to be homogeneous and have the same true quantitative effect and that the differences observed are residual, meaning that they are caused by inherent variability in biological processes, rather than some hidden subgroup property. If, however, we have reasons to believe that certain patients due to co-morbidity, co-medication, age or other factors will respond differently from others, then the spread in the data is caused not only by the residual effect but also by between patient differences due to

This chapter was previously published in "Machine learning in medicine-cookbook 2" as Chap. 9, 2014.

Electronic Supplementary Material The online version of this chapter (https://doi.org/10.1007/978-3-030-33970-8_33) contains supplementary material, which is available to authorized users.

some subgroup property. It may even be safe to routinely treat any patient effect as a random effect, unless there are good arguments no to do so. Random effects research models require a statistical approach different from that of fixed effects models.

With the fixed effects model the treatment differences are tested against the residual error, otherwise called the standard error. With the random effects models the treatment effects may be influenced not only by the residual effect but also by some unexpected, otherwise called random, factor, and so the treatment should no longer be tested against the residual effect. Because both residual and random effect constitute a much larger amount of uncertainty in the data, the treatment effect has to be tested against both of them. Random effects models is a very interesting class of models, but even a partial understanding is fairly difficult to achieve.

This chapter will address mixed random effects models in analysis-of-variance and give examples of studies qualifying for them. They are often called type 2 models if they include random exposure variables and type 3 models if they include both fixed and random exposure variables. Type 3 models are, otherwise, called mixed (effects) models.

Specific Scientific Question

In a parallel-group study of two treatments, each patient was measured weekly for 5 weeks. As repeated measures in one patient are more similar than unrepeated ones, a random interaction effect between week and patient was assumed.

Example

In a parallel-group study of two cholesterol reducing compounds, patients were measured weekly for 5 weeks. As repeated measures in one patient are more similar than unrepeated ones, we assumed that a random interaction variable between week and patient would appropriately adjust this effect.

Example   245

Patient_id	week	hdl-cholesterol (mmol/l)	treatment (0 or 1)
1	1	1,66	0
1	2	1,62	0
1	3	1,57	0
1	4	1,52	0
1	5	1,50	0
2	1	1,69	0
2	2	1,71	0
2	3	1,60	0
2	4	1,55	0
2	5	1,56	0

Only the first 2 patients of the data file is shown. The entire file entitled "fixedandrandomeffects" is in extras.springer.com. We will try and develop a mixed model (mixed means a model with both fixed and random predictors) for testing the data. Also, SPSS will be requested to produce a ZIP (compressed file that can be unzipped) file from the intervention study, which could then be used for making predictions about cholesterol values in future patients treated similarly. We will start by opening the intervention study's data file.

Command:
click Transform....click Random Number Generators....click Set Starting Point....click Fixed Value (2000000)....click OK....click Analyze....Mixed Linear....Generalized Mixed Linear Models....click Data Structure....click left mouse and drag patient_id to Subjects part of the canvas....click left mouse and drag week to Repeated Measures part of the canvas....click Fields and Effects.... click Target....check that the variable outcome is already in the Target window.... check that Linear model is marked....click Fixed Effects....drag treatment and week to Effect builder....click Random Effects....click Add Block....click Add a custom term....move week∗treatment (∗ is symbol multiplication and interaction) to the Custom term window....click Add term....click OK....click Model Options....click Save Fields....mark Predicted Values....click Export model.... type exportfixedandrandom....click Browse....in the appropriate folder enter in File name: mixed....click Run.

Fixed Coefficients

Target:outcome

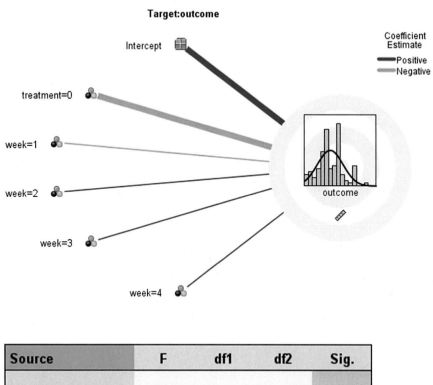

Source	F	df1	df2	Sig.
Corrected Model ▼	5,027	5	94	,000
treatment	23,722	1	94	,000
week	0,353	4	94	,841

Probability distribution:Normal
Link function:Identity

In the output sheet a graph is observed with the mean and standard errors of the outcome value displayed with the best fit Gaussian curve. The F-value of 23.722 indicates that one treatment is very significantly better than the other with p <0.0001. The thickness of the lines are a measure for level of significance, and so the significance of the 5 week is very thin and thus very weak. Week 5 is not shown.

Example   247

It is redundant, because it means absence of the other 4 weeks. If you click at the left bottom of the graph panel, a table comes up providing similar information in written form. The effect of the interaction variable is not shown, but implied in the analysis.

If we return to the data file page, we will observe that the software has produced a predicted value for each actually measured cholesterol value. The predicted and actual values are very much the same.

We will now use the ZIP file to make predictions about cholesterol values in future patients treated similarly.

week	treatment	patient_id
1	0	21
2	0	21
3	0	21
4	0	21
5	0	21
1	1	22
2	1	22
3	1	22
4	1	22
5	1	22

Command:
click Utilities....click Scoring Wizard....click Browse....click Select....Folder: enter the mixed ZIP file entitled "exportfixedandrandom"....click Select....in Scoring Wizard click Next....click Finish.

In the data file now the predicted cholesterol values are given.

week	treatment	patient_id	predicted cholesterol
1	0	21	1,88
2	0	21	1,96
3	0	21	1,94
4	0	21	1,91
5	0	21	1,89
1	1	22	2,12
2	1	22	2,20
3	1	22	2,18
4	1	22	2,15
5	1	22	2,13

Conclusion

The module Generalized mixed linear models provides the possibility to handle both fixed and random effects, and is, therefore appropriate to adjust data with repeated measures and presumably a strong correlation between the repeated measures. Also individual future patients treated similarly can be assessed for predicted cholesterol values using a ZIP file.

Note

More background theoretical and mathematical information of models with both fixed and random variables is given in:

1. Machine learning in medicine part one, Chap. 6, Mixed linear models, pp 65–76, 2013,
2. Statistics applied to clinical studies 5th edition, Chap. 56, Advanced analysis of variance, random effects and mixed effects models, pp 607–618, 2012,
3. SPSS for starters part one, Chap. 7, Mixed models, pp 25–29, 2010, and,
4. Machine learning in medicine part three, Chap. 9, Random effects, pp 81–94, 2013.

All of these references are from the same authors and have been edited by Springer Heidelberg Germany.

Chapter 34
Two-stage Least Squares (35 Patients)

General Purpose

The two stage least squares method assumes, that the independent variable (x-variable) is problematic, meaning that it is somewhat uncertain. An additional variable can be argued to provide relevant information about the problematic variable, and is, therefore, called instrumental variable, and included in the analysis. An example is given.

Background

Both path analysis and multistage least squares are adequate for simultaneously assessing both direct and indirect predictors. This makes interpretation less easy. Also, path analysis does not provide overall p-values.

Multistage regression is otherwise called multistage least squares. Its simplest version is two-stage least squares. It was invented by Philip G. Wright, professor of economics at Harvard University, Cambridge MA, 1928 (The tariff on animal and vegetable oils, McMillan New York). Multistage regression uses instrumental variables for improved estimation of problematic (i.e., somewhat uncertain) predictors (Angrist and Krueger, J Econ Perspect 2001; 15: 69). It is an alternative to traditional path analysis, which assumes, that predictor variables not only produce direct effects on the outcome, but also indirect effects through affecting concomitant predictor variables. With path analysis usual regression coefficients can not be applied,

This chapter was previously published in "Machine learning in medicine-cookbook 2" as Chap. 10, 2014.

Electronic Supplementary Material The online version of this chapter (https://doi.org/10.1007/978-3-030-33970-8_34) contains supplementary material, which is available to authorized users.

because they have the same unit as the outcome variable. Instead, standardized regression coefficients have to be used. This is what makes interpretation less easy. Also, path analysis does not provide overall p-values. In the current chapter, two stage least squares will be explained, as an alternative to traditional path analysis. A real data example will be used.

Primary Scientific Question

Non-compliance is a predictor of drug efficacy. Counseling causes improvement of patients' compliance and, therefore, indirectly improves the outcome drug efficacy.

$$y = \text{outcome variable (drug efficacy)}$$
$$x = \text{problematic variable (non} - \text{compliance)}$$
$$z = \text{instrumental variable(counseling)}$$

With two stage least squares the underneath stages are assessed.

$$\text{1st stage}$$
$$x = \text{intercept} + \text{regression coefficient times } z$$

With the help of the calculated intercept and regression coefficient from the above simple linear regression analysis improved x-values are calculated, e.g., for patient 1:

$$x_{\text{improved}} = \text{intercept} + \text{regression coefficient times } 8 = 27.68$$

$$\text{2nd stage}$$
$$y = \text{intercept} + \text{regression coefficient times } x_{\text{improved}}$$

Example

Patients' non-compliance is a factor notoriously affecting the estimation of drug efficacy. An example is given of a simple evaluation study that assesses the effect of non-compliance (pills not used) on the outcome, the efficacy of a novel laxative with numbers of stools per month as efficacy estimator (the y-variable). The data of the first 10 of the 35 patients are in the table below. The entire data file is in extras. springer.com, and is entitled "twostageleastsquares".

Example   251

Patient no	Instrumental variable (z)	Problematic predictor (x)	Outcome (y)
	Frequency counseling	Pills not used (non-compliance)	Efficacy estimator of new laxative (stools / month)
1.	8	25	24
2.	13	30	30
3.	15	25	25
4.	14	31	35
5.	9	36	39
6.	10	33	30
7.	8	22	27
8.	5	18	14
9.	13	14	39
10.	15	30	42

SPSS version 19 and up can be used for analysis. It uses the term explanatory variable for the problematic variable. Start by opening the data file.

Command:
Analyze....Regression....2 Stage Least Squares....Dependent: therapeutic efficacy....Explanatory: non-compliance.... Instrumental: counseling ....
click OK.

Model Description

		Type of Variable
Equation 1	y	dependent
	x	predictor
	z	instrumental

ANOVA

		Sum of Squares	df	Mean Square	F	Sig.
Equation 1	Regression	1408,040	1	1408,040	4,429	,043
	Residual	10490,322	33	317,889		
	Total	11898,362	34			

Coefficients

		Unstandardized Coefficients		Beta	t	Sig.
		B	Std. Error			
Equation 1	(Constant)	-49,778	37,634		-1,323	,195
	x	2,675	1,271	1,753	2,105	,043

The result is shown above. The non-compliance adjusted for counseling is a statistically significant predictor of laxative efficacy with $p = 0.043$. This p-value has been automatically been adjusted for multiple testing. When we test the model without the help of the instrumental variable counseling the p-value is larger and the effect is no more statistically significant as shown underneath.

Command:

Analyze....Regression....Linear....Dependent: therapeutic efficacy ....Independent: non-compliance....click OK.

ANOVA[b]

Model		Sum of Squares	df	Mean Square	F	Sig.
1	Regression	334,482	1	334,482	3,479	,071[a]
	Residual	3172,489	33	96,136		
	Total	3506,971	34			

a. Predictors: (Constant), non-compliance
b. Dependent Variable: drug efficacy

Coefficients[a]

Model		Unstandardized Coefficients		Standardized Coefficients	t	Sig.
		B	Std. Error	Beta		
1	(Constant)	15,266	7,637		1,999	,054
	non-compliance	,471	,253	,309	1,865	,071

a. Dependent Variable: drug efficacy

Conclusion

Two stage least squares with counseling as instrumental variable was more sensitive than simple linear regression with laxative efficacy as outcome and non-compliance as predictor. We should add that two stage least squares is at risk of overestimating the precision of the outcome, if the analysis is not adequately adjusted for multiple testing. However, in SPSS automatic adjustment for the purpose has been performed. The example is the simplest version of the procedure. And, multiple explanatory and instrumental variables can be included in the models.

Note

More background theoretical and mathematical information of two stage least squares analyses is given in Machine learning in medicine part two, Two-stage least squares, pp 9–15, Springer Heidelberg Germany, 2013, from the same authors.

Chapter 35
Autoregressive Models for Longitudinal Data (120 Mean Monthly Population Records)

General Purpose

Time series are encountered in every field of medicine. Traditional tests are unable to assess trends, seasonality, change points and the effects of multiple predictors, like treatment modalities, simultaneously. This chapter is to assess, whether autoregressive integrated moving average (ARIMA) methods are able to do all of that.

Background

A popular and widely used statistical method for time series forecasting is the ARIMA model. ARIMA is an acronym that stands for Auto Regressive Integrated Moving Average. It is a class of models that includes various temporal structures in time series data.

Traditionally time series data were analyzed without taking into account how "growth / decline over time" might have an effect on their analyses. Then, the statisticians Box and Jenkins (San Francisco: Holden-Day, 1970) presented a famous monograph called "Time Series Analysis: Forecasting and Control" in which they showed, that such data could be made stationary, i.e., steady over time. In this way, they could identify trends at a specific time period from a growth / decline that would be expected from previous data. More specifically, their approach involved considering a value Y at time point t and adding / subtracting based on the Y values at

This chapter was previously published in "Machine learning in medicine-cookbook 2" as Chap. 11, 2014.

Electronic Supplementary Material The online version of this chapter (https://doi.org/10.1007/978-3-030-33970-8_35) contains supplementary material, which is available to authorized users.

previous time points, and, also, adding / subtracting error terms from previous time points. ARIMA models are typically expressed like "ARIMA (p,d,q)", with the three terms p, d, and q defined as follows:

The term "p" means the number of preceding ("lagged") Y values that have to be added / subtracted to Y in the model, so as to make better predictions based on local periods of growth / decline in our data. This captures the "autoregressive" nature of ARIMA.

The term "d" represents the number of times that the data have to be "differenced" to produce a stationary signal (i.e., a signal that has a constant mean over time). This captures the "integrated" nature of ARIMA. If d = 0, this will mean, that our data does not tend to go up / down in the long term (i.e., the model is already "stationary"). In this case, you are, technically, just performing ARMA, not AR-I-MA. If p is 1, then it will mean, that the data is going up / down linearly. If p is 2, then it will mean, that the data is going up / down exponentially. More on this will be given below.

The term "q" represents the number of preceding/lagged values for the error term that are added/subtracted to Y. This captures the "moving average" part of ARIMA.

Specific Scientific Question

Monthly HbA1c levels in patients with diabetes type II are a good estimator for adequate diabetes control, and have been demonstrated to be seasonal with higher levels in the winter. A large patient population was followed for 10 year. The mean values are in the data. This chapter is to assess whether longitudinal summary statistics of a population can be used for the effects of seasons and treatment changes on populations with chronic diseases.

Note:
No conclusion can here be drawn about individual patients. Autoregressive models can also be applied with data sets of individual patients, and with multiple outcome variables like various health outcomes.

Example 257

Example

The underneath data are from the first year's observation data of the above diabetic patient data. The entire data file is in extras.springer.com, and is entitled "arimafile".

Date	HbA1	nurse	doctor	phone	self	meeting
01/01/1989	11,00	8,00	7,00	3	22	2
02/01/1989	10,00	8,00	9,00	3	27	2
03/01/1989	17,00	8,00	7,00	2	30	3
04/01/1989	7,00	8,00	9,00	2	29	2
05/01/1989	7,00	9,00	7,00	2	23	2
06/01/1989	10,00	8,00	9,00	3	27	2
07/01/1989	9,00	8,00	8,00	3	27	2
08/01/1989	10,00	8,00	7,00	3	30	2
09/01/1989	12,00	8,00	8,00	4	27	2
10/01/1989	13,00	9,00	11,00	3	32	2
11/01/1989	14,00	9,00	7,00	3	29	2
12/01/1989	23,00	10,00	11,00	5	39	3
01/01/1990	12,00	8,00	7,00	4	23	2
02/01/1990	8,00	8,00	6,00	2	25	3

Date = date of observation,
HbA1 = mean HbA1c of diabetes population,
nurse = mean number of diabetes nurse visits,
doctor = mean number of doctor visits,
phone = mean number of phone visits,
self = mean number of self-controls,
meeting = mean number of patient educational meetings

We will first assess the observed values along the time line. The analysis is performed using SPSS statistical software.

Command:
analyze....Forecast....Sequence Charts....Variables: enter HbA1c....Time Axis Labels: enter Date....click OK.

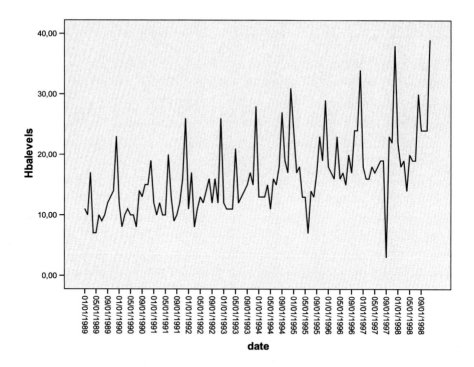

The above output sheets show the observed data. There are (1) numerous peaks, which are (2) approximately equally sized, and (3) there is an upward trend: (2) suggests periodicity which was expected from the seasonal pattern of HbA1c values, (3) is also expected, it suggests increasing HbA1c after several years due to beta-cell failure. Finally (4), there are several peaks that are not part of the seasonal pattern, and could be due to outliers.

ARIMA (autoregressive integrated moving average methodology) is used for modeling this complex data pattern. It uses the Export Modeler for outlier detection, and produces for the purpose XML (eXtended Markup Language) files for prediction modeling of future data.

Command:

Analyze....Forecast....Time Series Modeler....Dependent Variables: enter HbA1c....Independent Variables: enter nurse, doctor, phone, self control, and patient meeting....click Methods: Expert Modeler....click Criteria....Click Outlier Table....Select automatically ....Click Statistics Table....Select Parameter Estimates....mark Display forecasts....click Plots table....click Series, Observed values, Fit values....click Save....Predicted Values: mark Save....Export XML File: click Browse....various folders in your PC come up....in "File Name"of the appropriate folder enter "exportarima"....click Save....click Continue.... click OK.

Example   259

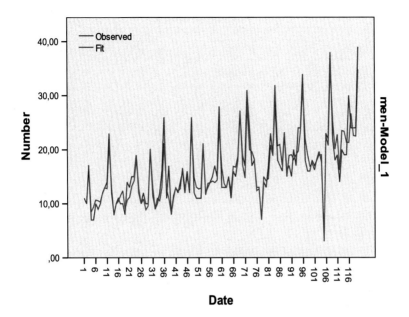

Date

The above graph shows that a good fit of the observed data is given by the ARIMA model, and that an adequate predictive model is provided. The upward trend is in agreement with beta-cell failure after several years.

The underneath table shows that 3 significant predictors have been identified. Also the goodness of fit of the ARIMA (p, d, q) model is given, where p = number of lags, d = the trend (one upward trend means d = 1), and q = number of moving averages (= 0 here). Both Stationary R square, and Ljung-Box tests are insignificant. A significant test would have meant poor fit. In our example, there is an adequate fit, but the model has identified no less than 7 outliers. Phone visits, nurse visits, and doctor visits were significant predictors at $p < 0.0001$, while self control and educational patient meetings were not so. All of the outliers are significantly more distant from the ARIMA model than could happen by chance. All of the p-values were very significant with $p < 0.001$ and < 0.0001.

Model Statistics

Model	Number of Predictors	Model Fit statistics Stationary R-squared	Ljung-Box Q(18) Statistics	DF	Sig.	Number of Outliers
men-Model_1	3	,898	17,761	18	,471	7

ARIMA Model Parameters

					Estimate	SE	t	Sig.
men-Model_1	men	Natural Log	Constant		-2,828	,456	-6,207	,000
	phone	Natural Log	Numerator	Lag 0	,569	,064	8,909	,000
	nurse	Natural Log	Numerator	Lag 0	1,244	,118	10,585	,000
	doctor	Natural Log	Numerator	Lag 0	,310	,077	4,046	,000
				Lag 1	-,257	,116	-2,210	,029
				Lag 2	-,196	,121	-1,616	,109
			Denominator	Lag 1	,190	,304	,623	,535

Outliers

			Estimate	SE	t	Sig.
men-Model_1	3	Additive	,769	,137	5,620	,000
	30	Additive	,578	,138	4,198	,000
	53	Additive	,439	,135	3,266	,001
	69	Additive	,463	,135	3,439	,001
	78	Additive	-,799	,138	-5,782	,000
	88	Additive	,591	,134	4,409	,000
	105	Additive	-1,771	,134	-13,190	,000

When returning to the data view screen, we will observe that SPSS has added HbA1 values (except for the first two dates due to lack of information) as a novel variable. The predicted values are pretty similar to the measured values, supporting the adequacy of the model.

We will now apply the XML file and the Apply Models modus for making predictions about HbA1 values in the next 6 months, assuming that the significant variables nurse, doctor, phone are kept constant at their overall means.

First add the underneath data to the original data file and rename the file, e.g., "arimafile2", and store it at an appropriate folder in your computer.

Date	HbA1	nurse	doctor	phone	self	meeting
01/01/1999		10,00	8,00	4,00		
01/02/1999		10,00	8,00	4,00		
01/03/1999		10,00	8,00	4,00		
01/04/1999		10,00	8,00	4,00		
01/05/1999		10,00	8,00	4,00		
01/06/1999		10,00	8,00	4,00		

Then open "arimafile2.sav and command:

Analyze....click Apply Models....click Reestimate from data....click First case after end of estimation period through a specified date....Observation: enter 01/06/1999....click Statistics: click Display Forecasts....click Save: Predicted Values mark Save....click OK.

The underneath table shows the predicted HbA1 values for the next 6 months and their upper and lower confidence limits (UCL and LCL).

Example   261

Forecast

Model		121	122	123	124	125	126
HbA1-Model_1	Forecast	17,69	17,30	16,49	16,34	16,31	16,30
	UCL	22,79	22,28	21,24	21,05	21,01	21,00
	LCL	13,49	13,19	12,58	12,46	12,44	12,44

For each model, forecasts start after the last non-missing in the range of the requested
estimation period, and end at the last period for which non-missing values of all the predictors
are available or at the end date of the requested forecast period, whichever is earlier.

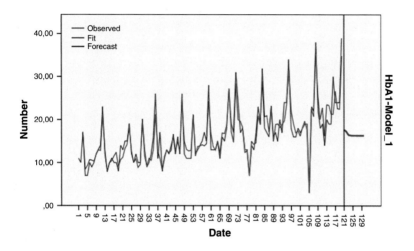

Also a graph of the HbA1 pattern after the estimation period is given as shown in
the above graph. When returning to the data view of the arimafile2, we will observe
that SPSS has added the predicted values as a novel variable.

Date	HbA1	nurse	doctor	phone	self	meeting	modeled HbA1	predicted HbA1
07/01/1998	19,00	11,00	8,00	5,00	28,00	4,00	21,35	21,35
08/01/1998	30,00	12,00	9,00	4,00	27,00	5,00	21,31	21,31
09/01/1998	24,00	13,00	8,00	5,00	30,00	5,00	26,65	26,65
10/01/1998	24,00	12,00	10,00	4,00	28,00	6,00	22,59	22,59
11/01/1998	24,00	11,00	8,00	5,00	26,00	5,00	22,49	22,49
12/01/1998	39,00	15,00	10,00	5,00	37,00	7,00	34,81	34,81
01/01/1999		10,00	8,00	4,00				17,69
01/02/1999		10,00	8,00	4,00				17,30
01/03/1999		10,00	8,00	4,00				16,49
01/04/1999		10,00	8,00	4,00				16,34
01/05/1999		10,00	8,00	4,00				16,31
01/06/1999		10,00	8,00	4,00				16,30

modeled HbA1 = calculated HbA1 values from the above arima model
Predicted HbA1 = the predicted HbA1 values using the XML file for future dates.

Conclusion

Autoregressive integrated moving average methods are appropriate for assessing trends, seasonality, and change points in a time series. In the example given no conclusion can be drawn about individual patients. Autoregressive models can, however, also be applied for data sets of individual patients. Also as a multivariate methodology it is appropriate for multiple instead of a single outcome variable like various health outcomes.

Note

More background theoretical and mathematical information of autoregressive models for longitudinal data is in Machine learning in medicine part two, Multivariate analysis of time series, pp 139–154, Springer Heidelberg Germany, 2013, from the same authors.

Chapter 36
Variance Components for Assessing the Magnitude of Random Effects (40 Patients)

General Purpose

If we have reasons to believe that in a study certain patients due to co-mobidity, co-medication and other factors will respond differently from others, then the spread in the data is caused not only by residual effect, but also by some subgroup property, otherwise called some random effect. Variance components analysis is able to assess the magnitudes of random effects as compared to that of the residual error of a study.

Examples are given.

Background

In a simple random sample, one observation is made on each of a number of separate individuals and the variation is assumed to be represented by independent and identically distributed random variables, one for each individual. This forms the basis of regression and other models widely used in biostatistics. However, there are two ways in which the assumption of a single random component corresponding to each individual might fail to be adequate. In the first, the random variation may have a more complex structure arising from several identifiable sources. The variation is then considered to have multiple components, which we call components of variance. This is the classical field of variance components and has a long history dating from the nineteenth century. The second way in which the assumption can fail is

This chapter was previously published in "Machine learning in medicine-cookbook 3" as Chap. 3, 2014.

Electronic Supplementary Material The online version of this chapter (https://doi.org/10.1007/978-3-030-33970-8_36) contains supplementary material, which is available to authorized users.

when the parameters describing the systematic part of the variation may themselves change randomly, for example, between individuals or groups of individuals.

Primary Scientific Question

Can a variance components analysis by including the random effect in the analysis reduce the unexplained variance in a study, and, thus, increase the accuracy of the analysis model as used.

Example

Variables			
PAT	treat	gender	cad
52,00	,00	,00	2,00
48,00	,00	,00	2,00
43,00	,00	,00	1,00
50,00	,00	,00	2,00
43,00	,00	,00	2,00
44,00	,00	,00	1,00
46,00	,00	,00	2,00
46,00	,00	,00	2,00
43,00	,00	,00	1,00
49,00	,00	,00	2,00
28,00	1,00	,00	1,00
35,00	1,00	,00	2,00

PAT = episodes of paroxysmal atrial tachycardias
treat = treatment modality (0 = placebo treatment, 1 = active treatment)
gender = gender (0 = female)
cad = presence of coronary artery disease (1 no, 2 = yes)

The first 12 of a 40 patient parallel-group study of the treatment of paroxysmal tachycardia with numbers of episodes of PAT as outcome is given above. The entire data file is in "variancecomponents", and is available at extras.springer.com. We had reason to believe that the presence of coronary artery disease would affect the outcome, and, therefore, used this variable as a random rather than fixed variable. SPSS statistical software was used for data analysis. Start by opening the data file in SPSS.

Example   265

Command:
Analyze....General Linear Model....Variance Components....Dependent Variable: enter "paroxtachyc"....Fixed Factor(s): enter "treat, gender"....Random Factor(s): enter "corartdisease"....Model: mark Custom....Model: enter "treat, gender, cad"....click Continue....click Options....mark ANOVA....mark Type III....mark Sums of squares....mark Expected mean squares....click Continue....click OK.

The output sheets are given underneath. The Variance Estimate table gives the magnitude of the Variance due to cad, and that due to residual error (unexplained variance, otherwise called Error). The ratio of the Var (cad) / [Var (Error) + Var (cad)] gives the proportion of variance in the data due to the random cad effect $(5.844/(28.426 + 5.844) = 0.206 = 20.6\%)$. This means that 79.4% instead of 100 % of the error is now unexplained.

Variance Estimates

Component	Estimate
Var(cad)	5,844
Var(Error)	28,426

Dependent
Variable: paroxtach
Method: ANOVA
(Type III Sum of
Squares)

The underneath ANOVA table gives the sums of squares and mean squares of different effects. E.g. the mean square of cad = 139.469, and that of residual effect = 28.426.

ANOVA

Source	Type III Sum of Squares	df	Mean Square
Corrected Model	727,069	3	242,356
Intercept	57153,600	1	57153,600
treat	515,403	1	515,403
gender	,524	1	,524
cad	139,469	1	139,469
Error	1023,331	36	28,426
Total	58904,000	40	
Corrected Total	1750,400	39	

Dependent Variable: paroxtach

The underneath Expected Mean Squares table gives the results of a special procedure, whereby variances of best fit quadratic functions of the variables are minimized to obtain the best unbiased estimate of the variance components. A little mental arithmetic is now required.

Expected Mean Squares

Source	Variance Component		
	Var(cad)	Var(Error)	Quadratic Term
Intercept	20,000	1,000	Intercept, treat, gender
treat	,000	1,000	treat
gender	,000	1,000	gender
cad	19,000	1,000	
Error	,000	1,000	

Dependent Variable: paroxtach
Expected Mean Squares are based on Type III Sums of Squares.
For each source, the expected mean square equals the sum of the coefficients in the cells times the variance components, plus a quadratic term involving effects in the Quadratic Term cell.

EMS (expected mean square) of cad (the random effect)
$$= 19 \times \text{Variance (cad)} + \text{Variance (Error)}$$
$$= 139.469$$

EMS of Error (the residual effect)
$$= 0 + \text{Variance (Error)}$$
$$= 28.426$$

EMS of cad $-$ Variance (Error)
$$= 19 \times \text{Variance (cad)}$$
$$= 139.469 - 28.426$$
$$= 110.043$$

Variance (cad)
$$= 110.043/19$$
$$= 5.844 \text{ (compare with the results of the above Variance Estimates table)}$$

It can, thus, be concluded that around 20% of the uncertainty is in the data is caused by the random effect.

Conclusion

If we have reasons to believe that in a study certain patients due to co-mobidity, co-medication and other factors will respond differently from others, then the spread in the data will be caused, not only by the residual effect, but also by the subgroup property, otherwise called the random effect. Variance components analysis, by including the random effect in the analysis, reduces the unexplained variance in a study, and, thus, increases the accuracy of the analysis model used.

Note

More background, theoretical and mathematical information of random effects models are given in Machine learning in medicine part three, Chap. 9, Random effects, pp 81–94, 2013, Springer Heidelberg Germany, from the same authors.

Chapter 37
Ordinal Scaling for Clinical Scores with Inconsistent Intervals (900 Patients)

General Purpose

Clinical studies often have categories as outcome, like various levels of health or disease. Multinomial regression is suitable for analysis (see Chap. 28). However, if one or two outcome categories in a study are severely underpresented, multinomial regression is flawed, and ordinal regression including specific link functions may provide a better fit for the data.

Background

In statistics, ordinal regression (also called "ordinal classification") is a type of regression analysis used for predicting an ordinal variable, i.e. a variable whose value exists on an arbitrary scale where only the relative ordering between different values is significant. More information about nominal, ordinal and scale variables is given in the Chaps. 9, 10 and 11. Ordinal regression can be considered an intermediate analytical model between regression and classification. Examples of ordinal regression are ordered logit and ordered probit regressions. Ordinal regression turns up often in the social sciences, for example in the modeling of human levels of preference (on a scale from, say, 1–5 for "very poor" to"excellent"), as well as in information retrieval. In machine learning, ordinal regression may also be called ranking learning. So far it is little used in health research.

This chapter was previously published in "Machine learning in medicine-cookbook 3"as Chap. 4, 2014.

Electronic Supplementary Material The online version of this chapter (https://doi.org/10.1007/978-3-030-33970-8_37) contains supplementary material, which is available to authorized users.

© Springer Nature Switzerland AG 2020

T. J. Cleophas, A. H. Zwinderman, *Machine Learning in Medicine – A Complete Overview*, https://doi.org/10.1007/978-3-030-33970-8_37

Primary Scientific Questions

This chapter is to assess how ordinal regression performs in studies where clinical scores have inconsistent intervals.

Example

In 900 patients the independent predictors for different degrees of feeling healthy were assessed. The predictors included were:

Variable	2	fruit consumption (times per week)
	3	unhealthy snacks (times per week)
	4	fastfood consumption (times per week)
	5	physical activities (times per week)
	6	age (number of years).

Feeling healthy (Variable 1) was assessed as mutually elusive categories:

1 very much so
2 much so
3 not entirely so
4 not so
5 not so at all.

Underneath are the first 10 patients of the data file. The entire data file is in extras. springer.com, and is entitled "ordinalscaling".

Variables					
1	2	3	4	5	6
4	6	9	12	6	34
4	7	24	3	6	35
4	3	5	9	6	30
4	5	14	6	3	36
4	9	9	12	12	62
2	2	3	3	6	31
3	3	26	6	3	57
5	9	38	6	6	36
4	5	8	9	6	28
5	9	25	12	12	28

First, we will perform a multinomial regression analysis using SPSS statistical software. Open the data file in SPSS.

Example   271

Command:

Analyze....Regression....Multinomial Logistic Regression....Dependent: enter feeling healthy....Covariates: enter fruitt/week, snacks.week, fastfood/week, physicalactivities/week, age in years....click OK.

Parameter Estimates

feeling healthy[a]		B	Std. Error	Wald	df	Sig.	Exp(B)	95% Confidence Interval for Exp (B)	
								Lower Bound	Upper Bound
very much so	Intercept	-1,252	,906	1,912	1	,167			
	fruit	,149	,069	4,592	1	,032	1,161	1,013	1,330
	snacks	,020	,017	1,415	1	,234	1,020	,987	1,055
	fastfood	-,079	,057	1,904	1	,168	,924	,827	1,034
	physical	-,013	,056	,059	1	,809	,987	,885	1,100
	age	-,027	,017	2,489	1	,115	,974	,942	1,007
much so	Intercept	-2,087	,863	5,853	1	,016			
	fruit	,108	,071	2,302	1	,129	1,114	,969	1,280
	snacks	-,001	,019	,004	1	,950	,999	,962	1,037
	fastfood	,026	,057	,212	1	,645	1,026	,919	1,147
	physical	-,005	,051	,009	1	,925	,995	,900	1,101
	age	-,010	,014	,522	1	,470	,990	,962	1,018
not entirely so	Intercept	2,161	,418	26,735	1	,000			
	fruit	,045	,039	1,345	1	,246	1,046	,969	1,130
	snacks	-,012	,011	1,310	1	,252	,988	,968	1,009
	fastfood	-,037	,027	1,863	1	,172	,964	,914	1,016
	physical	-,040	,025	2,518	1	,113	,961	,914	1,010
	age	-,028	,007	14,738	1	,000	,972	,959	,986
no so	Intercept	,781	,529	2,181	1	,140			
	fruit	,100	,046	4,600	1	,032	1,105	1,009	1,210
	snacks	-,001	,012	,006	1	,939	,999	,975	1,024
	fastfood	-,038	,034	1,225	1	,268	,963	,901	1,029
	physical	-,037	,032	1,359	1	,244	,963	,905	1,026
	age	-,028	,010	8,651	1	,003	,972	,954	,991

a. The reference category is: not so at all.

The above table gives the analysis results. Twenty-four p-values are produced, and a few of them are statistically significant at $p < 0.05$. For example, per fruit unit you may have 1.161 times more chance of feeling very healthy versus not healthy at all at $p = 0.032$. And per year of age you may have 0.972 times less chance of feeling not entirely healthy versus not healthy at all at $p = 0.0001$. We should add that the few significant p-values among the many insignificant ones could easily be due to type I errors (due to multiple testing). Also a flawed analysis due to inconsistent intervals has not yet been excluded. To assess this point a graph will be drawn.

Command:

Graphs....Legacy Dialogs....Bar....click Simple....mark Summary for groups of cases....click Define....Category Axis: enter "feeling healthy"....click OK.

The underneath graph is in the output sheet. It shows that, particularly the categories 1 and 2 are severely underpresented. Ordinal regression analysis with a complimentary log-log function gives little weight to small counts, and more weight to large counts, and may, therefore, better fit these data.

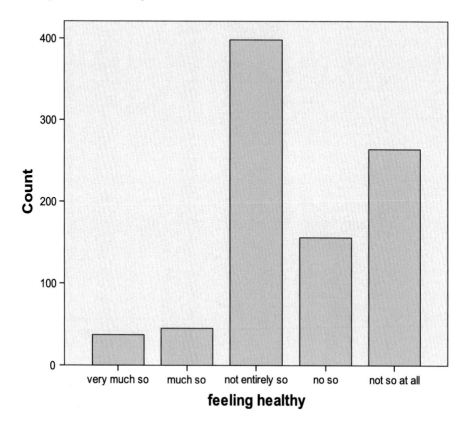

Command:
Analyze....Regression....Ordinal Regression....Dependent: enter feeling healthy....
Covariates: enter fruit/week, snacks.week, fastfood/week, physicalactivities/week, age in years....click Options....Link: click Complementary Log-log....click Continue....click OK.

Model Fitting Information

Model	-2 Log Likelihood	Chi-Square	df	Sig.
Intercept Only	2349,631			
Final	2321,863	27,768	5	,000

Link function: Complementary Log-log.

In the output sheets the model fitting table shows that the ordinal model provides an excellent fit for the data.

Parameter Estimates

		Estimate	Std. Error	Wald	df	Sig.	95% Confidence Interval	
							Lower Bound	Upper Bound
Threshold	[feelinghealthy = 1]	-2,427	,259	87,865	1	,000	-2,935	-1,920
	[feelinghealthy = 2]	-1,605	,229	49,229	1	,000	-2,053	-1,156
	[feelinghealthy = 3]	,483	,208	5,414	1	,020	,076	,890
	[feelinghealthy = 4]	,971	,208	21,821	1	,000	,564	1,379
Location	fruit	-,036	,018	3,907	1	,048	-,072	,000
	snacks	,004	,005	,494	1	,482	-,006	,013
	fastfood	,017	,013	1,576	1	,209	-,009	,042
	physical	,017	,012	1,772	1	,183	-,008	,041
	age	,015	,004	15,393	1	,000	,008	,023

Link function: Complementary Log-log.

The above table is also shown, and indicates that fruit and age are significant predictors of levels of feeling healthy. The less fruit/week, the more chance of feeling healthy versus not health at all ($p = 0.048$), the higher the age the more chance of feeling healthy versus not healthy at all ($p = 0.0001$).

Conclusion

Clinical studies often have categories as outcome, like various levels of health or disease. Multinomial regression is suitable for analysis, but, if one or two outcome categories in a study are severely underpresented, ordinal regression including specific link functions may better fit the data. The current chapter also shows that, unlike multinomial regression, ordinal regression tests the outcome categories as an overall function.

Note

More background, theoretical and mathematical information of multinomial regression is given in the Chap. 28.

Chapter 38
Loglinear Models for Assessing Incident Rates with Varying Incident Risks (12 Populations)

General Purpose

Data files that assess the effect of various predictors on frequency counts of morbidities/mortalities can be classified into multiple cells with varying incident risks (like, e.g., the incident risk of infarction). The underneath table gives an example:

In patients at risk of infarction with little soft drink consumption, and consumption of wine and other alcoholic beverages the incident risk of infarction equals 240/930 = 24.2 %, in those with lots of soft drinks, no wine, and no alcohol otherwise it is 285/1043 = 27.3 %.

soft drink (1 = little)	wine (0 = no)	alc beverages (0 = no)	infarcts number	population number
1,00	1,00	1,00	240	993
1,00	1,00	,00	237	998
2,00	1,00	1,00	236	1016
2,00	1,00	,00	236	1011
3,00	1,00	1,00	221	1004
3,00	1,00	,00	221	1003
1,00	,00	1,00	270	939
1,00	,00	,00	269	940
2,00	,00	1,00	274	979
2,00	,00	,00	273	966
3,00	,00	1,00	284	1041
3,00	,00	,00	285	1043

This chapter was previously published in "Machine learning in medicine-cookbook 3" as Chap. 5, 2014.

Electronic Supplementary Material The online version of this chapter (https://doi.org/10.1007/978-3-030-33970-8_38) contains supplementary material, which is available to authorized users.

© Springer Nature Switzerland AG 2020

T. J. Cleophas, A. H. Zwinderman, *Machine Learning in Medicine – A Complete Overview*, https://doi.org/10.1007/978-3-030-33970-8_38

The general loglinear model using Poisson distributions (see Statistics applied to clinical studies 5th edition, Chap. 23, Poisson regression, pp 267–275, Springer Heidelberg Germany, 2012, from the same authors) is an appropriate method for statistical testing. This chapter is to assess this method, frequently used by banks and insurance companies but little by clinicians so far.

Background

Until the late 1960's, contingency tables - two-way tables formed by cross classifying categorical variables - were typically analyzed by calculating chi-square values testing the hypothesis of independence. When tables consisted of more than two variables, researchers would compute the chi-squares for two-way tables and then again for multiple sub-tables formed from them in order to determine if associations and/or interactions were taking place among the variables. In the 1970's the analysis of crossclassified data changed quite dramatically with the publication of a series of papers on loglinear models by L.A. Goodman. Many other books appeared around that time building on Goodman's work (Bishop, Finberg & Holland 1975; Haberman 1975). Now researchers were introduced to a wide variety of models that could be fitted to crossclassified data. Thus, the introduction of the loglinear model provided them with a formal and rigorous method for selecting a model or models for describing associations between variables. A loglinear model is a mathematical model that takes the form of a function whose logarithm equals a linear combination of the parameters of the model, which makes it possible to apply (possibly multivariate) linear regression. That is, it has, thus, the general form of a linear regression.

Primary Scientific Question

Can general loglinear modeling identify subgroups with significantly larger incident risks than other subgroups.

Example

The example in the above table will be applied. We wish to investigate the effect of soft drink, wine, and other alcoholic beverages on the risk of infarction. The data file is in extras.springer.com, and is entitled "loglinear". Start by opening the file in SPSS statistical software.

Example   277

Command:

Analyze....Loglinear....General Loglinear Analysis....Factor(s): enter softdrink, wine, other alc beverages....click "Data" in the upper textrow of your screen.... click Weigh Cases....mark Weight cases by....Frequency Variable: enter "infarcts"....click OK....return to General Loglinear Analysis....Cell structure: enter "population".... Options....mark Estimates....click Continue....Distribution of Cell Counts: mark Poisson....click OK.

Parameter Estimates[b,c]

Parameter	Estimate	Std. Error	Z	Sig.	95% Confidence Interval	
					Lower Bound	Upper Bound
Constant	-1,513	,067	-22,496	,000	-1,645	-1,381
[softdrink = 1,00]	,095	,093	1,021	,307	-,088	,278
[softdrink = 2,00]	,053	,094	,569	,569	-,130	,237
[softdrink = 3,00]	0[a]	.	.	.	.	.
[wine = ,00]	,215	,090	2,403	,016	,040	,391
[wine = 1,00]	0[a]	.	.	.	.	.
[alcbeverages = ,00]	,003	,095	,029	,977	-,184	,189
[alcbeverages = 1,00]	0[a]	.	.	.	.	.
[softdrink = 1,00] * [wine = ,00]	-,043	,126	-,345	,730	-,291	,204
[softdrink = 1,00] * [wine = 1,00]	0[a]	.	.	.	.	.
[softdrink = 2,00] * [wine = ,00]	-,026	,126	-,209	,834	-,274	,221
[softdrink = 2,00] * [wine = 1,00]	0[a]	.	.	.	.	.
[softdrink = 3,00] * [wine = ,00]	0[a]	.	.	.	.	.
[softdrink = 3,00] * [wine = 1,00]	0[a]	.	.	.	.	.
[softdrink = 1,00] * [alcbeverages = ,00]	-,021	,132	-,161	,872	-,280	,237
[softdrink = 1,00] * [alcbeverages = 1,00]	0[a]	.	.	.	.	.
[softdrink = 2,00] * [alcbeverages = ,00]	,003	,132	,024	,981	-,256	,262
[softdrink = 2,00] * [alcbeverages = 1,00]	0[a]	.	.	.	.	.
[softdrink = 3,00] * [alcbeverages = ,00]	0[a]	.	.	.	.	.
[softdrink = 3,00] * [alcbeverages = 1,00]	0[a]	.	.	.	.	.
[wine = ,00] * [alcbeverages = ,00]	-,002	,127	-,018	,986	-,251	,246
[wine = ,00] * [alcbeverages = 1,00]	0[a]	.	.	.	.	.
[wine = 1,00] * [alcbeverages = ,00]	0[a]	.	.	.	.	.
[wine = 1,00] * [alcbeverages = 1,00]	0[a]	.	.	.	.	.
[softdrink = 1,00] * [wine = ,00] * [alcbeverages = ,00]	,016	,178	,089	,929	-,334	,366
[softdrink = 1,00] * [wine = ,00] * [alcbeverages = 1,00]	0[a]	.	.	.	.	.

[softdrink = 1,00] * [wine = 1,00] * [alcbeverages = , 00]	0ª	.	.	.	.	.
[softdrink = 1,00] * [wine = 1,00] * [alcbeverages = 1,00]	0ª	.	.	.	.	.
[softdrink = 2,00] * [wine = ,00] * [alcbeverages = ,00]	,006	,178	,036	,971	-,343	,356
[softdrink = 2,00] * [wine = ,00] * [alcbeverages = 1,00]	0ª	.	.	.	.	.
[softdrink = 2,00] * [wine = 1,00] * [alcbeverages = , 00]	0ª	.	.	.	.	.
[softdrink = 2,00] * [wine = 1,00] * [alcbeverages = 1,00]	0ª	.	.	.	.	.
[softdrink = 3,00] * [wine = ,00] * [alcbeverages = ,00]	0ª	.	.	.	.	.
[softdrink = 3,00] * [wine = ,00] * [alcbeverages = 1,00]	0ª	.	.	.	.	.
[softdrink = 3,00] * [wine = 1,00] * [alcbeverages = , 00]	0ª	.	.	.	.	.
[softdrink = 3,00] * [wine = 1,00] * [alcbeverages = 1,00]	0ª	.	.	.	.	.

a. This parameter is set to zero because it is redundant.
b. Model: Poisson
c. Design: Constant + softdrink + wine + alcbeverages + softdrink * wine + softdrink * alcbeverages + wine * alcbeverages + softdrink * wine * alcbeverages

The above pretty dull table gives some wonderful information. The soft drink classes 1 and 2 are not significantly different from zero. These classes have, thus, no greater risk of infarction than class 3. However, the regression coefficient of no wine is greater than zero at p = 0.016. No wine drinkers have a significantly greater risk of infarction than the wine drinkers have. No "other alcoholic beverages" did not protect from infarction better than the consumption of it. The three predictors did not display any interaction effects. This result would be in agreement with the famous French paradox.

Conclusion

Data files that assess the effect of various predictors on frequency counts of morbidities/mortalities can be classified into multiple cells with varying incident risks (like, e.g., the incident risk of infarction). The general loglinear model using Poisson distributions is an appropriate method for statistical testing. It can identify subgroups with significantly larger incident risks than other subgroups.

Note

More background, theoretical and mathematical information Poisson regression is given in Statistics applied to clinical studies 5th edition, Chap. 23, Poisson regression, pp 267–275, Springer Heidelberg Germany, 2012, from the same authors.

Chapter 39
Logit Loglinear and Hierarchical Loglinear Modeling for Outcome Categories (445 Patients)

General Purpose

Multinomial regression is adequate for identifying the main predictors of certain outcome categories, like different levels of injury or quality of life (QOL) (see also Chap. 28). An alternative approach is logit loglinear modeling. The latter method does not use continuous predictors on a case by case basis, but rather the weighted means of these predictors. This approach may allow for relevant additional conclusions from your data.

Background

Until the late 1960's, contingency tables - two-way tables formed by cross classifying categorical variables - were typically analyzed by calculating chi-square values testing the hypothesis of independence. When tables consisted of more than two variables, researchers would compute the chi-squares for two-way tables and then again for multiple sub-tables formed from them in order to determine if associations and/or interactions were taking place among the variables. In the 1970's the analysis of crossclassified data changed quite dramatically with the publication of a series of papers on loglinear models by L.A. Goodman. Many other books appeared around that time building on Goodman's work (Bishop, Finberg & Holland 1975; Haberman 1975). Now researchers were introduced to a wide variety of models that could be fitted to crossclassified data. Thus, the introduction of the loglinear

This chapter was previously published in "Machine learning in medicine-cookbook 3" as Chap. 6, 2014.

Electronic Supplementary Material The online version of this chapter (https://doi.org/10.1007/978-3-030-33970-8_39) contains supplementary material, which is available to authorized users.

model provided them with a formal and rigorous method for selecting a model or models for describing associations between variables. A loglinear model is a mathematical model that takes the form of a function whose logarithm equals a linear combination of the parameters of the model, which makes it possible to apply (possibly multivariate) linear regression. That is, it has, thus, the general form of a linear regression. In the Chap. 38 general loglinear modeling was explained. In this chapter logit loglinear modeling, and, in addition, hierarchical log-linear modeling will be addressed. First order interactions, and, in addition, second - third - fourth etc. order interactions will be computed for the purpose.

Primary Scientific Question

Does logit loglinear modeling allow for relevant additional conclusions from your categorical data as compared to polytomous/multinomial regression?

Example

age	gender	married	lifestyle	qol
55	1	0	0	2
32	1	1	1	2
27	1	1	0	1
77	0	1	0	3
34	1	1	0	1
35	1	0	1	1
57	1	1	1	2
57	1	1	1	2
35	0	0	0	1
42	1	1	0	2
30	0	1	0	3
34	0	1	1	1

Variable
1 age (years)
2 gender (0 = female)
3 married (0 = no)
4 lifestyle (0 = poor)
5 qol (quality of life levels 0 = low, 2 = high)

The above table show the data of the first 12 patiens of a 445 patient data file of qol (quality of life) levels and patient characteristics. The characteristics are the predictor variables of the qol levels (the outcome variable). The entire data file is in extras. springer.com, and is entitled "logitloglinear". We will first perform a traditional

Example   283

polynomial regression and then the logit loglinear model. SPSS statistical is used for analysis. Start by opening SPSS, and entering the data file.

Command:
Analyze....Regression....Multinomial Logistic Regression....Dependent: enter "qol".... Factor(s): enter "gender, married, lifestyle"....Covariate(s): enter "age".... click OK.

The underneath table shows the main results. The following conclusions are appropriate.

Parameter Estimates

qol[a]		B	Std. Error	Wald	df	Sig.	Exp(B)	95% Confidence Interval for Exp (B)	
								Lower Bound	Upper Bound
low	Intercept	28,027	2,539	121,826	1	,000			
	age	-,559	,047	143,158	1	,000	,572	,522	,626
	[gender=0]	,080	,508	,025	1	,875	1,083	,400	2,930
	[gender=1]	0[b]	.	.	0	.	.	.	.
	[married=0]	2,081	,541	14,784	1	,000	8,011	2,774	23,140
	[married=1]	0[b]	.	.	0	.	.	.	.
	[lifestyle=0]	-,801	,513	2,432	1	,119	,449	,164	1,228
	[lifestyle=1]	0[b]	.	.	0	.	.	.	.
medium	Intercept	20,133	2,329	74,743	1	,000			
	age	-,355	,040	79,904	1	,000	,701	,649	,758
	[gender=0]	,306	,372	,674	1	,412	1,358	,654	2,817
	[gender=1]	0[b]	.	.	0	.	.	.	.
	[married=0]	,612	,394	2,406	1	,121	1,843	,851	3,992
	[married=1]	0[b]	.	.	0	.	.	.	.
	[lifestyle=0]	-,014	,382	,001	1	,972	,987	,466	2,088
	[lifestyle=1]	0[b]	.	.	0	.	.	.	.

a. The reference category is: high.
b. This parameter is set to zero because it is redundant.

1. The unmarried subjects have a greater chance of QOL level 0 than the married ones (the b-value is positive here).
2. The higher the age, the less chance of QOL levels 0 and 1 (the b-values are negative here). If you wish, you may also report the odds ratios (Exp (B).

We will now perform a logit loglinear analysis.

Command:
Analyze.... Loglinear....Logit....Dependent: enter "qol"....Factor(s): enter "gender, married, lifestyle"....Cell Covariate(s): enter: "age"....Model: Terms in Model: enter: "gender, married, lifestyle, age"....click Continue....click Options....mark Estimates....mark Adjusted residuals....mark normal probabilities for adjusted residuals....click Continue....click OK.

The underneath table shows the observed frequencies per cell, and the frequencies to be expected, if the predictors had no effect on the outcome.

Cell Counts and Residuals[a],[b]

gender	married	lifestyle	qol	Observed Count	Observed %	Expected Count	Expected %	Residual	Standardized Residual	Adjusted Residual	Deviance
Male	Unmarried	Inactive	low	7	23,3%	9,111	30,4%	-2,111	-,838	-1,125	-1,921
			medium	16	53,3%	14,124	47,1%	1,876	,686	,888	1,998
			high	7	23,3%	6,765	22,6%	,235	,103	,127	,691
		Active	low	29	61,7%	25,840	55,0%	3,160	,927	2,018	2,587
			medium	5	10,6%	10,087	21,5%	-5,087	-1,807	-2,933	-2,649
			high	13	27,7%	11,074	23,6%	1,926	,662	2,019	2,042
	Married	Inactive	low	9	11,0%	10,636	13,0%	-1,636	-,538	-,826	-1,734
			medium	41	50,0%	43,454	53,0%	-2,454	-,543	-1,062	-2,183
			high	32	39,0%	27,910	34,0%	4,090	,953	2,006	2,958
		Active	low	15	23,8%	14,413	22,9%	,587	,176	,754	1,094
			medium	27	42,9%	21,336	33,9%	5,664	1,508	2,761	3,566
			high	21	33,3%	27,251	43,3%	-6,251	-1,590	-2,868	-3,308
Female	Unmarried	Inactive	low	12	26,1%	11,119	24,2%	,881	,303	,627	1,353
			medium	26	56,5%	22,991	50,0%	3,009	,887	1,601	2,529
			high	8	17,4%	11,890	25,8%	-3,890	-1,310	-1,994	-2,518
		Active	low	18	54,5%	19,930	60,4%	-1,930	-,687	-,978	-1,915
			medium	6	18,2%	5,799	17,6%	,201	,092	,138	,639
			high	9	27,3%	7,271	22,0%	1,729	,726	1,064	1,959
	Married	Inactive	low	15	18,5%	12,134	15,0%	2,866	,892	1,670	2,522
			medium	27	33,3%	29,432	36,3%	-2,432	-,562	-1,781	-2,158
			high	39	48,1%	39,434	48,7%	-,434	-,097	-,358	-,929
		Active	low	16	25,4%	17,817	28,3%	-1,817	-,508	-1,123	-1,855
			medium	24	38,1%	24,779	39,3%	-,779	-,201	-,882	-1,238
			high	23	36,5%	20,404	32,4%	2,596	,699	1,407	2,347

a. Model: Multinomial Logit
b. Design: Constant + qol + qol * gender + qol * married + qol * lifestyle + qol * age

The two graphs below show the goodnesses of fit of the model, which are obviously pretty good, as both expected versus observed counts (first graph below) and q-q plot (second graph below) show excellent linear relationships (q-q plots are further explained in Chap. 42).

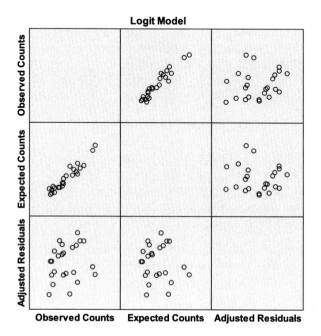

Logit Model

Example   285

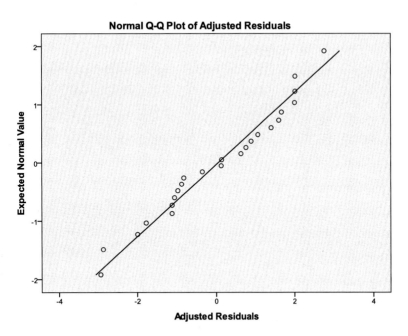

Normal Q-Q Plot of Adjusted Residuals

Note: the Q-Q plot (Q stands for quantile) shows here that the differences between observed and expected counts follow a normal distribution.

The next page table shows the results of the statistical tests of the data.

1. The unmarried subjects have a greater chance of QOL 1 (low QOL) than their married counterparts.
2. The poor lifestyle subjects have a greater chance of QOL 1 (low QOL) than their adequate-lifestyle counterparts.
3. The higher the age the more chance of QOL 2 (medium level QOL), which is neither very good nor very bad, nut rather in between (as you would expect).

We may conclude that the two procedures produce similar results, but the latter method provides some additional and relevant information about the lifestyle and age data.

Parameter Estimates[c,d]

Parameter		Estimate	Std. Error	Z	Sig.	95% Confidence Interval Lower Bound	95% Confidence Interval Upper Bound
Constant	[gender = 0] * [married = 0] * [lifestyle = 0]	-7,402[a]					
	[gender = 0] * [married = 0] * [lifestyle = 1]	-7,409[a]					
	[gender = 0] * [married = 1] * [lifestyle = 0]	-6,088[a]					
	[gender = 0] * [married = 1] * [lifestyle = 1]	-6,349[a]					
	[gender = 1] * [married = 0] * [lifestyle = 0]	-6,825[a]					
	[gender = 1] * [married = 0] * [lifestyle = 1]	-7,406[a]					
	[gender = 1] * [married = 1] * [lifestyle = 0]	-5,960[a]					
	[gender = 1] * [married = 1] * [lifestyle = 1]	-6,567[a]					
[qol = 1]		5,332	8,845	,603	,547	-12,004	22,667
[qol = 2]		4,280	10,073	,425	,671	-15,463	24,022
[qol = 3]		0[b]	.	.	.	.	.
[qol = 1] * [gender = 0]		,389	,360	1,079	,280	-,317	1,095
[qol = 1] * [gender = 1]		0[b]	.	.	.	.	.
[qol = 2] * [gender = 0]		-,140	,265	-,528	,597	-,660	,380
[qol = 2] * [gender = 1]		0[b]	.	.	.	.	.
[qol = 3] * [gender = 0]		0[b]	.	.	.	.	.
[qol = 3] * [gender = 1]		0[b]	.	.	.	.	.
[qol = 1] * [married = 0]		1,132	,283	4,001	,000	,578	1,687
[qol = 1] * [married = 1]		0[b]	.	.	.	.	.
[qol = 2] * [married = 0]		-,078	,294	-,267	,790	-,655	,498
[qol = 2] * [married = 1]		0[b]	.	.	.	.	.
[qol = 3] * [married = 0]		0[b]	.	.	.	.	.
[qol = 3] * [married = 1]		0[b]	.	.	.	.	.
[qol = 1] * [lifestyle = 0]		-1,004	,311	-3,229	,001	-1,613	-,394
[qol = 1] * [lifestyle = 1]		0[b]	.	.	.	.	.
[qol = 2] * [lifestyle = 0]		,016	,271	,059	,953	-,515	,547
[qol = 2] * [lifestyle = 1]		0[b]	.	.	.	.	.
[qol = 3] * [lifestyle = 0]		0[b]	.	.	.	.	.
[qol = 3] * [lifestyle = 1]		0[b]	.	.	.	.	.
[qol = 1] * age		,116	,074	1,561	,119	-,030	,261
[qol = 2] * age		,114	,054	2,115	,034	,008	,219
[qol = 3] * age		,149	,138	1,075	,282	-,122	,419

a. Constants are not parameters under the multinomial assumption. Therefore, their standard errors are not calculated.
b. This parameter is set to zero because it is redundant.
c. Model: Multinomial Logit
d. Design: Constant + qol + qol * gender + qol * married + qol * lifestyle + qol * age

Hierarchical Loglinear Regression

All of the results from the above logit loglinear analysis can also be obtained from a hierarchical loglinear analysis, but the latter can produce more. Not only first order interactions but also second - third - fourth etc order interactions can be readily computed. For analysis no menu commands are available in SPSS. However, the syntax commands to be given for the purpose are easy.

Command:
click File....click New....click Syntax....Syntax Editor....enter: hiloglinear qol(1,3) lifestyle (0,1)/criteria = delta (0)/design = qol∗lifestyle/ print=estim....click Run.... click All.

K-Way and Higher-Order Effects

	K	df	Likelihood Ratio		Pearson		Number of Iterations
			Chi-Square	Sig.	Chi-Square	Sig.	
K-way and Higher Order Effects[a]	1	5	35,542	,000	35,391	,000	0
	2	2	24,035	,000	23,835	,000	2
K-way Effects[b]	1	3	11,507	,009	11,556	,009	0
	2	2	24,035	,000	23,835	,000	0

a. Tests that k-way and higher order effects are zero.
b. Tests that k-way effects are zero.

Parameter Estimates

Effect	Parameter	Estimate	Std. Error	Z	Sig.	95% Confidence Interval	
						Lower Bound	Upper Bound
qol*lifestyle	1	-,338	,074	-4,580	,000	-,483	-,193
	2	,246	,067	3,651	,000	,114	,378
qol	1	-,206	,074	-2,789	,005	-,351	-,061
	2	,149	,067	2,208	,027	,017	,281
lifestyle	1	,040	,049	,817	,414	-,057	,137

The above tables in the output sheets show the most important results of the loglinear analysis.

1. There is a significant interaction "qol times lifestyle" at p = 0,0001, meaning that the qol levels in the inactive lifestyle group is different from those of the active lifestyle group.
2. There is also a significant qol effect at p = 0,005, meaning that medium and high qol is observed significantly more often than low qol.
3. There is no significant lifestyle effect, meaning that inactive and active lifestyles are equally distributed in the data.

For third order hierarchical loglinear modeling the underneath commands are required.

Command:
click File....click New....click Syntax....Syntax Editor....enter: hiloglinear qol(1,3) lifestyle (0,1) married(0,1)/criteria = delta (0)/design = qol∗lifestyle∗married/ print=estim....click Run....click All.

K-Way and Higher-Order Effects

	K	df	Likelihood Ratio		Pearson		Number of Iterations
			Chi-Square	Sig.	Chi-Square	Sig.	
K-way and Higher Order Effects[a]	1	11	120,711	,000	118,676	,000	0
	2	7	68,839	,000	74,520	,000	2
	3	2	15,947	,000	15,429	,000	3
K-way Effects[b]	1	4	51,872	,000	44,156	,000	0
	2	5	52,892	,000	59,091	,000	0
	3	2	15,947	,000	15,429	,000	0

a. Tests that k-way and higher order effects are zero.
b. Tests that k-way effects are zero.

Parameter Estimates

Effect	Parameter	Estimate	Std. Error	Z	Sig.	95% Confidence Interval	
						Lower Bound	Upper Bound
qol*lifestyle*married	1	-,124	,079	-1,580	,114	-,278	,030
	2	,301	,079	3,826	,000	,147	,456
qol*lifestyle	1	-,337	,079	-4,291	,000	-,491	-,183
	2	,360	,079	4,573	,000	,206	,514
qol*married	1	,386	,079	4,908	,000	,232	,540
	2	-,164	,079	-2,081	,037	-,318	-,010
lifestyle*married	1	-,038	,056	-,688	,492	-,147	,071
qol	1	-,110	,079	-1,399	,162	-,264	,044
	2	,110	,079	1,398	,162	-,044	,264
lifestyle	1	,047	,056	,841	,401	-,062	,156
married	1	-,340	,056	-6,112	,000	-,449	-,231

The above tables give the main results, and show that the analysis allows for some wonderful conclusions.

1. In the married subjects the combined effect of qol and lifestyle is different at p = 0,0001.
2. In the active lifestyle subjects qol scores are significantly different from those of the inactive lifestyle subjects at p = 0,0001.
3. In the married subjects the qol scores are significantly different from those of the unmarried ones at p = 0,037.
4. In the married subjects the lifestyle is not different from that of the unmarried subjects (p = 0,492).
5. The qol scores don't have significantly different counts (p = 0,162).
6. Lifestyles don't have significantly different counts (p = 0,401).
7. The married status is significantly more frequent than the unmarried status (p = 0,0001).

The many p-values need not necessarily be corrected for multiple testing, because of the hierarchical structure of the overall analysis. It start with testing first order models. If significant, then second order. If significant, then third order etc. For fourth order hierarchical loglinear modeling the underneath commands are required.

Command:
click File....click New....click Syntax....Syntax Editor....enter: hiloglinear qol(1,3) lifestyle (0,1) married (0,1) gender (0,1)/criteria = delta (0)/design = qol*lifestyle*married*gender/ print=estim....click Run....click All.

K-Way and Higher-Order Effects

	K	df	Likelihood Ratio		Pearson		Number of Iterations
			Chi-Square	Sig.	Chi-Square	Sig.	
K-way and Higher Order Effects[a]	1	23	133,344	,000	133,751	,000	0
	2	18	81,470	,000	90,991	,000	2
	3	9	25,896	,002	25,570	,002	3
	4	2	,042	,979	,042	,979	3
K-way Effects[b]	1	5	51,874	,000	42,760	,000	0
	2	9	55,573	,000	65,421	,000	0
	3	7	25,855	,001	25,528	,001	0
	4	2	,042	,979	,042	,979	0

a. Tests that k-way and higher order effects are zero.
b. Tests that k-way effects are zero.

Parameter Estimates

Effect	Parameter	Estimate	Std. Error	Z	Sig.	95% Confidence Interval	
						Lower Bound	Upper Bound
qol*lifestyle*married*gender	1	-,006	,080	-,074	,941	-,163	,151
	2	-,010	,080	-,127	,899	-,166	,146
qol*lifestyle*married	1	-,121	,080	-1,512	,130	-,278	,036
	2	,297	,080	3,726	,000	,141	,453
qol*lifestyle*gender	1	-,096	,080	-1,202	,229	-,254	,061
	2	,086	,080	1,079	,281	-,070	,242
qol*married*gender	1	,071	,080	,887	,375	-,086	,228
	2	-,143	,080	-1,800	,072	-,300	,013
lifestyle*married*gender	1	-,065	,056	-1,157	,247	-,176	,045
qol*lifestyle	1	-,341	,080	-4,251	,000	-,498	-,184
	2	,355	,080	4,455	,000	,199	,511
qol*married	1	,382	,080	4,769	,000	,225	,540
	2	-,162	,080	-2,031	,042	-,318	-,006
lifestyle*married	1	-,035	,056	-,623	,533	-,146	,075
qol*gender	1	-,045	,080	-,565	,572	-,203	,112
	2	,018	,080	,223	,823	-,138	,174
lifestyle*gender	1	-,086	,056	-1,531	,126	-,197	,024
married*gender	1	-,007	,056	-,123	,902	-,118	,104
qol	1	-,119	,080	-1,488	,137	-,276	,038
	2	,111	,080	1,390	,164	-,045	,267
lifestyle	1	,041	,056	,720	,472	-,070	,151
married	1	-,345	,056	-6,106	,000	-,455	-,234
gender	1	-,034	,056	-,609	,543	-,145	,076

The above tables show, that the results of the 4th order model are very much similar to that of the 3rd order model, and that the interaction gender∗lifestyle∗ married∗qol was not statistically significant. And, so, we can conclude here.

1. In the separate genders the combined effects of lifestyle, married status and quality of life were not significantly different.
2. In the married subjects the combined effect of qol and lifestyle is different at p = 0,0001.
3. In the active lifestyle subjects qol scores are significantly different from those of the inactive lifestyle at p = 0,0001.
4. The difference in married status is significant a p = 0,0001.
5. The qol scores don't have significantly different counts (p = 0,164).

Like with third order hierarchical loglinear modeling, the many p-values need not necessarily be corrected for multiple testing, because of its hierarchical structure. It starts with testing first order models. If significant, then second order. If significant, then third order etc.

Pearson chi-square test can answer questions like: is the risk of falling out of bed different between the departments of surgery and internal medicine. The analysis is very limited, because the interaction between two variables is assessed only. However, we may also be interested in the effect of the two variables separately.

Also, higher order contingency tables do exist. E.g., we may want to know, whether variables like ageclass, gender, and other patient characteristics interact with the former two variables. Pearson is unable to assess higher order contingency tables.

Hiloglinear modeling enables to assess both main variable effects, and higher order (=multidimensional) contingency tables. For SPSS hiloglinear modeling the syntax commands are given in this chapter.

Hiloglinear modeling is the basis of a very new and broad field of data analysis, concerned with the associations between multidimensional categorical inputs.

Conclusion

Multinomial regression is adequate for identifying the main predictors of certain outcome categories, like different levels of injury or quality of life An alternative approach is logit loglinear modeling. The latter method does not use continuous predictors on a case by case basis, but rather the weighted means. This approach allowed for relevant additional conclusions in the example given.

Note

More background, theoretical and mathematical information of polytomous/multi-nomial regression is given in the Chap. 28. More information of general loglinear modeling is in the Chap. 38, entitled "Loglinear models for assessing incident rates with varying incident risks".

Chapter 40
More on Polytomous Outcome Regressions (450 Patients)

General Purpose

If clinical studies have categories as outcome like for example various levels of health or disease, then linear regression is not adequate for analysis. Linear regression assumes continuous outcomes, where with each level severity increases by the same quantity. Outcome categories are very common in medical research. Examples include age classes, income classes, education levels, drug dosages, diagnosis groups, disease severities, etc. Statistics has generally difficulty to assess categories, and traditional models require either binary or continuous variables. Outcome categories are sometimes called polytomous outcomes. Various analytical methods have already been reviewed. Multinomial regression (Chap. 28) is adequate, if none of the outcome categories are underpresented. Random intercepts models (Chap. 30) often provides better power than multinomial regression. Ordinal regression (Chap. 37) is adequate, if one or two categories are underpresented. Logit loglinear regression (Chap. 39) analyzes all kinds of first and second order interactions of the predictors on the outcome categories. Hierarchical loglinear regression can analyze higher order interactions of the predictors on the outcome categories (Chap. 39). In this chapter negative binomial and Poisson regressions will be reviewed. These methods may be rather suited for binary outcomes than for polytomous outcomes, but they can, even so, be used for data with more than two outcome categories. The data are, then, assessed, as multivariate models with multiple dummy outcome variables.

Electronic Supplementary Material The online version of this chapter (https://doi.org/10.1007/978-3-030-33970-8_40) contains supplementary material, which is available to authorized users.

Background

In clinical research outcome categories like disease severity levels are very common, and statistics has great difficulty to analyze categories instead of continuously measured outcomes. Polytomous outcome regressions are regressions with categorical rather than continuous outcomes. Five methods of analysis are reviewed in this chapter. With multinomial regression the outcome categories are equally present in the data. With ordinal regression one or two outcome categories are underpresented. With negative binomial and Poisson regressions data are assessed as multivariate models with multiple dummy outcome variables. Random intercept regression is like multinomial but provides better power. With logit loglinear regression first and second order interactions of the predictors on the outcome categories are assessed. With hierarchical loglinear regression third and fourth order interactions of the predictors on the outcome categories are assessed. We should add, that data files with polytomous outcomes are rapidly pretty complex. Also many p-values are produced, including increasing numbers of false positive results due to type I errors of finding an effect, where there is none. However, with current big data, study files are generally large, and, therefore, often considered clinically relevant even so, particularly, if the results match prior hypotheses.

Primary Scientific Question

This chapter is to assess negative binomial and Poisson regressions for analyzing data with polytomous outcomes.. These methods may be rather suited for binary outcomes than for polytomous outcomes, but they can, even so, be used for data with more than two outcome categories.

Example

Multinomial regression is suitable for polytomous outcome analysis. However, if one or two outcome categories in a study are severely underpresented, multinomial regression is flawed, and ordinal regression including specific link functions will provide a better fit for the data. Strictly, ordinal data are, like nominal data, discrete data, however, with a stepping pattern, like severity scores, intelligence levels, physical strength scores. They are usually assessed with frequency tables and bar charts. Unlike scale data, that also have a stepping pattern, they do not necessarily have to have steps with equal intervals. This causes some categories to be underpresented compared to others. The effect of the levels of satisfaction with the doctor on the levels of quality of life (qol) is assessed. In 450 patients with coronary

Example   295

artery disease the satisfaction level of patients with their doctor was assumed to be an important predictor of patient qol (quality of life).

Variable

1 qol	2 treatment	3 counseling	4 sat doctor
4	3	1	4
2	4	0	1
5	2	1	4
4	3	0	4
2	2	1	1
1	2	0	4
4	4	0	1
4	3	0	1
4	4	1	4
3	2	1	4

1. qol	= quality of life score (1 = very low, 5 = vey high)
2. treatment	= treatment modality (1 = cardiac fitness, 2 = physiotherapy, 3 = wellness, 4 = hydrotherapy, 5 = nothing)
3. counseling	= counseling given (0 = no, 1 = yes)
4. sat doctor	= satisfaction with doctor (1 = very low, 5 = very high).

The above table gives the first 10 patients of a 450 patients study of the effects of doctors' satisfaction level and qol. The entire data file is in extras.springer.com, and is entitled "ordinalregression". It was previously used by the authors in SPSS for starters and 2nd levelers, Chap. 48, Springer Heidelberg Germany, 2016. Start by opening the data file in your computer with SPSS installed.

The table shows, that the frequencies of the qol scores are pretty heterogeneous with 111 patients very high scores and only 71 patients medium scores. This could mean that multinomial regression is somewhat flawed and that ordinal regression including specific link functions may provide a better fit for the data.

We will start with a traditional multinomial regression. For analysis the statistical model Multinomial Logistic Regression in the SPSS module Regression is required.

Command:
Analyze....Regression....Multinomial Regression....Dependent: enter qol.... Factor (s): enter treatment, counseling, sat (satisfaction) with doctor....click OK.

In the output sheets a reduced model, testing that all effects of a single predictor are zero, is shown. It is a pretty rough approach, and more details would be in place.

Likelihood Ratio Tests

Effect	Model Fitting Criteria	Likelihood Ratio Tests		
	-2 Log Likelihood of Reduced Model	Chi-Square	df	Sig.
Intercept	483,058[a]	,000	0	.
satdoctor	525,814	42,756	16	,000
treatment	496,384	13,326	12	,346
counseling	523,215	40,157	4	,000

The chi-square statistic is the difference in -2 log-likelihoods between the final model and a reduced model. The reduced model is formed by omitting an effect from the final model. The null hypothesis is that all parameters of that effect are 0.

a. This reduced model is equivalent to the final model because omitting the effect does not increase the degrees of freedom.

The next page table is in the output sheets. It shows that the effects of several factors on different qol scores are very significant, like the effect of counseling on very low qol, and the effects of satisfaction with doctor levels 1 and 2 on very low qol. However, other effects were insignificant, like the effects of treatments on very low qol, and the effects of satisfaction with doctor levels 3 and 4 on very low qol. In order to obtain a more general overview of what is going-on an ordinal regression will be performed.

Example 297

Parameter Estimates

qol score[a]		B	Std. Error	Wald	df	Sig.	Exp(B)	95% Confidence Interval for Exp (B)	
								Lower Bound	Upper Bound
very low	Intercept	-1,795	,488	13,528	1	,000			
	[treatment=1]	-,337	,420	,644	1	,422	,714	,314	1,626
	[treatment=2]	,573	,442	1,678	1	,195	1,773	,745	4,216
	[treatment=3]	,265	,428	,385	1	,535	1,304	,564	3,015
	[treatment=4]	0[b]	.	.	0	.	.	.	.
	[counseling=0]	1,457	,328	19,682	1	,000	4,292	2,255	8,170
	[counseling=1]	0[b]	.	.	0	.	.	.	.
	[satdoctor=1]	2,035	,695	8,579	1	,003	7,653	1,961	29,871
	[satdoctor=2]	1,344	,494	7,413	1	,006	3,834	1,457	10,089
	[satdoctor=3]	,440	,468	,887	1	,346	1,553	,621	3,885
	[satdoctor=4]	,078	,465	,028	1	,867	1,081	,435	2,687
	[satdoctor=5]	0[b]	.	.	0	.	.	.	.
low	Intercept	-2,067	,555	13,879	1	,000			
	[treatment=1]	-,123	,423	,084	1	,771	,884	,386	2,025
	[treatment=2]	,583	,449	1,684	1	,194	1,791	,743	4,320
	[treatment=3]	-,037	,462	,006	1	,936	,964	,389	2,385
	[treatment=4]	0[b]	.	.	0	.	.	.	.
	[counseling=0]	,846	,323	6,858	1	,009	2,331	1,237	4,392
	[counseling=1]	0[b]	.	.	0	.	.	.	.
	[satdoctor=1]	2,735	,738	13,738	1	,000	15,405	3,628	65,418
	[satdoctor=2]	1,614	,581	7,709	1	,005	5,023	1,607	15,698
	[satdoctor=3]	1,285	,538	5,704	1	,017	3,614	1,259	10,375
	[satdoctor=4]	,711	,546	1,697	1	,193	2,036	,699	5,933
	[satdoctor=5]	0[b]	.	.	0	.	.	.	.
medium	Intercept	-1,724	,595	8,392	1	,004			
	[treatment=1]	-,714	,423	2,858	1	,091	,490	,214	1,121
	[treatment=2]	,094	,438	,046	1	,830	1,099	,465	2,594
	[treatment=3]	-,420	,459	,838	1	,360	,657	,267	1,615
	[treatment=4]	0[b]	.	.	0	.	.	.	.
	[counseling=0]	,029	,323	,008	1	,929	1,029	,546	1,940
	[counseling=1]	0[b]	.	.	0	.	.	.	.
	[satdoctor=1]	3,102	,790	15,425	1	,000	22,244	4,730	104,594
	[satdoctor=2]	2,423	,632	14,714	1	,000	11,275	3,270	38,875
	[satdoctor=3]	1,461	,621	5,534	1	,019	4,309	1,276	14,549
	[satdoctor=4]	1,098	,619	3,149	1	,076	2,997	,892	10,073
	[satdoctor=5]	0[b]	.	.	0	.	.	.	.
high	Intercept	-,333	,391	,724	1	,395			
	[treatment=1]	-,593	,371	2,562	1	,109	,552	,267	1,142
	[treatment=2]	-,150	,408	,135	1	,713	,860	,386	1,916
	[treatment=3]	,126	,376	,113	1	,737	1,135	,543	2,371
	[treatment=4]	0[b]	.	.	0	.	.	.	.
	[counseling=0]	-,279	,284	,965	1	,326	,756	,433	1,320
	[counseling=1]	0[b]	.	.	0	.	.	.	.
	[satdoctor=1]	1,650	,666	6,146	1	,013	5,208	1,413	19,196
	[satdoctor=2]	1,263	,451	7,840	1	,005	3,534	1,460	8,554
	[satdoctor=3]	,393	,429	,842	1	,359	1,482	,640	3,432
	[satdoctor=4]	,461	,399	1,337	1	,248	1,586	,726	3,466
	[satdoctor=5]	0[b]	.	.	0	.	.	.	.

a. The reference category is: very high.
b. This parameter is set to zero because it is redundant.

The multinomial regression computes for each outcome category compared to a defined reference category the effect of each of the predictor variables separately without taking interactions into account. The ordinary regression, in contrast, computes the effect of the separate predictors on a single outcome as a variable consistent of categories with a stepping pattern.

For ordinal regression analysis the statistical model Ordinal Regression in the SPSS module Regression is required. The above example is used once more.

Command:
Analyze....Regression....Ordinal Regression....Dependent: enter qol....Factor(s): enter "treatment", "counseling", "sat with doctor"....click Options....Link: click Complementary Log-log....click Continue....click OK.

Model Fitting Information

Model	-2 Log Likelihood	Chi-Square	df	Sig.
Intercept Only	578,352			
Final	537,075	41,277	8	,000

Link function: Complementary Log-log.

Parameter Estimates

		Estimate	Std. Error	Wald	df	Sig.	95% Confidence Interval	
							Lower Bound	Upper Bound
Threshold	[qol = 1]	-2,207	,216	103,925	1	,000	-2,631	-1,783
	[qol = 2]	-1,473	,203	52,727	1	,000	-1,871	-1,075
	[qol = 3]	-,959	,197	23,724	1	,000	-1,345	-,573
	[qol = 4]	-,249	,191	1,712	1	,191	-,623	,124
Location	[treatment=1]	,130	,151	,740	1	,390	-,167	,427
	[treatment=2]	-,173	,153	1,274	1	,259	-,473	,127
	[treatment=3]	-,026	,155	,029	1	,864	-,330	,277
	[treatment=4]	0[a]	.	.	0	.	.	.
	[counseling=0]	-,289	,112	6,707	1	,010	-,508	-,070
	[counseling=1]	0[a]	.	.	0	.	.	.
	[satdoctor=1]	-,947	,222	18,214	1	,000	-1,382	-,512
	[satdoctor=2]	-,702	,193	13,174	1	,000	-1,081	-,323
	[satdoctor=3]	-,474	,195	5,935	1	,015	-,855	-,093
	[satdoctor=4]	-,264	,195	1,831	1	,176	-,646	,118
	[satdoctor=5]	0[a]	.	.	0	.	.	.

Link function: Complementary Log-log.
a. This parameter is set to zero because it is redundant.

The above tables are in the output sheets of the ordinal regression. The model fitting information table tells, that the ordinal model provides an excellent overall fit for the data. The parameter estimates table gives an *overall* function of all predictors on the outcome categories. Treatment is not a significant factor, but counseling, and the satisfaction with doctor levels 1–3 are very significant predictors of the quality of life of these 450 patients. The negative values of the estimates can be interpreted as follows: the less counseling, the less effect on quality of life, and the less satisfaction with doctor, the less quality of life.

Example   299

We will now apply negative binomial and Poisson regressions for the analysis of the above data. The first 10 patients from the above 450 patient file assessing the effect of various factors on qol scores (scores 1–5, very low to very high) is in the underneath table. Analyses have already been performed with multinomial regression and ordinal regression. Multinomial computed for each score levels of qol the effects of each of the predictor variable levels separately. Ordinal computed these effects on the outcome levels as a single overall outcome, the outcome is not 4 outcomes buth rather a five level single function. Next, a negative binomial and a Poisson regression will be used for analysis. Like Poisson negative binomial is not for categorical outcomes but rather binary outcomes, but it can be used for categorical outcomes. The data are then assessed as multivariate models with multiple dummy outcome variables.

qol	satdoctor	treatment	counseling
4	4	3	1
2	1	4	0
5	4	2	1
4	4	3	0
2	1	2	1
1	4	2	0
4	1	4	0
4	1	3	0
4	4	4	1
3	4	2	1

Command:
Analyze....Generalized Linear Models....Generalized Linear Models....mark Custom....Distribution: Negative binomial (1)....Link Function: Log....Response: Dependent Variable: qol score....Predictors: Factors: satdoctor, treatment, counseling....click Model....click Main Effects: enter satdoctor, treatment, counseling.... click Estimation: mark Robust Tests...click OK.

The underneath tables are in the output.

Model Information

Dependent Variable	qol score
Probability Distribution	Negative binomial (1)
Link Function	Log

Goodness of Fit[a]

	Value	df	Value/df
Deviance	82,834	441	,188
Scaled Deviance	82,834	441	
Pearson Chi-Square	69,981	441	,159
Scaled Pearson Chi-Square	69,981	441	
Log Likelihood[b]	-1032,531		
Akaike's Information Criterion (AIC)	2083,062		
Finite Sample Corrected AIC (AICC)	2083,471		
Bayesian Information Criterion (BIC)	2120,046		
Consistent AIC (CAIC)	2129,046		

Dependent Variable: qol score
Model: (Intercept), satdoctor, treatment, counseling

   a. Information criteria are in small-is-better form.

   b. The full log likelihood function is displayed and used in
      computing information criteria.

Tests of Model Effects

Source	Type III		
	Wald Chi-Square	df	Sig.
(Intercept)	2357,874	1	,000
satdoctor	16,226	4	,003
treatment	3,007	3	,391
counseling	24,063	1	,000

Dependent Variable: qol score
Model: (Intercept), satdoctor, treatment, counseling

Example   301

Parameter Estimates

Parameter	B	Std. Error	95% Wald Confidence Interval		Hypothesis Test		
			Lower	Upper	Wald Chi-Square	df	Sig.
(Intercept)	1,393	,0541	1,287	1,499	664,630	1	,000
[satdoctor=1]	-,277	,0868	-,448	-,107	10,212	1	,001
[satdoctor=2]	-,184	,0685	-,318	-,050	7,237	1	,007
[satdoctor=3]	-,122	,0656	-,251	,006	3,465	1	,063
[satdoctor=4]	-,036	,0617	-,157	,084	,350	1	,554
[satdoctor=5]	0[a]	.	.	.	.	.	.
[treatment=1]	,015	,0534	-,089	,120	,082	1	,775
[treatment=2]	-,092	,0631	-,216	,032	2,129	1	,145
[treatment=3]	-,024	,0578	-,138	,089	,175	1	,676
[treatment=4]	0[a]	.	.	.	.	.	.
[counseling=0]	-,212	,0433	-,297	-,127	24,063	1	,000
[counseling=1]	0[a]	.	.	.	.	.	.
(Scale)	1[b]						
(Negative binomial)	1[b]						

Dependent Variable: qol score
Model: (Intercept), satdoctor, treatment, counseling

a. Set to zero because this parameter is redundant.

b. Fixed at the displayed value.

Next, the Poisson model is applied.

Command:

Analyze....Generalized Linear Models....Generalized Linear Models....mark Custom....Distribution: Poisson....Link Function: Log....Response: Dependent Variable: qol score....Predictors: Factors: satdoctor, treatment, counseling....click Model.... click Main Effects: enter satdoctor, treatment, counseling....click Estimation: mark Robust Tests...click OK.

The underneath tables are in the output.

Model Information

Dependent Variable	qol score
Probability Distribution	Poisson
Link Function	Log

Goodness of Fit[a]

	Value	df	Value/df
Deviance	298,394	441	,677
Scaled Deviance	298,394	441	
Pearson Chi-Square	279,166	441	,633
Scaled Pearson Chi-Square	279,166	441	
Log Likelihood[b]	-807,965		
Akaike's Information Criterion (AIC)	1633,929		
Finite Sample Corrected AIC (AICC)	1634,338		
Bayesian Information Criterion (BIC)	1670,913		
Consistent AIC (CAIC)	1679,913		

Dependent Variable: qol score
Model: (Intercept), satdoctor, treatment, counseling

    a. Information criteria are in small-is-better form.

    b. The full log likelihood function is displayed and used in computing information criteria.

Tests of Model Effects

	Type III		
Source	Wald Chi-Square	df	Sig.
(Intercept)	2302,055	1	,000
satdoctor	21,490	4	,000
treatment	4,549	3	,208
counseling	30,512	1	,000

Dependent Variable: qol score
Model: (Intercept), satdoctor, treatment, counseling

Parameter Estimates

Parameter	B	Std. Error	95% Wald Confidence Interval		Hypothesis Test		
			Lower	Upper	Wald Chi-Square	df	Sig.
(Intercept)	1,415	,0503	1,316	1,513	792,213	1	,000
[satdoctor=1]	-,305	,0829	-,467	-,142	13,526	1	,000
[satdoctor=2]	-,206	,0639	-,331	-,081	10,368	1	,001
[satdoctor=3]	-,126	,0610	-,245	-,006	4,250	1	,039
[satdoctor=4]	-,044	,0567	-,155	,067	,597	1	,440
[satdoctor=5]	0[a]	.	.	.	.	.	.
[treatment=1]	,023	,0504	-,075	,122	,214	1	,643
[treatment=2]	-,106	,0607	-,225	,013	3,063	1	,080
[treatment=3]	-,019	,0544	-,126	,087	,127	1	,722
[treatment=4]	0[a]	.	.	.	.	.	.
[counseling=0]	-,235	,0425	-,318	-,152	30,512	1	,000
[counseling=1]	0[a]	.	.	.	.	.	.
(Scale)	1[b]						

Dependent Variable: qol score
Model: (Intercept), satdoctor, treatment, counseling
a. Set to zero because this parameter is redundant.
b. Fixed at the displayed value.

In the above output sheets it is observed, that the Akaike information index and other goodness of fit indices of the Poisson model are better than those of the negative binomial, but both provide pretty similar test statistics. However, the negative binomial adjusts for overdispersion, while Poisson does not. As overdispersion is a common phenomenon with categorical outcome data, this would mean, that the negative binomial model is here slightly more appropriate than the Poisson model. More information of the two methods using binary outcomes has been given in the Chap. 4.

Conclusion

Clinical studies often have categories (cats) as outcome, like various levels of health or disease. Multinomial regression is suitable for analysis, but, if one or two outcome categories in a study are severely underpresented, ordinal regression including specific link functions may better fit the data. The underneath table shows that in the example of this chapter the high qol cats were much more often present than the lower qol cats.

Command:
Analyze....Descriptive Statistics....Frequencies....Variable(s): enter "qol score"....
click OK.

qol score

		Frequency	Percent	Valid Percent	Cumulative Percent
Valid	very low	86	19,1	19,1	19,1
	low	73	16,2	16,2	35,3
	medium	71	15,8	15,8	51,1
	high	109	24,2	24,2	75,3
	very high	111	24,7	24,7	100,0
	Total	450	100,0	100,0	

The current chapter also shows that, unlike multinomial regression, ordinal regression tests the outcome categories as an overall function.

We should add that with loglinear models many null hypotheses are tested with these pretty complex models and that the risk of type one errors is large. If a more confirmative result is required, then multiplicity adjustments are required, and little statistical significance if any will be left in these kinds of analyses, Nonetheless, they are fascinating, and particularly with large samples often clinically relevant even so. An advantage of hierarchical loglinear modeling is that multiplicity adjustment is less necessary than it is with the other polytomous models.

SPSS Version 22 has started to provide an automated model for association analysis of multiple categorical inputs, and for producing multiway contingency tables. However, the syntax commands, already available in earlier versions, are pretty easy, and SPSS minimizes the risk of typos by providing already written commands.

A brief overview of analytic methods for polytomous outcome models is given underneath:

1. Multinomial regression (Chap. 28) is adequate, if none of the outcome categories are underpresented.
2. Random intercepts models (Chap. 30) often provides better power than multinomial regression.
3. Ordinal regression (Chap. 37) is adequate, if one or two categories are underpresented.
4. Logit loglinear regression (Chap. 39) analyzes all kinds of first and second order interactions of the predictors on the outcome categories.
5. Hierarchical loglinear regression can analyze higher order interactions of the predictors on the outcome categories (Chap. 39).
6. In this chapter negative binomial and Poisson regressions have been reviewed.

Although all of the methods may sometimes produce somewhat similar results, this is not necessarily so, dependent on the fit of the data given. We should add that the methods are currently widely applied. Is it recommendable, therefore, for novices to take appropriate notice of all of the methods.

Note

More background, theoretical and mathematical information of ordinal regression and ordinal data is given in the Chaps. 11 and 37. More information about the principles of hierarchical loglinear regressions, otherwise called hiloglinear regressions are in the Chap. 52, SPSS for starters and 2nd levelers, Springer Heidelberg Germany, 2015, from the same authors, and in the Chap. 39 of the current edition.

Chapter 41
Heterogeneity in Clinical Research: Mechanisms Responsible (20 Studies)

General Purpose

In clinical research similar studies often have different results. This may be due to differences in patient-characteristics and trial-quality-characteristics such as the use of blinding, randomization, and placebo-controls. This chapter is to assess whether 3-dimensional scatter plots and regression analyses with the treatment results as outcome and the predictors of heterogeneity as exposure are able to identify mechanisms responsible.

Background

Mounting evidence suggests that there is frequently considerable variation in the risk of the outcome of interest in clinical trial populations. These differences in risk will often cause clinically important heterogeneity in treatment effects across the trial population, such that the balance between treatment risks and benefits may differ substantially between large identifiable patient subgroups; the "average" benefit observed in the summary result may even be non-representative of the treatment effect for a typical patient in the trial. Conventional subgroup analyses, which examine whether specific patient characteristics modify the effects of treatment, may be unable to detect variations in treatment benefit (and harm) across risk groups, because they do not account for the fact that patients have multiple characteristics simultaneously that affect the likelihood of treatment benefit.

This chapter was previously published in "Machine learning in medicine-cookbook 3" as Chap. 7, 2014.

Electronic Supplementary Material The online version of this chapter (https://doi.org/10.1007/978-3-030-33970-8_41) contains supplementary material, which is available to authorized users.

© Springer Nature Switzerland AG 2020
T. J. Cleophas, A. H. Zwinderman, *Machine Learning in Medicine – A Complete Overview*, https://doi.org/10.1007/978-3-030-33970-8_41

With multiple studies meta-analysis-methodologies including multiple group chi-squares, Cochran Q-tests, I square tests (Modern Meta-analysis, Springer Heidelberg Germany, 2017, from the same authors) can be applied to estimate the amount of heterogeneity between studies. However, with a single study, this is impossible, but scatter plots, and regression analyses with the treatment results as outcome and the assumed predictors of heterogeneity as exposure are sometimes able to identify mechanisms of heterogeneity.

Primary Scientific Question

Are scatter plots and regression models able to identify the mechanisms responsible for heterogeneity in clinical research.

Example

Variables			
1	2	3	4
% ADEs	study size	age	investigator type
21,00	106	1	1
14,40	578	1	1
30,40	240	1	1
6,10	671	0	0
12,00	681	0	0
3,40	28411	1	0
6,60	347	0	0
3,30	8601	0	0
4,90	915	0	0
9,60	156	0	0
6,50	4093	0	0
6,50	18820	0	0
4,10	6383	0	0
4,30	2933	0	0
3,50	480	0	0
4,30	19070	1	0
12,60	2169	1	0
33,20	2261	0	1
5,60	12793	0	0
5,10	355	0	0

ADEs = adverse drug effects
age 0 = young, 1 = elderly
investigator type, 0 = pharmacists, 1 = clinicians

Example   309

In the above 20 studies the % of admissions to hospital due to adverse drug effects were assessed. The studies were very heterogeneous, because the percentages admissions due to adverse drug effects varied from 3.3 to 33.2. In order to identify possible mechanisms responsible, a scatter plot was first drawn. The data file is in extras.springer.com and is entitled "heterogeneity".

Start by opening the data file in SPSS statistical software.

Command:
click Graphs....click Legacy Dialogs....click Scatter/Dot....click 3-D Scatter....click Define....Y-Axis: enter percentage (ADEs)....X Axis: enter study-magnitude....Z Axis: enter clinicians =1....Set Markers by: enter elderly = 1....click OK.

The underneath figure is displayed, and it gives a 3-dimensional graph of the outcome (% adverse drug effects) versus study size versus investigator type (1 = clinician, 0 = pharmacist). A 4th dimension is obtained by coloring the circles (green = elderly, blue = young). Small studies tended to have larger results. Also clinician studies (clinicians = 1) tended to have larger results, while studies in elderly had both large and small effects.

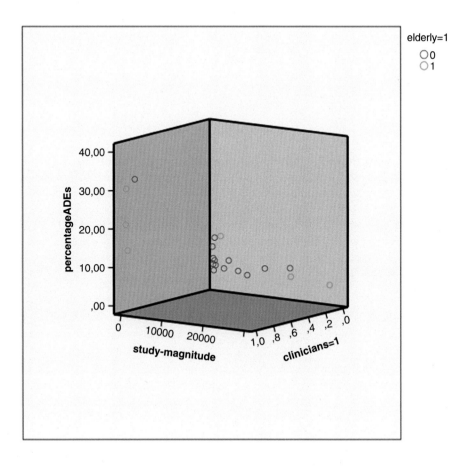

In order to test whether the observed trends were statistically significant, a linear regression is performed.

Command:

Analyze....Regression....Linear....Dependent: enter "percentage ADEs".... Independent(s): enter "study-magnitude, elderly = 1, clinicians = 1"....click OK.

Coefficients^a

Model		Unstandardized Coefficients		Standardized Coefficients		
		B	Std. Error	Beta	t	Sig.
1	(Constant)	6,924	1,454		4,762	,000
	study-magnitude	-7,674E-5	,000	-,071	-,500	,624
	elderly=1	-1,393	2,885	-,075	-,483	,636
	clinicians=1	18,932	3,359	,887	5,636	,000

a. Dependent Variable: percentageADEs

The output sheets show the above table. The investigator type is the only statistically significant predictor of % of ADEs. Clinicians observed significantly more ADE admissions than did pharmacists at $p < 0.0001$. This is in agreement with the above graph

Conclusion

In clinical research similar studies often have different results. This may be due to differences in patient-characteristics and trial-quality-characteristics such as the use of blinding, randomization, and placebo-controls. This chapter shows that 3-dimensional scatter plot are able to identify the mechanisms responsible. Linear regression analyses with the treatment results as outcome and the predictors of heterogeneity as exposure are able to rule out heterogeneity due to chance. This is particularly important, when no clinical explanation is found or when heterogeneity seems to be clinically irrelevant.

Note

More background, theoretical and mathematical information of heterogeneous studies and meta-regression is in Statistics applied to clinical studies 5th edition, Chap. 33, Meta-analysis, review and update of methodologies, pp 379–390, and Chap. 34, Meta-regression, pp 391–397, Springer Heidelberg Germany, both from the same authors as the current work.

Chapter 42
Performance Evaluation of Novel Diagnostic Tests (650 and 588 Patients)

General Purpose

Both logistic regression and c-statistics can be used to evaluate the performance of novel diagnostic tests (see also Machine learning in medicine part two, Chap. 6, pp 45–52, Logistic regression for assessment of novel diagnostic tests against controls, Springer Heidelberg Germany, 2013, from the same authors). This chapter is to assess whether one method can outperform the other.

Background

When outcomes are binary, the c-statistic (equivalent to the area under the Receiver of an Operating Characteristic (ROC) curve) is a standard measure of the predictive accuracy of a logistic regression model. Both logistic regression with the presence of disease as outcome and test scores of as predictor and c-statistics can be used for comparing the performance of qualitative diagnostic tests. However, c-statistics may perform less well with very large areas under the curve, and it assesses relative risks while in practice absolute risk levels may be more important

This chapter was previously published in "Machine learning in medicine-cookbook 3" as Chap. 8, 2014.

Electronic Supplementary Material The online version of this chapter (https://doi.org/10.1007/978-3-030-33970-8_42) contains supplementary material, which is available to authorized users.

Primary Scientific Question

Is logistic regression with the odds of disease as outcome and test scores as covariate a better alternative for concordance (c)-statistics using the area under the curve of ROC (receiver operated characteristic) curves.

Example

In 650 patients with peripheral vascular disease a noninvasive vascular lab test was performed. The results of the first 10 patients are underneath.

test score	presence of peripheral vascular disease (0 = no, 1 = yes)
1,00	,00
1,00	,00
2,00	,00
2,00	,00
3,00	,00
3,00	,00
3,00	,00
4,00	,00
4,00	,00
4,00	,00

The entire data file is in extras.springer.com, and is entitled "vascdisease1". Start by opening the data file in SPSS.

Then Command:
Graphs....Legacy Dialogs....Histogram....Variable(s): enter "score"....Row(s): enter "disease"....click OK.

The underneath figure shows the output sheet. On the x-axis we have the vascular lab scores, on the y-axis "how often". The scores in patients with (1) and without (0) the presence of disease according to the gold standard (angiography) are respectively in the lower and upper graph.

Example 313

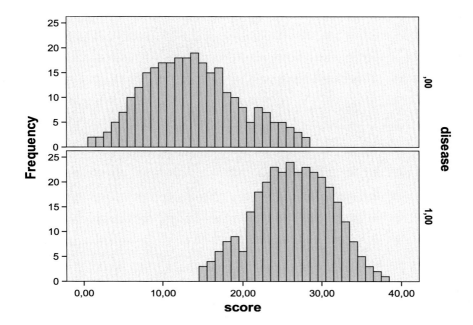

The second data file is obtained from a parallel-group population of 588 patients after the noninvasive vascular test has been improved. The first 10 patients are underneath.

test score	presence of peripheral vascular disease (0 = no, 1 = yes)
1,00	,00
2,00	,00
2,00	,00
3,00	,00
3,00	,00
3,00	,00
4,00	,00
4,00	,00
4,00	,00
4,00	,00

The entire data file is in extras.springer.com, and is entitled "vascdisease2". Start by opening the data file in SPSS.

Then Command:
Graphs....Legacy Dialogs....Histogram....Variable(s): enter "score"....Row(s): enter "disease"....click OK.

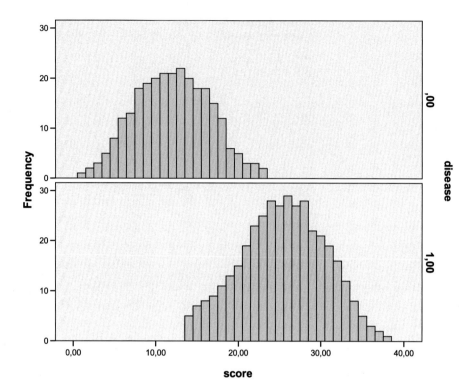

The above figure is in the output sheet.

The first test (upper figure) seems to perform less well than the second test (lower figure), because there may be more risk of false positives (the 0 disease curve is more skewed to the right in the upper than in the lower figure).

Binary Logistic Regression

Binary logistic regression is used for assessing this question. The following reasoning is used. If we move the threshold for a positive test to the right, then the proportion of false positive will decrease. The steeper the logistic regression line the faster this will happen. In contrast, if we move the threshold to the left, the proportion of false negatives will decrease. Again, the steeper the logistic regression line, the faster it will happen. And so, the steeper the logistic regression line, the fewer false negatives and false positives and thus the better the diagnostic test.

For both data files the above analysis is performed.

Command:

Analyze.... Regression.....Binary logistic.... Dependent variable: disease.... Covariate: score.....OK.

The output sheets show the best fit regression equations.

Example   315

Variables in the Equation

		B	S.E.	Wald	df	Sig.	Exp(B)
Step 1ª	VAR00001	,398	,032	155,804	1	,000	1,488
	Constant	-8,003	,671	142,414	1	,000	,000

a. Variable(s) entered on step 1: VAR00001.

Variables in the Equation

		B	S.E.	Wald	df	Sig.	Exp(B)
Step 1ª	VAR00001	,581	,051	130,715	1	,000	1,789
	Constant	-10,297	,915	126,604	1	,000	,000

a. Variable(s) entered on step 1: VAR00001.

Data file 1: log odds of having the disease $= -8.003 + 0.398$ times the score.
Data file 2: log odds of having the disease $= -10.297 + 0.581$ times the score.

The regression coefficient of data file 2 is much steeper than that of data file 1, 0.581 and 0.398.

Both regression equations produce highly significant regression coefficients with standard errors of respectively 0.032 and 0.051 and p-values of < 0.0001. The two regression coefficients are tested for significance of difference using the z – test (the z-test is in Chap. 2 of Statistics on a Pocket Calculator part 2, pp 3–5, Springer Heidelberg Germany, 2012, from the same authors):

$$z = (0.398 - 0.581)/\sqrt{(0.0.32^2 + 0.051^2)} = -0.183/0.060 = -3.05,$$

which corresponds with a p-value of < 0.01.

Obviously, test 2 produces a significantly steeper regression model, which means that it is a better predictor of the risk of disease than test 1. We can, additionally, calculate the odds ratios of successfully testing with test 2 versus test 1. The odds of disease with test 1 equals $e^{0.398} = 1.488$, and with test 2 it equals $e^{0.581} = 1.789$. The odds ratio $= 1.789/1.488 = 1.202$, meaning that the second test produces a 1.202 times better chance of rightly predicting the disease than test 1 does.

C-statistics
C-statistics is used as a contrast test. Open data file 1 again.

Command:
Analyze....ROC Curve....Test Variable: enter "score"....State Variable: enter "disease"....Value of State Variable: type "1"....mark ROC Curve....mark Standard Error and Confidence Intervals....click OK.

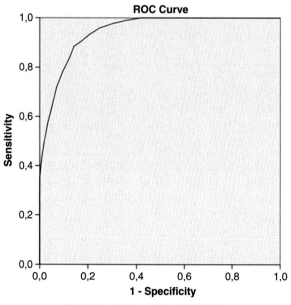

Diagonal segments are produced by ties.

Area Under the Curve

Test Result Variable(s):score

Area	Std. Error[a]	Asymptotic Sig.[b]	Asymptotic 95% Confidence Interval	
			Lower Bound	Upper Bound
,945	,009	,000	,928	,961

The test result variable(s): score has at least one tie between the positive actual state group and the negative actual state group. Statistics may be biased.

a. Under the nonparametric assumption
b. Null hypothesis: true area = 0.5

Subsequently the same procedure is followed for data file 2.

Example 317

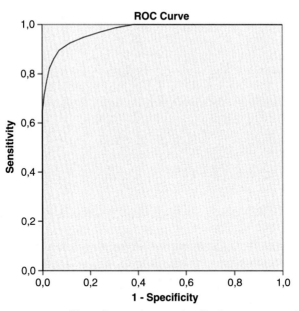

Diagonal segments are produced by ties.

Area Under the Curve

Test Result Variable(s):score

Area	Std. Error[a]	Asymptotic Sig.[b]	Asymptotic 95% Confidence Interval	
			Lower Bound	Upper Bound
,974	,005	,000	,965	,983

The test result variable(s): score has at least one tie between the positive actual state group and the negative actual state group. Statistics may be biased.

a. Under the nonparametric assumption
b. Null hypothesis: true area = 0.5

The Area under curve of data file 2 is larger than that of data file 1. The test 2 seems to perform better. The z-test can again be used to test for significance of difference.

$$z = (0.974 - 0.945)/\sqrt{(0.009^2 + 0.005^2)} = 2.90$$
$$p = < 0.01.$$

Conclusion

Both logistic regression with the presence of disease as outcome and test scores of as predictor and c-statistics can be used for comparing the performance of qualitative diagnostic tests. However, c-statistics performs less well with very large areas under the curve, and it assesses relative risks while in practice absolute risk levels are more important

Note

More background, theoretical and mathematical information of logistic regression and c-statistics is in Machine learning in medicine part two, Chap. 6, pp 45–52, Logistic regression for assessment of novel diagnostic tests against controls, Springer Heidelberg Germany, 2013, from the same authors.

Chapter 43
Quantile-Quantile Plots, a Good Start for Looking at your Medical Data (50 Cholesterol Measurements and 58 Patients)

General Purpose

A good place to start looking at your data before analysis is a data plot, e.g., a scatter plot or histogram. It can help you decide whether the data are normal (bell shape, Gaussian), and give you a notion of outlier data and skewness. Another approach is using a normality test like the chi-square goodness of fit, the Shapiro-Wilkens, or the Kolmogorov Smirnov tests (see Testing clinical trials for randomness, Chap. 42, in: Statistics applied to clinical studies 5th edition, Springer Heidelberg Germany, 2012, from the same authors), but these tests often have little power, and, therefore, do not adequately identify departures from normality. This chapter is to assess the performance of another and probably better method, the Q-Q (quantile-quantile) plot.

Background

In statistics and probability, quantiles are cut points dividing the range of a probability distribution into continuous intervals with equal probabilities, or dividing the observations in a sample in the same way. There is one fewer quantile than the number of groups created. Thus quartiles are the three cut points that will divide a dataset into four equal-sized groups. Common quantiles have special names: for instance quartile, decile (creating 10 groups).

As an example, in the graph below a normal probability distribution with on the x-axis individual data of a random sample and on the y-axis "how often" is given. Four equal areas under the curve are drawn:

Electronic Supplementary Material The online version of this chapter (https://doi.org/10.1007/978-3-030-33970-8_43) contains supplementary material, which is available to authorized users.

T. J. Cleophas, A. H. Zwinderman, *Machine Learning in Medicine – A Complete Overview*, https://doi.org/10.1007/978-3-030-33970-8_43

$-\infty$ to Q_1,
Q_1 to Q_2,
Q_2 to Q_3,
Q_3 to ∞.

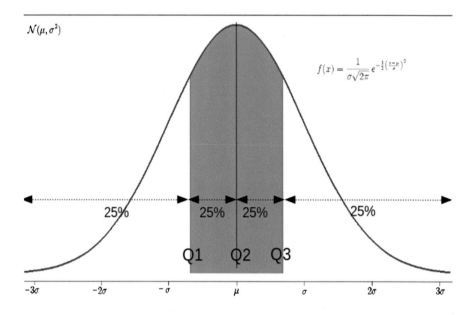

There is one fewer quantile than the number of groups created. The groups created are termed halves, thirds, quarters, etc., though sometimes the terms for the quantile are used for the groups created, rather than for the cut points. The Q-Q plot, or quantile-quantile plot, is a graphical tool to help us assess if a set of data plausibly came from some theoretical distribution such as a normal or exponential. If both sets of quantiles came from the same distribution, we should see the points forming a line that's roughly straight.

Specific Scientific Question

Are Q-Q plots of medical records capable of identifying normality and departures from normality. Random samples of hdl cholesterol and ages are used for examples.

Q-Q Plots for Assessing Departures from Normality

hdl cholesterol values (mmol/l)
3,80
4,20
4,27
3,70
3,76
4,11
4,24
4,20
4,24
3,63

The above table gives the first 10 values of a 50 value data file of hdl cholesterol measurements. The entire file is in the SPSS file entitled "q-q plot", and is available on the internet at extras.springer.com. SPSS statistical software is applied. Start by opening the data file in SPSS.

Command:
click   Graphs...Legacy   Dialogs...Histogram...Variable: enter hdlcholesterol...click OK.

A histogram with individual hdl cholesterol values on the x-axis and "how often" on the y-axis is given in the output sheet: 50 hdl cholesterol values are classified in percentages (%) or quantiles (= frequencies = numbers of observations/50 here). E. g., one value is between 2,5 and 3,0, two values are between 3,0 and 3,5, etc. The pattern tends to be somewhat bell shape, but there is obvious outlier frequencies close to 3 mmol/l and close to 4 mmol/l. Also some skewness to the right is observed, and the values around 4 mmol/l look a little bit like Manhattan rather than Gaussian.

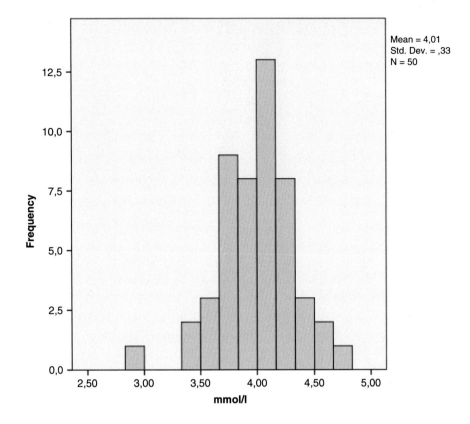

A Q-Q plot (quantile-quantile plot) can be helpful do decide what type of data we have here. First, the best fit normal curve is construed, e.g., based on the mean and standard deviation of the data. A graph of it is easy to produce in SPSS.

Command:
click Graphs...Legacy Dialogs...Histogram...Variable: enter hdlcholesterol ...mark: Display normal curve...click OK.

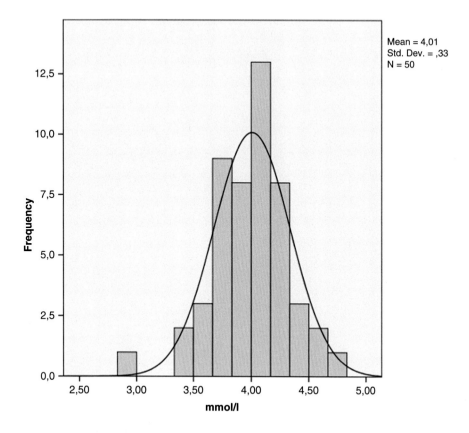

SPSS uses the curve to calculate the values for a Q-Q plot.

Command:
Analyze...Descriptive Statistics...Q-Q plots...Variables: enter hdlcholesterol... click OK.

The underneath plot is construed of the observed x-values versus the same x-values taken from the above best fit normal curve. If our data perfectly matched the best fit Gaussian curve, then all of the x-values would be on the 45° diagonal line. However, we have outliers. The x-value close to 3 mmol/l is considerably left from the diagonal, and thus smaller than expected. The value close to 4 mmol/l is obviously on the right side of the diagonal, and thus larger than expected. Nonetheless, The remainder of the observed values very well fit the diagonal, and it seems adequate to conclude that normal statistical test for analysis of these data will be appropriate.

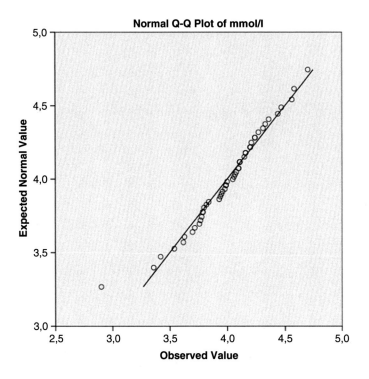

Q-Q Plots as Diagnostics for Fitting Data to Normal (and Other Theoretical) Distributions

Age (years)
85,00
89,00
50,00
63,00
76,00
57,00
86,00
56,00
76,00
66,00

The above table gives the first 10 values of a 58 value data file of patients with different ages. The entire file is in the SPSS file entitled "q-q plot", and is available on the internet at extras.springer.com. SPSS statistical software is applied. Start by opening the data file in SPSS.

Command:
Analyze...Descriptive Statistics...Q-Q plots...Variables: enter age...click OK.

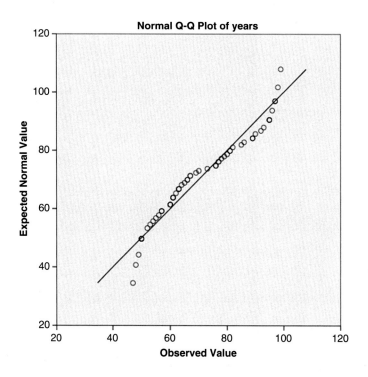

In the output sheets is the above graph. It shows a pattern with the left end below the diagonal line and the right end above it. Also the overall pattern seems to be somewhat undulating with the initially an increasing slope, and then a decreasing slope. The possible interpretations of these patterns are the following.

1. Left end below and right end above the diagonal may indicate a bells shape with long tails (overdispersion).
2. In contrast, left end above and right end below indicates short tails.
3. An increasing slope from left to right may indicate skewness to the right.
4. In contrast, a decreasing slope suggests skewness to the left.
5. The few cases with largest departures from the diagonal may of course also be interpreted as outliers.

The above Q-Q plot can hardly be assumed to indicate Gaussian data. The histogram confirms this.

Command:
click Graphs...Legacy Dialogs...Histograms...Variables: enter age...click OK.

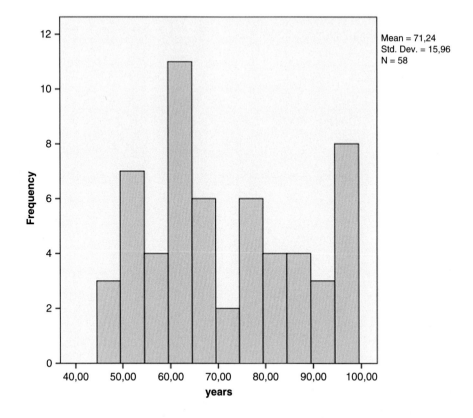

The histogram given in the output sheets seems to confirm that this is so. The Q-Q plot method is somewhat subjective, but an excellent alternative to underpowered goodness of fit tests, and provides better information regarding normality than simple data plots or histograms do, because each datum assessed against its best fit normal distribution counterpart. We should add that SPSS and other software also offer the construction of Q-Q plots using other than normal distributions.

Conclusion

Q-Q plots are adequate assess whether your data have a Gaussian-like pattern. Non-Gaussian patterns and outliers are visualized, and often an interpretation can be given of them. The Q-Q plot method is similar to the less popular P-P (probability-probability) plot method, which has cumulative probabilities (= areas under curve left from the x-value), instead of the x-values on the x-axis and their expected counterparts on the y-axis. They are a little bit harder to understand.

Note

More background, theoretical and mathematical information of frequency distributions and goodness of fit testing is in the Chap. 42, pp 469–478, Testing clinical trials for randomness, in: Statistics applied to clinical studies 5th edition, Springer Heidelberg Germany, 2012, from the same authors as the current work.

Chapter 44
Rate Analysis of Medical Data Better than Risk Analysis (52 Patients)

General Purpose

For the assessment of medical treatments clinical event analysis with logistic regression is often performed. Treatment modalities are used as predictor and the logodds of the event as outcome. However, instead of the logodds of event, counted rates of events can be computed and statistically tested. This may produce better sensitivity of testing, because their standard errors are smaller.

Background

Incidence risk is a measure of disease occurrence over a defined period of time. It is a proportion, therefore takes values from 0 to 1 (0% to 100%). Incidence rate takes into account the time an individual is at risk of disease. Incidence risk and incidence rate are often confused. In addition, there is a serious difference in meaning between the two. Risk is a proportion of new cases in a given population, while rate is the proportion of new cases in a given population during a limited time of observation. Rate, obviously, takes the time as a limiting factor into account, while risk does not. With statistical tests, if you account less, you will prove less, and your p-values will rise.

Electronic Supplementary Material The online version of this chapter (https://doi.org/10.1007/978-3-030-33970-8_44) contains supplementary material, which is available to authorized users.

Specific Scientific Question

Does rate analysis of medical events provide better sensitivity of testing than traditional risk analysis.

Example

We will use an example also used in the Chap. 10 of SPSS for starters part two, pp 43–48, Poisson regression, Springer Heidelberg Germany, 2012, from the same authors. In a parallel-group study of 52 patients the presence of torsade de pointes was measured during two treatment modalities.

treatment modality	presence torsade de pointes
,00	1,00
,00	1,00
,00	1,00
,00	1,00
,00	1,00
,00	1,00
,00	1,00
,00	1,00
,00	1,00
,00	1,00

The first 10 patients are above. The entire data file is in extras.springer.com, and is entitled "rates". SPSS statistical software will be used for analysis. First, we will perform a traditional binary logistic regression with torsade de pointes as outcome and treatment modality as predictor.

Command:
Analyze...Regression...Binary Logistic...Dependent: torsade... Covariates: treatment...click OK.

Variables in the Equation

		B	S.E.	Wald	df	Sig.	Exp(B)
Step 1[a]	VAR00001	1,224	,626	3,819	1	,051	3,400
	Constant	-,125	,354	,125	1	,724	,882

a. Variable(s) entered on step 1: VAR00001.

Example   331

The above table shows that the treatment modality does not significantly predict the presence of torsades de pointes. The numbers of torsades in one group is not significantly different from the other group.

A rate analysis is performed subsequently.

Command:

Generalized Linear Models . . .mark Custom. . .Distribution: Poisson . . .Link Function: Log. . .Response: Dependent Variable: torsade. . .Predictors: Main Effect: treatment. . .Estimation: mark Robust Tests. . .click OK.

Parameter Estimates

| Parameter | B | Std. Error | 95% Wald Confidence Interval | | Hypothesis Test | | |
			Lower	Upper	Wald Chi-Square	df	Sig.
(Intercept)	-,288	,1291	-,541	-,035	4,966	1	,026
[VAR00001=,00]	-,470	,2282	-,917	-,023	4,241	1	,039
[VAR00001=1,00]	0^a	.	.	.	.	.	.
(Scale)	1^b						

Dependent Variable: torsade
Model: (Intercept), VAR00001

a. Set to zero because this parameter is redundant.

b. Fixed at the displayed value.

The predictor treatment modality is now statistically significant at p = 0.039. And so, using the Poisson distribution in Generalized Linear Models, we found that treatment one performed significantly better in predicting numbers of torsades de pointe than did treatment zero at 0.039. We will check with a 3-dimensional graph of the data if this result is in agreement with the data as observed.

Command:

Graphs. . .Legacy Dialog. . .3-D Bar: X-Axis mark: Groups of Cases, Z-Axis mark: Groups of Cases. . .Define 3-D Bar: X Category Axis: treatment, Z Category Axis: torsade. . .OK.

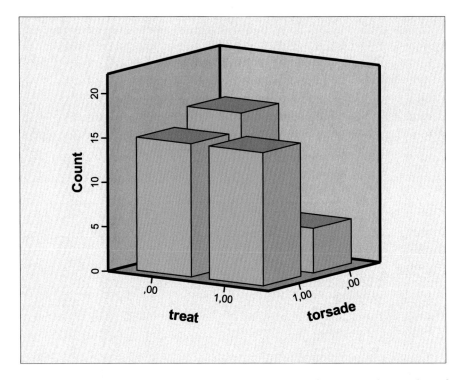

The above graph shows that in the 0-treatment (placebo) group the number of patients with torsades de pointe is virtually equal to that of the patients without. However, in the 1-treatment group it is smaller. The treatment seems to be efficacious.

Conclusion

Rate analysis using Poisson regression is different from logistic regression, because it uses a log transformed dependent variable. For the analysis of rates Poisson regression is very sensitive and, thus, better than standard logistic regression.

Note

More background, theoretical and mathematical information of rate analysis is given in Chap. 10 of SPSS for starters part two, pp 43–48, Poisson regression, Springer Heidelberg Germany, 2012, from the same authors.

Chapter 45
Trend Tests Will Be Statistically Significant if Traditional Tests Are Not (30 and 106 Patients)

General Purpose

Incremental dosages of medicines usually cause incremental treatment efficacies. This chapter is to assess whether trend tests are more sensitive than traditional ANOVAs for continuous outcome data (analyses of variance) and chi-square tests for binary outcome data to demonstrate the incremental efficacies.

Background

One way analysis of variance with 3 groups of patients with continuous outcome data assesses between-groups sum of squares with $3 - 1 = 2$ degrees of freedom, while for a trend test of these data a single linear regression of y- versus x-variable is applied with just 1 degree of freedom. Therefore, the trend testing is here likely to provide better sensitivity and a better p-value of differences in the data. Similarly, with binary outcome data the Pearson chi-square test of a 2×2 interaction matrix has 2 degrees of freedom while the linear-by-linear association test commonly used for trend testing here has again just 1 degree of freedom, and is therefore, likely to provide better statistics and a better p-value of difference in the data.

Electronic Supplementary Material The online version of this chapter (https://doi.org/10.1007/ 978-3-030-33970-8_45) contains supplementary material, which is available to authorized users.

T. J. Cleophas, A. H. Zwinderman, *Machine Learning in Medicine – A Complete Overview*, https://doi.org/10.1007/978-3-030-33970-8_45

Specific Scientific Questions

In patients with hypertension do incremental treatment dosages cause incremental beneficial effect on blood pressure? We will use the examples previously used in the Chaps. 9 and 12 of SPSS for starters part one, pp 33–34, and 43–46, entitled "Trend test for continuous data" and "trend tests for binary data", Springer Heidelberg Germany, 2010, from the same authors.

Example 1

In a parallel group study of 30 patients with hypertension 3 incremental antihypertensive treatment dosages are assessed. The first 13 patients of the data file is given underneath. The entire data file is in extras.springer.com, and is entitled "trend.sav".

Variable	
1	2
1,00	113,00
1,00	131,00
1,00	112,00
1,00	132,00
1,00	114,00
1,00	130,00
1,00	115,00
1,00	129,00
1,00	122,00
2,00	118,00
2,00	109,00
2,00	127,00
2,00	110,00

Var 1 = treatment dosage (Var = variable)
Var 2 = treatment response (mean blood pressure after treatment)

We will first perform a one-way ANOVA (see also Chap.8, SPSS for starters part one, entitled "One way ANOVA, Kruskall-Wallis", pp 29-31, Springer Heidelberg Germany, 2012, from the same authors) to see, if there are any significant differences in the data. If not, we will perform a trend test using simple linear regression.

Command:
Analyze...Compare Means...One-way ANOVA...dependent list: mean blood pressure after treatment... factor: treatment dosage...click OK.

ANOVA

treatment response

	Sum of Squares	df	Mean Square	F	Sig.
Between Groups	246,667	2	123,333	2,035	,150
Within Groups	1636,000	27	60,593		
Total	1882,667	29			

The output table shows that there is no significant difference in efficacy between the treatment dosages, and so, sadly, this is a negative study. However, a trend test having just 1 degree of freedom has more sensitivity than a usual one-way ANOVA, and it could, therefore, be statistically significant even so.

Command:

Analyze...regression...linear...dependent = mean blood pressure after treatment... independent = treatment dosage...click OK.

ANOVA[b]

Model		Sum of Squares	df	Mean Square	F	Sig.
1	Regression	245,000	1	245,000	4,189	,050[a]
	Residual	1637,667	28	58,488		
	Total	1882,667	29			

a. Predictors: (Constant), treatment dosage
b. Dependent Variable: treatment response

The above output table shows that treatment dosage is a significant predictor of treatment response wit a p-value of 0.050. There is, thus, a significantly incremental response with incremental dosages.

Example 2

In a parallel group study of 106 patients with hypertension 3 incremental antihypertensive treatment dosages are assessed. The first 13 patients of the data file is given underneath. The entire data file is in extras.springer.com, and is entitled "trend.sav".

responder	treatment
(1= yes, 0 = no)	1 = low, 2 = medium, 3 = high dosage)
1,00	1,00
1,00	1,00
1,00	1,00
1,00	1,00
1,00	1,00
1,00	1,00
1,00	1,00
1,00	1,00
1,00	1,00
1,00	1,00
1,00	2,00
1,00	2,00
1,00	2,00

Command:

Analyze...Descriptive Statistics...Crosstabs...Row(s): enter responders... Column(s): enter treatment...click Cell(s)...Counts: mark Observed...Percentage: mark Columns...click continue...click OK

The underneath contingency table shows that with incremental dosages the % of responders incrementally rises from 40% to 51.3 and then to 64.3%.

			treatment			Total
			1,00	2,00	3,00	
responder	,00	Count	15	19	15	49
		% within treatment	60,0%	48,7%	35,7%	46,2%
	1,00	Count	10	20	27	57
		% within treatment	40,0%	51,3%	64,3%	53,8%
Total		Count	25	39	42	106
		% within treatment	100,0%	100,0%	100,0%	100,0%

Subsequently, a chi-square test will be performed to assess whether the cells are significantly different from one another.

Command:

Analyze...Descriptive Statistics...Crosstabs... Row(s): enter responders... Column(s): enter treatment...click Statistics...Chi-square...click OK.

Example 2   337

Chi-Square Tests

	Value	df	Asymp. Sig. (2-sided)
Pearson Chi-Square	3,872[a]	2	,144
Likelihood Ratio	3,905	2	,142
Linear-by-Linear Association	3,829	1	,050
N of Valid Cases	106		

a. 0 cells (,0%) have expected count less than 5. The minimum expected count is 11,56.

The output table shows that the Pearson chi-square value for multiple groups testing is not significant with a value of 3.872 and a p-value of 0.144, and we need to conclude that there is no significant difference between the cells. Subsequently, a chi-square test for trends is required for that purpose. Actually, the "linear-by-linear association" from the same table is appropriate. It has approximately the same chi-square value, but it has only 1 degree of freedom, and, therefore it reaches statistical significance with a p-value of 0.050. There is, thus, a significant incremental trend of responding with incremental dosages. As an alternative the trend in this example can also be tested using logistic regression with responding as outcome variable and treatment as independent variable.

Command:
Analyze...Regression...Binary Logistic Regression...Dependent: enter responder...Covariates: enter treatment...click OK.

Variables in the Equation

		B	S.E.	Wald	df	Sig.	Exp(B)
Step 1[a]	treatment	,500	,257	3,783	1	,052	1,649
	Constant	-,925	,587	2,489	1	,115	,396

a. Variable(s) entered on step 1: treatment.

The output sheet shows that the p-value of the logistic model is virtually identical to the p-value of chi-square test for trends, 0.052 and 0.050.

Conclusion

The examples in this chapter show that both with continuous and binary outcome variables trend tests are more sensitive to demonstrate significant effects in dose response studies than traditional statistical tests.

Note

More background, theoretical and mathematical information of trend tests are given in the Chap. 27, Trend-testing, pp 313–318, in: Statistics applied to clinical studies 5th edition, Springer Heidelberg Germany, 2012, from the same authors.

Chapter 46
Doubly Multivariate Analysis of Variance for Multiple Observations from Multiple Outcome Variables (16 Patients)

General Purpose

Doubly multivariate ANOVA (analysis of variance) is for studies with multiple paired observations and more than a single outcome variable. An example is in the SPSS statistical software tutorial case studies: in a diet study of overweight patients the triglyceride and weight values were the outcome variables and they were measured repeatedly during several months of follow up. This chapter is to explain advantages, as compared to traditional methods, in preventing type I errors from being inflated, and accounting multiple effects simultaneously.

Background

One way analysis of variance (ANOVA) is for analysis of studies with multiple unpaired observations (i.e. 1 subject is observed once) and a single outcome variable (see Chap. 8, One way anova and Kruskal-Wallis, pp 29–31, in: SPSS for starters part one, Springer Heidelberg Germany, 2010, from the same authors).

Repeated measures ANOVA is for studies with multiple paired observations (i.e. more than a single observation per subject) and also with a single outcome variable (see Chap. 6, Repeated measures anova, pp 21–24, in: SPSS for starters part one, Springer Heidelberg Germany, 2010, from the same authors).

Multivariate ANOVA is for studies with multiple unpaired observations and more than a single outcome variable (see Chap.4, Multivariate anova, pp 13-20, in: SPSS for starters part two, Springer Heidelberg Germany, 2012, from the same authors).

Electronic Supplementary Material The online version of this chapter (https://doi.org/10.1007/978-3-030-33970-8_46) contains supplementary material, which is available to authorized users.

T. J. Cleophas, A. H. Zwinderman, *Machine Learning in Medicine – A Complete Overview*, https://doi.org/10.1007/978-3-030-33970-8_46

Finally, doubly multivariate ANOVA (MANOVA) is for studies with multiple paired observations and more than a single outcome variable. Underneath are schematic presentations.

1. 1 Way ANOVA

Group	n patients	outcome		
		mean	standard deviation (SD)	
1	n	"	"	"
2	n			
3	n			

2. Repeated Measures ANOVA

Person	outcomes			
	treatment 1	treatment 2	treatment 3	SD^2
1	"	"	"	"
2				
3				
4				

3. Multivariate ANOVA (MANOVA)

Group	outcome	
	$mean_1$	$mean_2$
1	"	"
2		
3		

4. Doubly MANOVA (tr = treatment)

Person	outcomes					
	tr 1	tr 2	tr 3	tr 1	tr 2	tr 3
1	"	"	"	"	"	"
2						
3						
4						

Specific Scientific Question

Can doubly multivariate analysis be used to simultaneously assess the effects of three different sleeping pills on two outcome variables, (1) hours of sleep and (2) morning body temperatures (in patients with sleep deprivation morning body temperature is lower than in those without sleep deprivation).

Example   341

Example

In 16 patients a three period crossover study of three sleeping pills (treatment levels) were studied. The underneath table give the data of the first 8 patients. The entire data file is entitled "doubly.sav", and is in extras.springer.com. Two outcome variables are measured at three levels each. This study would qualify for a doubly multivariate analysis, because we multiple paired outcomes and multiple measures of each of the outcomes.

hours			age	gen	temp		
a	b	c			a	b	c
6,10	6,80	5,20	55,00	0,00	35,90	35,30	36,80
7,00	7,00	7,90	65,00	0,00	37,10	37,80	37,00
8,20	9,00	3,90	74,00	0,00	38,30	34,00	39,10
7,60	7,80	4,70	56,00	1,00	37,50	34,60	37,70
6,50	6,60	5,30	44,00	1,00	36,40	35,30	36,70
8,40	8,00	5,40	49,00	1,00	38,30	35,50	38,00
6,90	7,30	4,20	53,00	0,00	37,00	34,10	37,40
6,70	7,00	6,10	76,00	0,00	36,80	36,10	36,90

hours = hours of sleep on sleeping pill
a, b, c = different sleeping pills (levels of treatment)
age = patient age
gen = gender
temp = different morning body temperatures on sleeping pill

SPSS statistical software will be used for data analysis. We will start by opening the data file in SPSS.

Then Command:

Analyze...General Linear Models...Repeated Measures...Within-Subject Factor Name: type treatment...Number of Levels: type 3...click Add...Measure Name: type hours...click Add...Measure Name: type temp...click Add...click Define ...Within-Subjects Variables(treatment): enter hours a, b, c, and temp a, b, c... Between-Subjects Factor(s): enter gender...click Contrast...Change Contrast ...Contrast...select Repeated...click Change...click Continue...click Plots... Horizontal Axis: enter treatment...Separate Lines: enter gender...click Add...click Continue...click Options...Display Means for: enter gender*treatment ...mark Estimates of effect size...mark SSCP matrices...click Continue...click OK.

The underneath table is in the output sheets.

Multivariate Tests[b]

Effect			Value	F	Hypothesis df	Error df	Sig.	Partial Eta Squared
Between Subjects	Intercept	Pillai's Trace	1,000	3,271E6	2,000	13,000	,000	1,000
		Wilks' Lambda	,000	3,271E6	2,000	13,000	,000	1,000
		Hotelling's Trace	503211,785	3,271E6	2,000	13,000	,000	1,000
		Roy's Largest Root	503211,785	3,271E6	2,000	13,000	,000	1,000
	gender	Pillai's Trace	,197	1,595[a]	2,000	13,000	,240	,197
		Wilks' Lambda	,803	1,595[a]	2,000	13,000	,240	,197
		Hotelling's Trace	,245	1,595[a]	2,000	13,000	,240	,197
		Roy's Largest Root	,245	1,595[a]	2,000	13,000	,240	,197
Within Subjects	treatment	Pillai's Trace	,562	3,525[a]	4,000	11,000	,044	,562
		Wilks' Lambda	,438	3,525[a]	4,000	11,000	,044	,562
		Hotelling's Trace	1,282	3,525[a]	4,000	11,000	,044	,562
		Roy's Largest Root	1,282	3,525[a]	4,000	11,000	,044	,562
	treatment * gender	Pillai's Trace	,762	8,822[a]	4,000	11,000	,002	,762
		Wilks' Lambda	,238	8,822[a]	4,000	11,000	,002	,762
		Hotelling's Trace	3,208	8,822[a]	4,000	11,000	,002	,762
		Roy's Largest Root	3,208	8,822[a]	4,000	11,000	,002	,762

a. Exact statistic
b. Design: Intercept + gender
Within Subjects Design: treatment

Doubly multivariate analysis has multiple paired outcomes and multiple measures of these outcomes. For analysis of such data both between and within subjects tests are performed. We are mostly interested in the within subject effects of the treatment levels, but the above table starts by showing the not so interesting gender effect on hours of sleep and morning temperatures. They are not significantly different between the genders. More important is the treatment effects. The hours of sleep and the morning temperature are significantly different between the different treatment levels at $p = 0.044$. Also these significant effects are different between males and females at $p = 0.002$.

Tests of Within-Subjects Contrasts

Source	Measure	treatment	Type III Sum of Squares	df	Mean Square	F	Sig.	Partial Eta Squared
treatment	hours	Level 1 vs. Level 2	,523	1	,523	6,215	,026	,307
		Level 2 vs. Level 3	62,833	1	62,833	16,712	,001	,544
	temp	Level 1 vs. Level 2	49,323	1	49,323	15,788	,001	,530
		Level 2 vs. Level 3	62,424	1	62,424	16,912	,001	,547
treatment * gender	hours	Level 1 vs. Level 2	,963	1	,963	11,447	,004	,450
		Level 2 vs. Level 3	,113	1	,113	,030	,865	,002
	temp	Level 1 vs. Level 2	,963	1	,963	,308	,588	,022
		Level 2 vs. Level 3	,054	1	,054	,015	,905	,001
Error(treatment)	hours	Level 1 vs. Level 2	1,177	14	,084			
		Level 2 vs. Level 3	52,637	14	3,760			
	temp	Level 1 vs. Level 2	43,737	14	3,124			
		Level 2 vs. Level 3	51,676	14	3,691			

The above table shows, whether differences between levels of treatment were significantly different from one by comparison with the subsequent levels (contrast tests). The effects of treatment levels 1 versus (vs) 2 on hours of sleep were different at $p = 0.026$, levels 2 vs 3 at $p = 0.001$. The effects of treatments levels 1 vs 2 on morning temperatures were different at $p = 0.001$, levels 2 vs 3 on morning temperatures were also different at $p = 0.001$. The effects on hours of sleep of treatment levels 1 vs 2 accounted for the differences in gender remained very significant at $p = 0.004$.

Example   343

gender * treatment

Measure	gender	treatment	Mean	Std. Error	95% Confidence Interval	
					Lower Bound	Upper Bound
hours	,00	1	6,980	,268	6,404	7,556
		2	7,420	,274	6,833	8,007
		3	5,460	,417	4,565	6,355
	1,00	1	7,350	,347	6,607	8,093
		2	7,283	,354	6,525	8,042
		3	5,150	,539	3,994	6,306
temp	,00	1	37,020	,284	36,411	37,629
		2	35,460	,407	34,586	36,334
		3	37,440	,277	36,845	38,035
	1,00	1	37,250	,367	36,464	38,036
		2	35,183	,526	34,055	36,311
		3	37,283	,358	36,515	38,051

The above table shows the mean hours of sleep and mean morning temperatures for the different subsets of observations. Particularly, we observe the few hours of sleep on treatment level 3, and the highest morning temperatures at the same level. The treatment level 2, in contrast, pretty many hours of sleep and, at the same time, the lowest morning temperatures (consistent with longer periods of sleep). The underneath figures show the same.

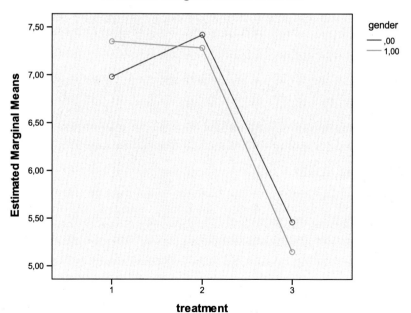

Estimated Marginal Means of hours

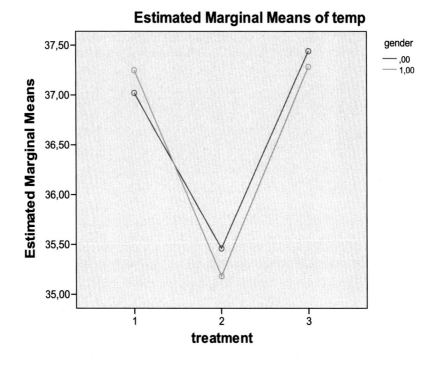

Estimated Marginal Means of temp

Conclusion

Doubly multivariate ANOVA is for studies with multiple paired observations and more than a single outcome variable. For example, in a study with two or more different outcome variables the outcome values are measured repeatedly during a period of follow up or in a study with two or more outcome variables the outcome values are measured at different levels, e.g., different treatment dosages or different compounds. The multivariate approach prevents the type I errors from being inflated, because we only have one test and, so, the p-values need not be adjusted for multiple testing (see Chap. 3, Multiple treatments, pp 19–27, and Chap. 4, Multiple endpoints, pp 29–36, both in: Machine learning in medicine part three, Springer Heidelberg Germany, from the same authors). Also, the multivariate test battery accounts for multiple effects simultaneously.

Note

Additional background, theoretical and mathematical information of multiple variables data files as reviewed in this chapter are the following:

Chapter 8, One way anova and Kruskal-Wallis, pp 29–31, in: SPSS for starters part
   one, Springer Heidelberg Germany, 2010, from the same authors),
Chapter 6, Repeated measures anova, pp 21–24, in: SPSS for starters part one,
   Springer Heidelberg Germany, 2010, from the same authors),
Chapter 4, Multivariate anova, pp 13–20, in: SPSS for starters part two, Springer
   Heidelberg Germany, 2012, from the same authors.

The advantages of multivariate analyses as compared to univariate analyses are
discussed in the Chap. 3, Multiple treatrments, pp 19–27, and the Chap. 4, Multiple
endpoints, pp 29–36, both in: Machine learning in medicine part three, Springer
Heidelberg Germany, 2013, from the same authors.

Chapter 47
Probit Models for Estimating Effective Pharmacological Treatment Dosages (14 Tests)

General Purpose

Probit regression is, just like logistic regression, for estimating the effect of predictors on yes/no outcomes. If your predictor is multiple pharmacological treatment dosages, then probit regression may be more convenient than logistic regression, because your results will be reported in the form of response rates instead of odds ratios. The dependent variable of the two methods log odds (otherwise called logit) and log prob (otherwise called probit) are closely related to one another. Log prob (probability), is the z-value corresponding to its area under the curve value of the normal distribution. It can be shown that the log odds of responding $\approx (\pi / \sqrt{3})$ x log prob of responding (see Chap. 7, Machine learning in medicine part three, Probit regression, pp 63–68, 2013, Springer Heidelberg Germany, from the same authors).

Background

In statistics, a probit model is a type of regression where the dependent variable can take only two values, for example married or not married. The word is a "portman teau" word, a word coming from probability + unit. The purpose of the model is to estimate the probability that an observation with particular characteristics will fall into a specific one of the categories; moreover, classifying observations based on their predicted probabilities is a type of binary classification model.

A probit model is a popular specification for an ordinal or a binary response model. As such it treats the same set of problems as does logistic regression using similar techniques. The probit model, which employs a probit link function, is most

Electronic Supplementary Material The online version of this chapter (https://doi.org/10.1007/978-3-030-33970-8_47) contains supplementary material, which is available to authorized users.

often estimated using the standard maximum likelihood procedure, such an estimation being called a probit regression. The probit model is usually credited to Chester Bliss, 1934, a biologist from Springfield Ohio known for his contributions to statistics.

Specific Scientific Question

This chapter will assess whether probit regression is able to find response rates of different dosages of mosquito repellents.

Example

Simple Probit Regression

repellent nonchem	repellent chem	mosquitos gone	n mosquitos
1	,02	1000	18000
1	,03	1000	18500
1	,03	3500	19500
1	,04	4500	18000
1	,07	9500	16500
1	,09	17000	22500
1	,10	20500	24000

In 14 test sessions the effect measured as the numbers of mosquitos gone after administration of different dosages of a chemical repellent was assessed. The first 7 sessions are in the above table. The entire data file is entitled probit.sav, and is in extras.springer.com. Start by opening the data file in SPSS statistical software.

Command:
Analyze....Regression....Probit Regression....Response Frequency: enter "mosquitos gone"....Total Observed: enter "n mosquitos"....Covariate(s): enter "chemical"....Transform: select "natural log"....click OK.

Example   349

Chi-Square Tests

		Chi-Square	df[a]	Sig.
PROBIT	Pearson Goodness-of-Fit Test	7706,816	12	,000[b]

a. Statistics based on individual cases differ from statistics based on aggregated cases.
b. Since the significance level is less than ,150, a heterogeneity factor is used in the calculation of confidence limits.

In the output sheets the above table shows that the goodness of fit tests of the data is significant, and, thus, the data do not fit the probit model very well. However, SPSS is going to produce a heterogeneity correction factor and we can proceed. The underneath shows that chemical dilution levels are a very significant predictor of proportions of mosquitos gone.

Parameter Estimates

	Parameter	Estimate	Std. Error	Z	Sig.	95% Confidence Interval	
						Lower Bound	Upper Bound
PROBIT[a]	chemical (dilution)	1,649	,006	286,098	,000	1,638	1,660
	Intercept	4,489	,017	267,094	,000	4,472	4,506

a. PROBIT model: PROBIT(p) = Intercept + BX (Covariates X are transformed using the base 2.718 logarithm.)

Cell Counts and Residuals

	Number	chemical (dilution)	Number of Subjects	Observed Responses	Expected Responses	Residual	Probability
PROBIT	1	-3,912	18000	1000	448,194	551,806	,025
	2	-3,624	18500	1000	1266,672	-266,672	,068
	3	-3,401	19500	3500	2564,259	935,741	,132
	4	-3,124	18000	4500	4574,575	-74,575	,254
	5	-2,708	16500	9500	8405,866	1094,134	,509
	6	-2,430	22500	17000	15410,676	1589,324	,685
	7	-2,303	24000	20500	18134,992	2365,008	,756
	8	-3,912	22500	500	560,243	-60,243	,025
	9	-3,624	18500	1500	1266,672	233,328	,068
	10	-3,401	19000	1000	2498,508	-1498,508	,132
	11	-3,124	20000	5000	5082,861	-82,861	,254
	12	-2,708	22000	10000	11207,821	-1207,821	,509
	13	-2,430	16500	8000	11301,162	-3301,162	,685
	14	-2,303	18500	13500	13979,056	-479,056	,756

The above table shows that according to chi-square tests the differences between observed and expected proportions of mosquitos gone is several times statistically significant.

It does, therefore, make sense to make some inferences using the underneath confidence limits table.

Confidence Limits

	Probability	95% Confidence Limits for chemical (dilution)			95% Confidence Limits for log(chemical (dilution))[b]		
		Estimate	Lower Bound	Upper Bound	Estimate	Lower Bound	Upper Bound
PROBIT[a]	,010	,016	,012	,020	-4,133	-4,453	-3,911
	,020	,019	,014	,023	-3,968	-4,250	-3,770
	,030	,021	,016	,025	-3,863	-4,122	-3,680
	,040	,023	,018	,027	-3,784	-4,026	-3,612
	,050	,024	,019	,029	-3,720	-3,949	-3,557
	,060	,026	,021	,030	-3,665	-3,882	-3,509
	,070	,027	,022	,031	-3,617	-3,825	-3,468
	,080	,028	,023	,032	-3,574	-3,773	-3,430
	,090	,029	,024	,034	-3,535	-3,726	-3,396
	,100	,030	,025	,035	-3,500	-3,683	-3,365
	,150	,035	,030	,039	-3,351	-3,506	-3,232
	,200	,039	,034	,044	-3,233	-3,368	-3,125
	,250	,044	,039	,048	-3,131	-3,252	-3,031
	,300	,048	,043	,053	-3,040	-3,150	-2,943
	,350	,052	,047	,057	-2,956	-3,059	-2,860
	,400	,056	,051	,062	-2,876	-2,974	-2,778
	,450	,061	,055	,067	-2,799	-2,895	-2,697
	,500	,066	,060	,073	-2,722	-2,819	-2,614
	,550	,071	,064	,080	-2,646	-2,745	-2,529
	,600	,077	,069	,087	-2,569	-2,672	-2,442
	,650	,083	,074	,095	-2,489	-2,598	-2,349
	,700	,090	,080	,105	-2,404	-2,522	-2,251
	,750	,099	,087	,117	-2,313	-2,441	-2,143
	,800	,109	,095	,132	-2,212	-2,351	-2,022
	,850	,123	,106	,153	-2,094	-2,248	-1,879
	,900	,143	,120	,183	-1,945	-2,120	-1,699
	,910	,148	,124	,191	-1,909	-2,089	-1,655
	,920	,154	,128	,200	-1,870	-2,055	-1,608
	,930	,161	,133	,211	-1,827	-2,018	-1,556
	,940	,169	,138	,224	-1,780	-1,977	-1,497
	,950	,178	,145	,239	-1,725	-1,931	-1,430
	,960	,190	,153	,259	-1,661	-1,876	-1,352
	,970	,206	,164	,285	-1,582	-1,809	-1,255
	,980	,228	,179	,324	-1,477	-1,719	-1,126
	,990	,269	,206	,397	-1,312	-1,579	-,923

a. A heterogeneity factor is used.
b. Logarithm base = 2.718.

E.g., one might conclude that a 0,143 dilution of the chemical repellent causes 0,900 (=90%) of the mosquitos to have gone. And 0,066 dilution would mean that 0,500 (=50%) of the mosquitos disappeared.

Multiple Probit Regression

Like multiple logistic regression using multiple predictors, probit regression can also be applied with multiple predictors. We will add as second predictor to the above example the nonchemical repellents ultrasound (=1) and burning candles (= 2) (see uppermost table of this chapter).

Example   351

Command:
Analyze....Regression....Probit Regression....Response Frequency: enter "mosquitos gone"....Total Observed: enter "n mosquitos"....Covariate(s): enter "chemical".... Transform: select "natural log"....click OK.

Chi-Square Tests

		Chi-Square	df[a]	Sig.
PROBIT	Pearson Goodness-of-Fit Test	3863,489	11	,000[b]

a. Statistics based on individual cases differ from statistics based on aggregated cases.
b. Since the significance level is less than ,150, a heterogeneity factor is used in the calculation of confidence limits.

Again, the goodness of fit is not what it should be, but SPSS adds a correction factor for heterogeneity. The underneath shows the regression coefficients for the multiple model. the no chemical repellents have significantly different effects on the outcome.

Parameter Estimates

Parameter		Estimate	Std. Error	Z	Sig.	95% Confidence Interval	
						Lower Bound	Upper Bound
PROBIT[a]	chemical (dilution)	1,654	,006	284,386	,000	1,643	1,665
Intercept[b]	ultrasound	4,678	,017	269,650	,000	4,661	4,696
	burning candles	4,321	,017	253,076	,000	4,304	4,338

a. PROBIT model: PROBIT(p) = Intercept + BX (Covariates X are transformed using the base 2.718 logarithm.)
b. Corresponds to the grouping variable repellentnonchemical.

Cell Counts and Residuals

	Number	repellentnonc hemical	chemical (dilution)	Number of Subjects	Observed Responses	Expected Responses	Residual	Probability
PROBIT	1	1	-3,912	18000	1000	658,233	341,767	,037
	2	1	-3,624	18500	1000	1740,139	-740,139	,094
	3	1	-3,401	19500	3500	3350,108	149,892	,172
	4	1	-3,124	18000	4500	5630,750	-1130,750	,313
	5	1	-2,708	16500	9500	9553,811	-53,811	,579
	6	1	-2,430	22500	17000	16760,668	239,332	,745
	7	1	-2,303	24000	20500	19388,521	1111,479	,808
	8	2	-3,912	22500	500	355,534	144,466	,016
	9	2	-3,624	18500	1500	871,485	628,515	,047
	10	2	-3,401	19000	1000	1824,614	-824,614	,096
	11	2	-3,124	20000	5000	3979,458	1020,542	,199
	12	2	-2,708	22000	10000	9618,701	381,299	,437
	13	2	-2,430	16500	8000	10202,854	-2202,854	,618
	14	2	-2,303	18500	13500	12873,848	626,152	,696

In the above Cell Counts table, it is shown that according to the chi-square tests the differences of observed and expected proportions of mosquitos gone were statistically significant several times. The next page table gives interesting results. E. g., a 0,128 dilution of the chemical repellent causes 0,900 (=90%) of the mosquitos to have gone in the ultrasound tests.

And 0,059 dilution would mean that 0,500 (=50%) of the mosquitos disappeared.

The results of burning candles were less impressive. 0,159 dilution caused 90 % of the mosquitos to disappear, 0,073 dilution 50%.

Confidence Limits

	nonchemical	Probability	95% Confidence Limits for chemical (dilution)			95% Confidence Limits for log(chemical (dilution))[b]		
			Estimate	Lower Bound	Upper Bound	Estimate	Lower Bound	Upper Bound
PROBIT[a]	ultrasound	,010	,014	,011	,018	-4,235	-4,486	-4,042
		,020	,017	,014	,020	-4,070	-4,296	-3,895
		,030	,019	,015	,022	-3,966	-4,176	-3,801
		,040	,021	,017	,024	-3,887	-4,086	-3,731
		,050	,022	,018	,025	-3,823	-4,013	-3,673
		,060	,023	,019	,027	-3,769	-3,951	-3,624
		,070	,024	,020	,028	-3,721	-3,896	-3,581
		,080	,025	,021	,029	-3,678	-3,848	-3,542
		,090	,026	,022	,030	-3,639	-3,804	-3,506
		,100	,027	,023	,031	-3,603	-3,763	-3,473
		,150	,032	,027	,036	-3,455	-3,597	-3,337
		,200	,036	,031	,040	-3,337	-3,467	-3,227
		,250	,039	,035	,044	-3,236	-3,356	-3,131
		,300	,043	,038	,048	-3,146	-3,258	-3,043
		,350	,047	,042	,052	-3,062	-3,169	-2,961
		,400	,051	,046	,056	-2,982	-3,085	-2,882
		,450	,055	,049	,061	-2,905	-3,006	-2,803
		,500	,059	,053	,066	-2,829	-2,929	-2,725
		,550	,064	,058	,071	-2,753	-2,853	-2,646
		,600	,069	,062	,077	-2,675	-2,777	-2,564
		,650	,075	,067	,084	-2,596	-2,700	-2,478
		,700	,081	,073	,092	-2,512	-2,620	-2,387
		,750	,089	,079	,102	-2,421	-2,534	-2,287
		,800	,098	,087	,114	-2,320	-2,440	-2,174
		,850	,111	,097	,130	-2,202	-2,332	-2,042
		,900	,128	,111	,153	-2,054	-2,197	-1,874
		,910	,133	,115	,160	-2,018	-2,165	-1,833
		,920	,138	,119	,167	-1,979	-2,129	-1,789
		,930	,144	,124	,175	-1,936	-2,091	-1,740
		,940	,151	,129	,185	-1,889	-2,048	-1,686
		,950	,160	,135	,197	-1,834	-1,999	-1,623
		,960	,170	,143	,212	-1,770	-1,942	-1,550
		,970	,184	,154	,232	-1,691	-1,871	-1,459
		,980	,205	,169	,262	-1,587	-1,778	-1,339
		,990	,241	,196	,317	-1,422	-1,632	-1,149

Example   353

Confidence Limits

nonchemical	Probability	95% Confidence Limits for chemical (dilution)			95% Confidence Limits for log(chemical (dilution))[b]		
		Estimate	Lower Bound	Upper Bound	Estimate	Lower Bound	Upper Bound
burning candles	,010	,018	,014	,021	-4,019	-4,247	-3,841
	,020	,021	,017	,025	-3,854	-4,058	-3,693
	,030	,024	,019	,027	-3,750	-3,939	-3,599
	,040	,025	,021	,029	-3,671	-3,850	-3,528
	,050	,027	,023	,031	-3,607	-3,777	-3,469
	,060	,029	,024	,033	-3,553	-3,716	-3,420
	,070	,030	,026	,034	-3,505	-3,662	-3,376
	,080	,031	,027	,036	-3,462	-3,614	-3,336
	,090	,033	,028	,037	-3,423	-3,571	-3,300
	,100	,034	,029	,038	-3,387	-3,531	-3,267
	,150	,039	,034	,044	-3,239	-3,367	-3,128
	,200	,044	,039	,049	-3,121	-3,240	-3,015
	,250	,049	,044	,054	-3,020	-3,132	-2,916
	,300	,053	,048	,059	-2,930	-3,037	-2,826
	,350	,058	,052	,065	-2,845	-2,950	-2,741
	,400	,063	,057	,070	-2,766	-2,869	-2,658
	,450	,068	,061	,076	-2,688	-2,793	-2,578
	,500	,073	,066	,082	-2,613	-2,718	-2,497
	,550	,079	,071	,089	-2,537	-2,644	-2,415
	,600	,085	,076	,097	-2,459	-2,571	-2,331
	,650	,093	,082	,106	-2,380	-2,495	-2,244
	,700	,101	,089	,116	-2,295	-2,417	-2,151
	,750	,110	,097	,129	-2,205	-2,333	-2,049
	,800	,122	,106	,144	-2,104	-2,240	-1,936
	,850	,137	,119	,165	-1,986	-2,133	-1,802
	,900	,159	,136	,195	-1,838	-1,999	-1,633
	,910	,165	,140	,203	-1,802	-1,966	-1,592
	,920	,172	,145	,213	-1,763	-1,932	-1,548
	,930	,179	,151	,223	-1,720	-1,893	-1,499
	,940	,188	,157	,236	-1,672	-1,850	-1,444
	,950	,198	,165	,251	-1,618	-1,802	-1,381
	,960	,211	,175	,270	-1,554	-1,745	-1,308
	,970	,229	,187	,296	-1,475	-1,675	-1,217
	,980	,254	,206	,334	-1,371	-1,582	-1,096
	,990	,299	,238	,404	-1,206	-1,436	-,906

a. A heterogeneity factor is used.
b. Logarithm base = 2.718.

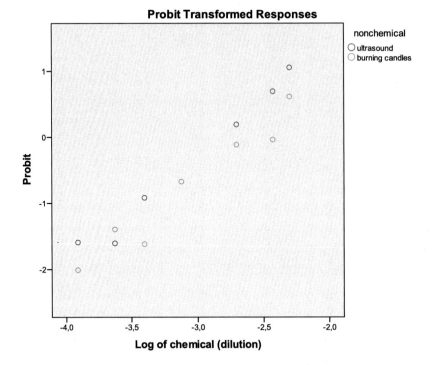

Probit Transformed Responses

The above figure supports the adequacy of the multiple variables probit model, with two similarly sloped linear patterns (the blue and the green one) of "chemical repellent levels" versus "mosquitos gone levels" regressions.

Conclusion

Probit regression is, just like logistic regression, for estimating the effect of predictors on yes/no outcomes. If your predictor is multiple pharmacological treatment dosages, then probit regression may be more convenient than logistic regression, because your results will be reported in the form of response rates instead of odds ratios. This chapter shows that probit regression is able to find response rates of different dosages of mosquito repellents.

Note

More background, theoretical and mathematical information of probit regression is given in the Chap. 7, Machine learning in medicine part three, Probit regression, pp 63–68, 2013, Springer Heidelberg Germany, from the same authors).

Chapter 48
Interval Censored Data Analysis for Assessing Mean Time to Cancer Relapse (51 Patients)

General Purpose

In survival studies time to first outpatient clinic check instead of time to event is, usually, measured. This analysis assumes that time to first outpatient check is equal to time to relapse. However, instead of a time to relapse an interval is given, in which the relapse has occurred, and so this variable is somewhat loose. This chapter is to assess whether mean time to relapse can be appropriately inferenced from a generalized linear model with an interval censored link function.

Background

Often in survival studies time to first outpatient clinic check is measured instead of time to event. Somewhere in the interval between the last and current visit an event may have taken place. For simplicity such data are often analyzed using the proportional hazard model of Cox (Chap.17, Cox regression, pp. 209-212, in: Statistics applied to clinical studies 5th edition, Springer Heidelberg Germany, 2012, from the same authors). However, this analysis is not entirely appropriate. It assumes that time to first outpatient check is equal to time to relapse. However, instead of a time to relapse an interval is given, in which the relapse has occurred, and so this variable is somewhat more loose than the usual variable time to event. An appropriate statistic for the current variable would be the mean time to relapse inferenced from a generalized linear model with an interval censored link function, rather than the proportional hazard method of Cox.

Electronic Supplementary Material The online version of this chapter (https://doi.org/10.1007/978-3-030-33970-8_48) contains supplementary material, which is available to authorized users.

T. J. Cleophas, A. H. Zwinderman, *Machine Learning in Medicine – A Complete Overview*, https://doi.org/10.1007/978-3-030-33970-8_48

Specific Scientific Question

This chapter is to assess whether an appropriate statistic for the variable "time to first check" in survival studies would be the mean time to relapse, as inferenced from a generalized linear model with an interval censored link function.

Example

In 51 patients in remission their status at the time-to-first-outpatient-clinic-control was checked (mths = months).

treatment (0 and 1)	time to first check (mths)	result (0 = remission 1 = relapse)
1	11	0
0	12	1
0	9	1
1	12	0
0	12	0
1	12	0
1	5	1
1	12	0
1	12	0
0	12	0

The first 10 patients are above. The entire data file is entitled "intervalcensored. sav", and is in extras.springer.com. Cox regression was applied. Start by opening the data file in SPSS statistical software.

Command:
Analyze....Survival....Cox Regression....Time: time to first check....Status: result....Define Event....Single value: type 1....click Continue....Covariates: enter treatment....click Categorical....Categorical Covariates: enter treatment.... click Continue....click Plots....mark Survival....Separate Lines for: enter treatment....click Continue....click OK.

Variables in the Equation

	B	SE	Wald	df	Sig.	Exp(B)
treatment	.919	.477	3.720	1	.054	2.507

Example 357

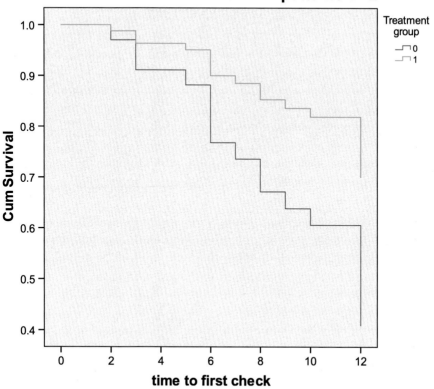

The above table is in the output. It shows that treatment is not a significant predictor for relapse. In spite of the above Kaplan-Meier curves, suggesting the opposite, the treatments are not significantly different from one another because p > 0.05. However, the analysis so far is not entirely appropriate. It assumes that time to first outpatient check is equal to time to relapse. However, instead of a time to relapse an interval is given between 2 and 12 months in which the relapse has occurred, and so this variables is somewhat more loose than the usual variable time to event. An appropriate statistic for the current variable would be the mean time to relapse inferenced from a generalized linear model with an interval censored link function, rather than the proportional hazard method of Cox.

Command:
Analyze.... click Generalized Linear Models.... click once again Generalized Linear Models.... Type of Model.... mark Interval censored survival.... click Response.... Dependent Variable: enter Result.... Scale Weight Variable: enter "time to first check".... click Predictors.... Factors: enter "treatment".... click Model.... click once again Model: enter once again "treatment".... click Save.... mark Predicted value of mean of response.... click OK.

Parameter Estimates

| Parameter | B | Std. Error | 95% Wald Confidence Interval | | Hypothesis Test | | |
			Lower	Upper	Wald Chi-Square	df	Sig.
(Intercept)	.467	.0735	.323	.611	40.431	1	.000
[treatment=0]	-.728	.1230	-.969	-.487	35.006	1	.000
[treatment=1]	0ᵃ	.	.	.	.	.	.
(Scale)	1ᵇ						

Dependent Variable: Result
Model: (Intercept), treatment
a. Set to zero because this parameter is redundant.
b. Fixed at the displayed value.

The generalized linear model shows, that, after censoring the intervals, the treatment 0 is, compared to treat 1, a very significant better maintainer of remission. When we return to the data, we will observe as a novel variable, the mean predicted probabilities of persistent remission for each patient. This is shown underneath for the first 10 patients. For the patients on treatment 1 it equals 79,7 %, for the patients on treatment 0 it is only 53,7 %. And so, treatment 1 performs, indeed, a lot better than does treatment 0 (mths = months).

treatment (0 and 1)	time to first check (mths)	result (0 = remission 1 = relapse)	Mean Predicted_1
1	11	0	.797
0	12	1	.537
0	9	1	.537
1	12	0	.797
0	12	0	.537
1	12	0	.797
1	5	1	.797
1	12	0	.797
1	12	0	.797
0	12	0	.537

Conclusion

This chapter assesses whether an appropriate statistic for the variable "time to first check" in survival studies is the mean time to relapse, as inferenced from a generalized linear model with an interval censored link function. The current example shows that, in addition, more sensitivity of testing is obtained with p-values of 0.054 versus 0.0001. Also, predicted probabilities of persistent remission or risk of relapse for different treatment modalities are given. This method is an important tool for analyzing such data.

Note

More background, theoretical and mathematical information of survival analyses is given in Chap. 17, Cox regression, pp. 209–212, in: Statistics applied to clinical studies 5th edition, Springer Heidelberg Germany, 2012, from the same authors.

Chapter 49
Structural Equation Modeling (SEM) with SPSS Analysis of Moment Structures (Amos) Software for Cause Effect Relationships in Pharmacodynamic Studies I (35 Patients)

General Purpose

This chapter is to assess, whether the Amos (analysis of moment structures) add-on module of SPSS statistical software, frequently used in econo-/sociometry, but little used in medicine, is able to perform an SEM (structural equation modeling) analysis of pharmacodynamic data.

Background

In clinical efficacy studies the outcome is often influenced by multiple causal factors, like drug - noncompliance, frequency of counseling, and many more factors. Structural equation modeling (SEM) was only recently formally defined by Pearl (In: Causality, reason, and inference, Cambridge University Press, Cambridge UK 2000). This statistical methodology includes

(1) factor analysis (see also Chap. 14, Factor analysis, pp 167–181, in: Machine learning in medicine part one, Springer Heidelberg Germany, 2013, from the same authors),

(2) path analysis (see also Chap. 2, Multistage regression, in: SPSS for starters part two, pp 3–6, Springer Heidelberg Germany, 2012 from the same authors),

(3) regression analysis (see also Chap. 14, Linear regression, basic approach, in: Statistics applied to clinical studies 5th edition, pp 161–176, Springer Heidelberg Germany, 2012, from the same authors).

Electronic Supplementary Material The online version of this chapter (https://doi.org/10.1007/978-3-030-33970-8_49) contains supplementary material, which is available to authorized users.

An SEM model looks like a complex regression model, but it is more. It extends the prior hypothesis of correlation to that of causality, and this is accomplished by a network of variables tested versus one another with standardized rather than unstandardized regression coefficients.

The network is commonly named a Bayesian network, otherwise called a DAG (directed acyclic graph), (see also Chap. 16, Bayesian networks, pp 163–170, in: Machine learning in medicine part 2, Springer Heidelberg Germany, 2013, from the same authors), which is a probabilistic graphical model of nodes (the variables) and connecting arrows presenting the conditional dependencies of the nodes.

This chapter is to assess whether the Amos (analysis of moment structures) module of SPSS statistical software, so far little used in medicine, is able to perform an SEM analysis of pharmacodynamic data. A free trial download of the Amos module is available at www.jmp.com.

Specific Scientific Question

Can SEM modeling in Amos (Analysis of Moment Structures) demonstrate direct and indirect effects of non-compliance and counseling on treatment efficacy.

Example

We will use the same example as the one used in Chap. 2, Multistage regression, in: SPSS for starters part two, pp 3–6, Springer Heidelberg Germany, 2012 from the same authors.

stool stools / month	counseling counselings / month	noncompliance drug noncompliances / month
24,00	8,00	25,00
30,00	13,00	30,00
25,00	15,00	25,00
35,00	10,00	31,00
39,00	9,00	36,00
30,00	10,00	33,00
27,00	8,00	22,00
14,00	5,00	18,00
39,00	13,00	14,00
42,00	15,00	30,00

The first 10 patients of the 35 patient data file is above. The entire data file is in extras.springer.com, and is entitled "amos1.sav". We will first perform traditional linear regressions. Start by opening the data file.

Example   363

Command:

Analyze....Regression....Linear....Dependent: enter "stool"....Independent(s): enter "counseling and non-compliance"....click OK.

Coefficients^a

Model		Unstandardized Coefficients		Standardized Coefficients	t	Sig.
		B	Std. Error	Beta		
1	(Constant)	2,270	4,823		,471	,641
	counseling	1,876	,290	,721	6,469	,000
	non-compliance	,285	,167	,190	1,705	,098

a. Dependent Variable: ther eff

The above table is given on the output sheet, and shows that, with p = 0.10 as cut-off for statistical significance both variables are significant.

Command:

Analyze....Regression....Linear....Dependent: enter "counseling"....Independent(s): enter "non-compliance"....click OK.

Coefficients^a

Model		Unstandardized Coefficients		Standardized Coefficients	t	Sig.
		B	Std. Error	Beta		
1	(Constant)	4,228	2,800		1,510	,141
	non-compliance	,220	,093	,382	2,373	,024

a. Dependent Variable: counseling

The above table shows that non-compliance is also a significant predictor of counseling. This would mean that non-compliance works two ways: it predicts therapeutic efficacy directly and indirectly through counseling. However, the indirect way is not taken into account in the one step linear regression. We will now use the Amos add-on module for further analysis.

Command:

Analyze....click IBM SPSS Amos

The work area of Amos appears. The menu is in the second upper row. The toolbar is on the left. In the empty area on the right you can draw your networks.

click File....click Save as....Browse the folder you selected in your personal computer, and enter Amos1....click Save.

In the first upper row the title Amos1 has appeared, in the bottom rectangle left from the empty area the title Amos1 has also appeared.

click Diagram....left click "Draw Observed" and drag to empty area....click the green rectangle and a colorless rectangle appears....left click it and a red rectangle appears....do this 2 more times and have the rectangles at different places....click Diagram again....left click "Draw Unobserved" and drag to right part of empty area....click the green ellipse....a colorless ellipse appears, and later a red and finally black ellipse.

The underneath figure shows how your screen will look by now. There are four rectangle nodes for observed variables, and one oval node for an unobserved, otherwise called latent, variable.

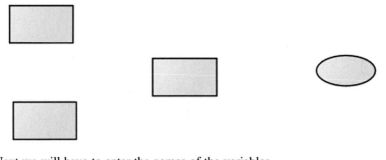

Next we will have to enter the names of the variables.

Command:
right click in the left upper rectangle....click Object Properties....Variable name: type "noncompliance"....close dialog box....the name is now in the rectangle.... do the same for the other two rectangles and type in the ellipse the term others (it indicates the remainder of variables not taken into account in the current model, together with the variables present the outcome is explained by 100%).

Next arrows have to be added to the diagram.

Command:
click Diagram....click Draw Path for arrows....click Draw Covariance for double-headed arrow.

Example   365

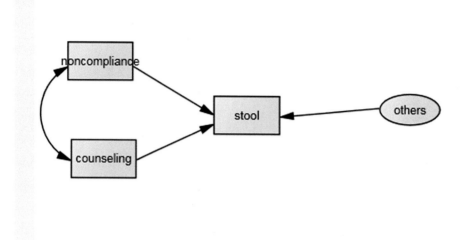

The above figure is now in the empty area. In order to match the "others" variables in the ellipse with the three other variables of the model, they a regression weight, like the value 1, has to be added.

right click at the arrow of the ellipse....click Object Properties....click Parameters....Regression weights: enter 1....close dialog box.

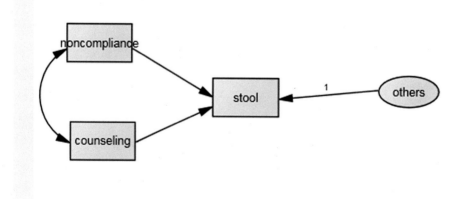

The empty area now has the value 1.

click from menu View....Analysis Properties....Output....mark "Minimization history, Standardized estimates, and Squared multiple correlations"....close dialog box....click Analyze....Calculate Estimates.

A new path diagram button has appeared in the upper white rectangle left from the empty area. Click it

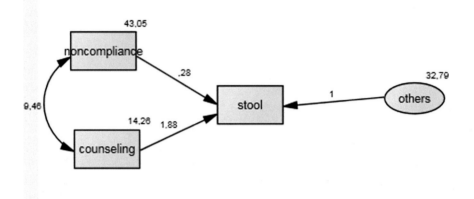

Unstandardized regression coefficients are now in the model, that of counseling versus stool equals 1.88, that of noncompliance versus stool equals 0.28. These values are identical to the values obtained by ordinary multiple linear regression as shown in the previous tabs. However, for path analysis standardized values are more important.

In order to view the standardized values, click in the third white rectangle left from the empty area "Standardized estimates".

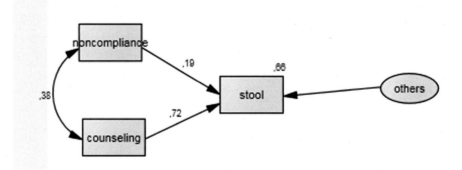

Now we observe the standardized regression coefficients. They are identical to the standardized regression coefficients as computed by the ordinary linear regression models as shown in the previous tabs:

0.19 noncompliance versus stool
0.72 counseling versus stool
0.38 noncompliance versus counseling.

What advantage does this path analysis give us as compared to traditional regression modeling. The advantage is that multiple regression coefficients, as they are standardized, can be simply added up after weighting in order to estimate the entire strength of prediction. Single path analysis gives a standardized regression coefficient of 0.19. This underestimates the real effect of non-compliance. Two step path analysis is more realistic and shows that the add-up path statistic is larger and equals

$$0.19 + 0.38 \times 0.72 = 0.46$$

The two-path statistic of 0.46 is a lot better than the single path statistic of 0.19 with an increase of 60%.

Conclusion

SEM is adequate for cause effect assessments in pharmacology, and, in addition, it is very easy to use. Arbuckle, the author of IBM SPSS Amos 19 User's Guide noted, that it may open the way to data analysis to nonstatisticians, because it avoids mathematics, and, like other machine learning software, e.g., SPSS modeler (see the Chaps. 61, 64, 65), Knime (see the Chaps. 7, 8, 70, 71, 74), and Weka (see the Chap.70), it makes extensively use of beautiful graphs to visualize procedures and results instead.

The current chapter gives only the simplest applications of SEM modeling. SEM modeling can also handle binary data using chi-square tests, include multiple models in a single analysis, replace more complex multivariate analysis of variance with similar if not better power.

Note

More background, theoretical and mathematical information of structural equation models like path analysis, factor analysis, and regression models are in

(1) the Chap. 14, Factor analysis, pp 167–181, in: Machine learning in medicine part 1, Springer Heidelberg Germany, 2013,

(2) the Chap. 2, Multistage regression, in: SPSS for starters part 2, pp 3–6, Springer Heidelberg Germany, 2012,
(3) the Chap. 14, Linear regression, basic approach, in: Statistics applied to clinical studies 5th edition, pp 161–176, Springer Heidelberg Germany, 2012, all of them from the same authors.

Chapter 50
Structural Equation Modeling (SEM) with SPSS Analysis of Moment Structures (Amos) Software for Cause Effect Relationships in Pharmacodynamic Studies II (35 Patients)

General Purpose

Just like the Chap. 49, this chapter is to assess whether the Amos (analysis of moment structures) add-on module of SPSS statistical software, frequently used in econo-/sociometry but little used in medicine, is able to perform an SEM analysis of pharmacodynamic data.

Background

In clinical efficacy studies the outcome is often influenced by multiple causal factors, like drug - noncompliance, frequency of counseling, and many more factors. Structural equation modeling (SEM) was only recently formally defined by Pearl (In: Causality, reason, and inference, Cambridge University Press, Cambridge UK 2000). This statistical methodology includes

(1) factor analysis (see also Chap. 14, Factor analysis, pp 167–181, in: Machine learning in medicine part one, Springer Heidelberg Germany, 2013, from the same authors),

(2) path analysis (see also Chap. 2, Multistage regression, in: SPSS for starters part two, pp 3–6, Springer Heidelberg Germany, 2012 from the same authors),

(3) regression analysis (see also Chap. 14, Linear regression, basic approach, in: Statistics applied to clinical studies 5th edition, pp 161–176, Springer Heidelberg Germany, 2012, from the same authors).

Electronic Supplementary Material The online version of this chapter (https://doi.org/10.1007/978-3-030-33970-8_50) contains supplementary material, which is available to authorized users.

T. J. Cleophas, A. H. Zwinderman, *Machine Learning in Medicine – A Complete Overview*, https://doi.org/10.1007/978-3-030-33970-8_50

An SEM model looks like a complex regression model, but it is more. It extends the prior hypothesis of correlation to that of causality, and this is accomplished by a network of variables tested versus one another with standardized rather than unstandardized regression coefficients.

The network is commonly named a Bayesian network, otherwise called a DAG (directed acyclic graph), (see also Chap. 16, Bayesian networks, pp 163–170, in: Machine learning in medicine part 2, Springer Heidelberg Germany, 2013, from the same authors), which is a probabilistic graphical model of nodes (the variables) and connecting arrows presenting the conditional dependencies of the nodes.

This chapter is to assess whether the Amos (analysis of moment structures) add-on module of SPSS statistical software, so far little used in medicine, is able to perform an SEM analysis of pharmacodynamic data.

Primary Scientific Question

Can SEM modeling in Amos (analysis of moment structures) demonstrate direct and indirect effects of non-compliance and counseling on treatment efficacy and quality of life.

Example

We will use the same example as the one used in Chap. 3, Multivariate analysis using path statistics, in: SPSS for starters part 2, pp 7–11, Springer Heidelberg Germany, 2012 from the same authors.

stool stools /month	counseling counselings /month	noncompliance drug noncompliances /month	qol quality of life score
24,00	8,00	25,00	69,00
30,00	13,00	30,00	110,00
25,00	15,00	25,00	78,00
35,00	10,00	31,00	103,00
39,00	9,00	36,00	103,00
30,00	10,00	33,00	102,00
27,00	8,00	22,00	76,00
14,00	5,00	18,00	75,00
39,00	13,00	14,00	99,00
42,00	15,00	30,00	107,00

Example   371

The first 10 patients of the 35 patient data file is above. The entire data file is in extras.springer.com, and is entitled "amos2.sav".

We will use SEM modeling for estimating variances and covariances in these data.

Variance $= \Sigma \left[(x - x_{mean})^2 \right]$.

It is a measure for the spread of the data of the variable x.

$$\text{Covariance} = \Sigma \left[(x_1 - x_{1mean}) \, (x_2 - x_{2mean}) \right].$$

It is a measure for the strength of association between the two variables x_1 and x_2. If the covariances are significantly larger than zero, this would mean that there is a significant association between them.

Command:

Analyze....click IBM SPSS Amos

The work area of Amos appears. The menu is in the second upper row. The toolbar is on the left. In the empty area on the right you can draw your networks.

click File....click Save as....Browse the folder you selected in your personal computer, and enter amos2....click Save.

In the first upper row the title amos2 has appeared, in the bottom rectangle left from the empty area the title amos2 has also appeared.

click Diagram....left click "Draw Observed" and drag to empty area....click the green rectangle and a colorless rectangle appears....left click it and a red rectangle appears....do this 3 more times and have the rectangles at different places

The underneath figure shows how your screen will look by now. There are four rectangle nodes for observed variables.

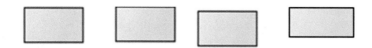

Next we will have to enter the names of the variables.

Command:

right click in the left upper rectangle....click Object Properties....Variable name: type "noncompliance"....close dialog box....the name is now in the rectangle.... do the same for the other three rectangles.

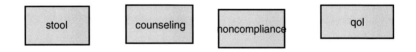

Next arrows have to be added to the diagram.

Command:
click Diagram. . . .click Draw Covariances.

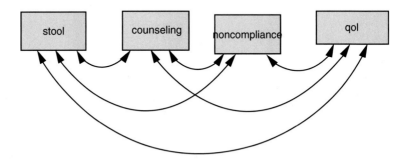

The above figure is now in the empty area. We will subsequently perform the analysis.

Command:
Analyze. . . .Calculate Estimates. . . .click File. . . .click Save as. . . .Browse for the folder of your choice and enter a name. . . .click Save. . . .click the new path diagram button that has appeared in the upper white rectangle left from the empty area.

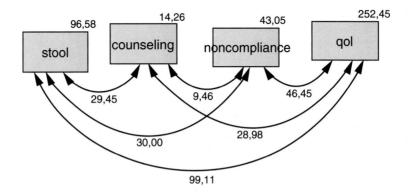

Unstandardized covariances of the variables are now in the graph and variances of the variables are in the right upper corner of the nodes.

We will also view the text output.

Example   373

Command:
click View....click Text output.

Covariances: (Group number 1 - Default model)

			Estimate	S.E.	C.R.	P	Label
stool	<-->	counseling	29,449	8,125	3,624	***	
counseling	<-->	noncompliance	9,461	4,549	2,080	,038	
noncompliance	<-->	qol	46,454	19,574	2,373	,018	
stool	<-->	noncompliance	30,003	12,197	2,460	,014	
counseling	<-->	qol	28,980	11,428	2,536	,011	
stool	<-->	qol	99,109	31,718	3,125	,002	

Variances: (Group number 1 - Default model)

	Estimate	S.E.	C.R.	P	Label
stool	96,576	23,423	4,123	***	
counseling	14,261	3,459	4,123	***	
noncompliance	43,050	10,441	4,123	***	
qol	252,462	61,231	4,123	***	

The above table shows the same values as the graph did, but p-values are added to the covariances. All of them except stool versus counseling were statistically significant with p-values from 0.002 to 0.038, meaning that all of these variables were closer associated with one another than could happen by chance.

Unstandardized covariances of variables with different units are not appropriate, and, therefore, Amos also produces standardized values (= unstandardized divided by their own standard errors).

click View....click Analysis Properties....click Output tab....mark Standardized estimates....close dialog box....choose Analyze....click Calculate Estimates....click the path diagram button....click standardized estimates in third white rectangle left from the empty area.

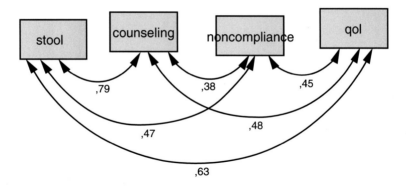

The standardized covariances is given.
Finally, we will view the standardized results as table.

click View. . . .click Text Output.

Variables

Name	Label	Observed	Variance Estimate	SE
stool		✓	96,58	23,42
counseling		✓	14,26	3,46
noncompliance		✓	43,05	10,44
qol		✓	252,46	61,23

Regression weights

Dependent	Independent	Estimate	SE	Standardized

Covariances

Variable 1	Variable 2	Estimate	SE	Correlation
stool	counseling	29,45	8,13	,79
counseling	noncompliance	9,46	4,55	,38
noncompliance	qol	46,45	19,57	,45
stool	noncompliance	30,00	12,20	,47
counseling	qol	28,98	11,43	,48
stool	qol	99,11	31,72	,63

The standardized covariances are in the column entitled Correlation.

Conclusion

SEM modeling can estimate covariances with their standard error and p-values. Significant p-values mean that the association of the variables is statistically significant and that the paired data are thus closer to one another than could happen by chance. The analyses of covariances is a basic methodology of SEM modeling used for testing and making clinical inferences like the presence of meaningful cause effect relationships like pharmacodynamic relationships. Unfortunately, overall statistics cannot be computed, but, instead, overall goodness of fit tests are given, that do, however, not prove whether a model is statistically significant from a null hypothesis, but does show, whether it provides better or worse information than any other DAG (directed acyclic graph) model as obtained from the same data.

Note

More background, theoretical and mathematical information of structural equation models like path analysis, factor analysis, and regression models are in

(1) Chap.14, Factor analysis, pp 167-181, in: Machine learning in medicine part 1, Springer Heidelberg Germany, 2013, in
(2) the Chap. 2, Multistage regression, in: SPSS for starters part two, pp 3-6, Springer Heidelberg Germany, 2012, and in
(3) the Chap. 14, Linear regression, basic approach, in: Statistics applied to clinical studies 5th edition, pp 161-176, Springer Heidelberg Germany, 2012, all of them from the same authors.

Chapter 51
Firth's Bias-adjusted Estimates for Biased Logistic Data Models (23 Challenger Launchings)

General Purpose

With logistic regressions, if sample sizes are small or strongly related to one of the binary outcomes, the estimated correlation coefficients may be biased. The same problem will, of course, occur, if your binary data are assessed in the form of contingency tables. This chapter is to assess Firth's method as a possible solution for the purpose.

Background

Firth's penalized likelihood approach is a method of addressing issues of separability, small sample sizes, and bias of the parameter estimates. A real data example is used to perform some comparisons between results from using the Firth method to results from the usual unconditional, conditional, and exact conditional logistic regression analyses. Firth was professor in statistics at University of Warwick UK, and published his method entitled Bias reduction in exponential family nonlinear models (Biometrika 2009; 96: 793). When the sample size is large enough, the unconditional estimates and the Firth penalized-likelihood estimates should be nearly the same. The example given underneath shows, that Firth's penalized likelihood approach compares favorably with unconditional, conditional, and exact conditional logistic regression; however, this is not an exhaustive analysis of Firth's method.

Electronic Supplementary Material The online version of this chapter (https://doi.org/10.1007/978-3-030-33970-8_51) contains supplementary material, which is available to authorized users.

Specific Scientific Question

This chapter is to assess Firth's method as a possible solution for analyzing clinical data with binary outcomes and a strong relationship of the predictor with one of the outcomes.

Example

Haim Bar from Cornell University Ithaca NY used the faulty 0-ring example to explain Firth's method (Cornell Statistical Consulting Unit, StatNews #82 February 2012). The faulty 0-ring example involves the Space shuttle Challenger program. Like most design-related disasters, the catastrophic failure of a pair of 0-rings in the space shuttle Challenger May 2012 was the result of more than just a poor design by the contractors for the ship's solid rocket booster. The famous 0-ring dataset assessed the presence/absence of 0-rings in launches of space shuttles. And one such absence proved to be fatal for the crew of the Challenger shuttle program. Interestingly, of 23 launchings 7 failed to produce 0-rings, while in these seven launchings four of them took place at a temperature below 66^0 F. In contrast, of the launchings at a temperature equal or above 66^0 F all of them produced 0-rings.

		0-ring present (1)	absent (0)
temperature	$< 66^0$ F (1)	4 (a)	0 (b)
	$> 66^0$ F (0)	16 (c)	3 (d)

A traditional chi-square test produced an insignificant effect.
Chi-square = 0.726, and p = 1.000.
A 1-sided Fisher exact test produced an insignificant effect as well with p = 0.547.
The underneath data are the actual data. Launching temperatures in °Fahrenheit (F), and presence of 0-rings are given. The results are pretty special. In particular, it is noticed that launching temperatures with the presence of 0-ring were never under 66°.

Example   379

launching temperatures	presence 0-ring (1,00)	launching temperature < 66⁰ F(1,00)
70,00	0,00	0,00
57,00	0,00	1,00
63,00	0,00	1,00
70,00	0,00	0,00
53,00	0,00	1,00
75,00	0,00	0,00
58,00	0,00	1,00
66,00	1,00	0,00
69,00	1,00	0,00
68,00	1,00	0,00
67,00	1,00	0,00
72,00	1,00	0,00
73,00	1,00	0,00
70,00	1,00	0,00
78,00	1,00	0,00
67,00	1,00	0,00
67,00	1,00	0,00
75,00	1,00	0,00
70,00	1,00	0,00
81,00	1,00	0,00
76,00	1,00	0,00
79,00	1,00	0,00
76,00	1,00	0,00

In contrast, absence of 0-rings were observed in 4/7 launchings with launching temperatures under 66°. Usually, a binary logistic regression with the log odds of low temperature as predictor and presence of 0-ring as outcome would seem appropriate for statistical testing these data. However, binary logistic regression is better adequate with symmetry of the two interventional groups. For convenience the data are in an SPSS data file and are saved in extras.springer.com entitled "Firthdata". Open your data in your computer mounted with SPSS statistical software.

Command:

Analyze....Regression....Binary Logistic Regression....Dependent: presence of 0-ring....Covariates: launchingtemp....click OK.

Variables in the Equation

		B	S.E.	Wald	df	Sig.	Exp(B)
Step 1ᵃ	VAR00001	-,232	,108	4,601	1	,032	,793
	Constant	15,043	7,379	4,156	1	,041	3412315,418

a. Variable(s) entered on step 1: VAR00001.

The above table is in the output of a standard binary logistic regression with logodds of the presence of an 0-ring as outcome and launching temperatures as predictor. The outcome is statistically significant at p = 0.032. The temperature predicts the presence of 0-rings. However, this result is not entirely appropriate given the asymmetry of the proportions of low temperatures in the 0-ring presence and absence launchings.

Next, a Firth's bias-adjusted estimate will be performed. It uses a so- called penalized likelihood function instead of a standard maximum likelihood estimate. It is a computationally laborious method, and a computer program is required other than SPSS statistical software, for example R, Mathlab, SAS statistical software. these programs also require considerable knowledge of syntax. We will use the Free Statistics and Forecasting software program from WESSA (WESSA.net/rwasp_logisticregression.wasp) based on the R program.

For the purpose enter the above program, and click "Bias-Reduced Logistic Regression-Free Statistics Software (Calculator). the enter from the above data the first two columns, and command "Compute".

A new window is opened and gives (1) a summary of computational transactions, (2) the coefficients of the bias-reduced logistic regression and (3) a summary of bias-reduced logistic regression. Also many logistic regression fittings are produced, based on penalization with Jeffreys invariant rather than derived from the aymptotic bias of estimated coefficients. Finally, drawings of ROC plots, and sensitivity and specificity results are in the output sheets. Underneath only summaries are given.

Summary of computational transaction	
Raw Input	view raw input (R code)
Raw Output	view raw output of R engine
Computing time	1 seconds
R Server	Big Analytics Cloud Computing Center

Coefficients of Bias-Reduced Logistic Regression				
Variable	Parameter	S.E.	t-stat	2-sided p-value
(Intercept)	11.9495445379743	6.25544800689536	1.91026198679972	0.0698512587833005
X	-0.186042338011932	0.0915823985708808	-2.03142023920615	0.0550595604490489

Summary of Bias-Reduced Logistic Regression	
Deviance	20.5253520625057
Penalized deviance	14.4443763162055
Residual Degrees of Freedom	21
ROC Area	0.78125
Hosmer–Lemeshow test	
Chi-square	NaN
Degrees of Freedom	8
P(>Chi)	NaN

Obviously, the traditional logistic regression produced a p-value of 0.032, while the Firth's bias-adjusted analysis produced a p-value of 0.055. The Firth analysis was less sensitive than the traditional logistic model. However, this is as expected. In statistics if you take into account more, for example symmetry of exposure groups, then you are likely to prove less. So, your p-value should rise.

Conclusion

With logistic regressions, if sample sizes are small or strongly related to one of the binary outcomes, the estimated correlation coefficients may be biased. The same problem will, of course, occur, if your binary data are assessed in the form of contingency tables. This chapter is to assess Firth's method as a possible solution for the purpose. Firth's method is a penalized likelihood approach. It is a method of addressing issues of separability, small sample sizes, and bias of the parameter estimates. A real data example is used to perform some comparisons between results from the Firth method to those from the usual unconditional, conditional, and exact conditional logistic regression methods. When the sample size is large enough, the unconditional estimates and the Firth penalized-likelihood estimates should be virtually the same.

Launching temperatures seem to be a predictor for the presence of 0 rings. This is supported by the underneath three dimensional graph. It shows, that the presence of low launching temperatures is associated with the absence of 0-rings, and the absence of low launching temperature is associated with many 0-ring launchings. Given the strong asymmetry between the numbers of low and higher temperature launchings, a traditional chi-square or logistics regression is not entirely appropriate, because a prior assumption is symmetry.

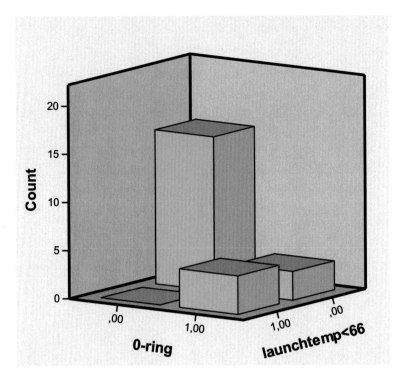

The current chapter shows, that a Firth's bias-adjusted logistic regression is more appropriate. As for the result, we should add, that, as expected, the p-value of the Firth's method was slightly less sensitive than that of the traditional logistic regression.

Note

More background, theoretical and mathematical information of binary logistic regression is available in the Chap. 19 of the current edition, and in the edition Statistics applied to clinical studies 5th edition, Chaps. 17 and 31, entitled "Logistic and Cox regression, Markov models, Laplace transformations", and "Time-dependent factor analysis", pp 199-218, and pp 353–364, Springer Heidelberg Germany 2012, from the same authors.

Chapter 52
Omics Research (125 Patients, 24 Predictor Variables)

General Purpose

Omics is a neologism and term related to the suffix -oma, frequently applied in medicine in nouns, that emphasize tumors or swellings. Omics refers to current names of scientific fields in biology ending on omics, including terms like

genomics,
transcriptomics,
proteonomics,
metabolomics,
lipidomics,
glucomics,
foodomics.

Most fields are in early stage of development, and a common characteristic is, that they involve big data requiring multivariate statistics. This and the next chapters will particularly focus on canonical big data models, and will use for the purpose canonical correlation analysis as well as sparse canonical correlations, the principles of which have already addressed in the Chaps. 23 and 27. These methods are suitable for statistically analyzing multivariate big data models and perform adequately, even if the numbers of predictor variables are much larger than those of the participating subjects like often observed with, for example, genetic data.

Electronic Supplementary Material The online version of this chapter (https://doi.org/10.1007/978-3-030-33970-8_52) contains supplementary material, which is available to authorized users.

Background

Multiomics refers to a biological analysis approach in which data sets involve multiple "omics", covering the study of "omes" such as the genome, proteome, transcriptome, epigenome, and microbiome. "Functional omics" aim at identifying the functions of as many variables as possible of a given "ome" field, and combines different -omics fields such as transcriptomics and proteomics with one another. A Masters degree entitled "Functional Omics" has started this year at the Imperial College London UK. The omics terminology is helpful in order to provide a better structure of big data studies. At the same time, everything is very much in a preliminary stage, and, methodologies for analyzing big data are very limited. Currently, papers addressing canonical statistics (see also Chap. 27) are fashion. But the 85 chapters of the current edition underline that machine learning offers many more relevant analytical methodologies. Nonetheless, canonical correlations and particularly sparse canonical correlations will be an eye opener, if you have data where the numbers of predictor variables in a study is a multiple of the numbers of participants. Canonical correlations is a multivariate analytic method related to Manova (multivariate analysis of variance). Manova (multivariate analysis of variance) is based on both multiple predictors and outcomes. Examples were already given in the Chap. 27. It can not only include multiple predictors and outcomes, but also optimal scalings enabling big data analyses. In addition, unlike latent variables methods (Chap. 22), it is scientifically rigid, because no subjective decision about the structure of the latent variables has to be taken. This chapter and the next one will address canonical correlations and regressions more broadly, and will be use for the purpose three versions of canonical networks, (1) a small data model, (2) a big data model, (3) a big data model with optimal scaling.

Condensed Terminology

canonical correlation analysis = multivariate analysis of correlation = analysis of multiple x and multiple y variables = it measures the strength of association between two canonical variates

variate = random variable = here "set of random variables obeying a given probabilistic law"

canonical variate (CV) = weighted sum of variables in an analysis of the above set of variables obeying a given probabilistic law

canonical weights = a and b values as indicated below, they are chosen such that the correlation is maximized (like the b values of a simple linear regression).

canonical root = pair of canonical variates

orthogonality of canonical variates = independence of one another

redundancy = proportion of variance in one set explained by the variance in the other set = it measures the magnitude of relationships between the two canonical variates as compared

Wilk's lambda = U value = test statistic of significance of canonical correlation coefficient

Bartlett's V = test statistic of significance of canonical correlation coefficient

eigenvectors = squared correlation coefficients that can be interpreted as amounts of certainty in the data explained by CV_x s about CV_y s.

dependent variables = outcome variables

predictor variables = covariates

Specific Scientific Question

This chapter and the next one will address canonical correlations and regressions more broadly, and will be use for the purpose three versions of canonical networks, (1) a small data model, (2) a big data model, (3) a big data model with optimal scaling.

Canonical Networks, Small Data Model

A simple example of a canonical network with two datasets of respectively three predictor (x) variables and two outcome (y) variables is given underneath. The ovals are variables with left from CVx1 the dataset 1 with three predictor variables (variable 1, 2, 3) and right from CVx1 in dataset 2 two outcome variables (variable 4, 5). The arrows are positive linear correlations.

CVx1 is the left canonical variate of the first root.
CVy1 is the right canonical variate of the first root.
CVx2 is the left canonical variate of the second root.
CVy2 is the right canonical variate of the second root.

Multiple x and y variables can be used to construct a canonical model using CVs

$$CVx_1 = a_1 \, x_1 + a_2 \, x_2 + a_3 \, x_3$$
$$CVy_1 = b_1 \, y_1 + b_2 \, y_2$$

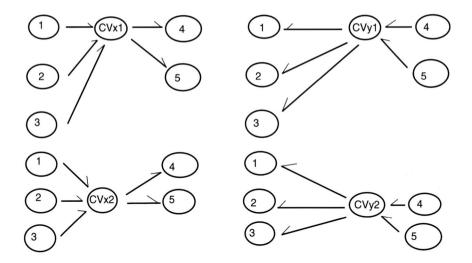

Canonical variates are variables like the latent factor of a factor analysis. However, canonical variates are linearly determined by all of the predictor and all of the outcome variables in a network, rather than by a subjectively selected subgroup of them. This makes canonical correlations scientifically more rigorous than factor analysis is. The linear correlation between the x and y variables in the first root is called the *first-root* canonical correlation. It covers much of the variability in the data from five variables. However, as observable from the above graphs, that all work simultaneously, some variability is left in the model, and in the *second-root* CVx2 is tested against CVy2. This does not produce as strong a canonical correlation as did the first root, but often some rest variability is present and this can be estimated from the eigenvalues of the canonical correlation of the roots. Eigenvalues are squared correlation coefficients that can be interpreted as amounts of certainty in the data explained by CVx variables about CVy variables.

Canonical Networks, Big Data Model

A 125 patients' data-file was supposed to include 28 variables consistent of both patients' microarray highly expressed gene expression levels (24 variables) and their drug efficacy scores (4 variables). All of the gene expression levels were standardized by scoring them on 11 points linear scales (0–10). The data-file was in SPSS statistical software and was entitled "optscalingfactorplscanonical-125". It is saved at "extras.springer.com". We will first perform a traditional manova. Open the file in your computer mounted with SPSS statistical software.

Command:

Analyze....General Linear Model....Multivariate....Dependent Variables: enter the four drug efficacy score....Covariates: enter the 24 genes....click OK.

The underneath table is in the output. The above table of multivariate tests is in the output. It shows, that manova can be considered, just like analysis of variance (anova), as a regression model with intercepts and regression coefficients. Just like anova, it is based on normal distributions, and the results as given indicate, that the model is adequate for the data. Generally, Pillai's method gives the best robustness. We can conclude that, with $p = 0.05$ as cut-off for statistical significance only the genes 16, and 17 are significant predictors of four drug efficacy outcome scores adjusted for one another.

However, we do not know the relative importance of one outcome variable versus the other. Separate anovas would be needed for that purpose. Also, unlike anova, manova does not give overall p-values, but rather separate p-values for separate covariates. However, in the given example, the genes are considered as a cluster of genes forming a single functional unit. Also, the outcome variables are considered as a cluster presenting different dimensions or aspects of drug efficacy. And, so, we are, particularly, interested in the combined effect of the set of covariates on the set of outcomes, rather than we are in modeling the separate variables. Instead of manova some latent variables models could have been constructed of the data, but latent variables are subjective, and a canonical regression is not, and may be a better choice.

Multivariate Tests[b]

Effect		Value	F	Hypothesis df	Error df	Sig.
Intercept	Pillai's Trace	,015	,364[a]	4,000	97,000	,834
	Wilks' Lambda	,985	,364[a]	4,000	97,000	,834
	Hotelling's Trace	,015	,364[a]	4,000	97,000	,834
	Roy's Largest Root	,015	,364[a]	4,000	97,000	,834
geneone	Pillai's Trace	,013	,317[a]	4,000	97,000	,866
	Wilks' Lambda	,987	,317[a]	4,000	97,000	,866
	Hotelling's Trace	,013	,317[a]	4,000	97,000	,866
	Roy's Largest Root	,013	,317[a]	4,000	97,000	,866
genetwo	Pillai's Trace	,011	,261[a]	4,000	97,000	,902
	Wilks' Lambda	,989	,261[a]	4,000	97,000	,902
	Hotelling's Trace	,011	,261[a]	4,000	97,000	,902
	Roy's Largest Root	,011	,261[a]	4,000	97,000	,902
genethree	Pillai's Trace	,043	1,078[a]	4,000	97,000	,372
	Wilks' Lambda	,957	1,078[a]	4,000	97,000	,372
	Hotelling's Trace	,044	1,078[a]	4,000	97,000	,372
	Roy's Largest Root	,044	1,078[a]	4,000	97,000	,372
genefour	Pillai's Trace	,021	,522[a]	4,000	97,000	,719
	Wilks' Lambda	,979	,522[a]	4,000	97,000	,719
	Hotelling's Trace	,022	,522[a]	4,000	97,000	,719
	Roy's Largest Root	,022	,522[a]	4,000	97,000	,719
genesixteen	Pillai's Trace	,147	4,193[a]	4,000	97,000	,004
	Wilks' Lambda	,853	4,193[a]	4,000	97,000	,004
	Hotelling's Trace	,173	4,193[a]	4,000	97,000	,004
	Roy's Largest Root	,173	4,193[a]	4,000	97,000	,004
geneseventeen	Pillai's Trace	,254	8,250[a]	4,000	97,000	,000
	Wilks' Lambda	,746	8,250[a]	4,000	97,000	,000
	Hotelling's Trace	,340	8,250[a]	4,000	97,000	,000
	Roy's Largest Root	,340	8,250[a]	4,000	97,000	,000
geneeighteen	Pillai's Trace	,066	1,710[a]	4,000	97,000	,154
	Wilks' Lambda	,934	1,710[a]	4,000	97,000	,154
	Hotelling's Trace	,071	1,710[a]	4,000	97,000	,154
	Roy's Largest Root	,071	1,710[a]	4,000	97,000	,154
genenineteen	Pillai's Trace	,073	1,915[a]	4,000	97,000	,114
	Wilks' Lambda	,927	1,915[a]	4,000	97,000	,114
	Hotelling's Trace	,079	1,915[a]	4,000	97,000	,114
	Roy's Largest Root	,079	1,915[a]	4,000	97,000	,114
genetwentyfour	Pillai's Trace	,082	2,161[a]	4,000	97,000	,079
	Wilks' Lambda	,918	2,161[a]	4,000	97,000	,079
	Hotelling's Trace	,089	2,161[a]	4,000	97,000	,079
	Roy's Largest Root	,089	2,161[a]	4,000	97,000	,079
genetwentyfive	Pillai's Trace	,021	,508[a]	4,000	97,000	,730
	Wilks' Lambda	,979	,508[a]	4,000	97,000	,730
	Hotelling's Trace	,021	,508[a]	4,000	97,000	,730
	Roy's Largest Root	,021	,508[a]	4,000	97,000	,730
genetwentysix	Pillai's Trace	,036	,898[a]	4,000	97,000	,469
	Wilks' Lambda	,964	,898[a]	4,000	97,000	,469
	Hotelling's Trace	,037	,898[a]	4,000	97,000	,469
	Roy's Largest Root	,037	,898[a]	4,000	97,000	,469
genetwentyseven	Pillai's Trace	,078	2,054[a]	4,000	97,000	,093
	Wilks' Lambda	,922	2,054[a]	4,000	97,000	,093
	Hotelling's Trace	,085	2,054[a]	4,000	97,000	,093
	Roy's Largest Root	,085	2,054[a]	4,000	97,000	,093
genethirtyone	Pillai's Trace	,060	1,545[a]	4,000	97,000	,195
	Roy's Largest Root	,037	,898[a]	4,000	97,000	,469

genetwentyseven	Pillai's Trace	,078	2,054[a]	4,000	97,000	,093
	Wilks' Lambda	,922	2,054[a]	4,000	97,000	,093
	Hotelling's Trace	,085	2,054[a]	4,000	97,000	,093
	Roy's Largest Root	,085	2,054[a]	4,000	97,000	,093
genethirtyone	Pillai's Trace	,060	1,545[a]	4,000	97,000	,195
	Wilks' Lambda	,940	1,545[a]	4,000	97,000	,195
	Hotelling's Trace	,064	1,545[a]	4,000	97,000	,195
	Roy's Largest Root	,064	1,545[a]	4,000	97,000	,195
genethirtytwo	Pillai's Trace	,011	,271[a]	4,000	97,000	,896
	Wilks' Lambda	,989	,271[a]	4,000	97,000	,896
	Hotelling's Trace	,011	,271[a]	4,000	97,000	,896
	Roy's Largest Root	,011	,271[a]	4,000	97,000	,896
genethirtythree	Pillai's Trace	,004	,105[a]	4,000	97,000	,980
	Wilks' Lambda	,996	,105[a]	4,000	97,000	,980
	Hotelling's Trace	,004	,105[a]	4,000	97,000	,980
	Roy's Largest Root	,004	,105[a]	4,000	97,000	,980
genethirtyfour	Pillai's Trace	,054	1,383[a]	4,000	97,000	,246
	Wilks' Lambda	,946	1,383[a]	4,000	97,000	,246
	Hotelling's Trace	,057	1,383[a]	4,000	97,000	,246
	Roy's Largest Root	,057	1,383[a]	4,000	97,000	,246
genethirtyseven	Pillai's Trace	,028	,696[a]	4,000	97,000	,596
	Wilks' Lambda	,972	,696[a]	4,000	97,000	,596
	Hotelling's Trace	,029	,696[a]	4,000	97,000	,596
	Roy's Largest Root	,029	,696[a]	4,000	97,000	,596
genethirtyeight	Pillai's Trace	,037	,921[a]	4,000	97,000	,455
	Wilks' Lambda	,963	,921[a]	4,000	97,000	,455
	Hotelling's Trace	,038	,921[a]	4,000	97,000	,455
	Roy's Largest Root	,038	,921[a]	4,000	97,000	,455
genethirtynine	Pillai's Trace	,068	1,777[a]	4,000	97,000	,140
	Wilks' Lambda	,932	1,777[a]	4,000	97,000	,140
	Hotelling's Trace	,073	1,777[a]	4,000	97,000	,140
	Roy's Largest Root	,073	1,777[a]	4,000	97,000	,140
geneforty	Pillai's Trace	,010	,253[a]	4,000	97,000	,907
	Wilks' Lambda	,990	,253[a]	4,000	97,000	,907
	Hotelling's Trace	,010	,253[a]	4,000	97,000	,907
	Roy's Largest Root	,010	,253[a]	4,000	97,000	,907
genefortyone	Pillai's Trace	,047	1,184[a]	4,000	97,000	,323
	Wilks' Lambda	,953	1,184[a]	4,000	97,000	,323
	Hotelling's Trace	,049	1,184[a]	4,000	97,000	,323
	Roy's Largest Root	,049	1,184[a]	4,000	97,000	,323
genefortytwo	Pillai's Trace	,022	,540[a]	4,000	97,000	,707
	Wilks' Lambda	,978	,540[a]	4,000	97,000	,707
	Hotelling's Trace	,022	,540[a]	4,000	97,000	,707
	Roy's Largest Root	,022	,540[a]	4,000	97,000	,707
genefortyfive	Pillai's Trace	,052	1,336[a]	4,000	97,000	,262
	Wilks' Lambda	,948	1,336[a]	4,000	97,000	,262
	Hotelling's Trace	,055	1,336[a]	4,000	97,000	,262
	Roy's Largest Root	,055	1,336[a]	4,000	97,000	,262
genefifty	Pillai's Trace	,036	,896[a]	4,000	97,000	,469
	Wilks' Lambda	,964	,896[a]	4,000	97,000	,469
	Hotelling's Trace	,037	,896[a]	4,000	97,000	,469
	Roy's Largest Root	,037	,896[a]	4,000	97,000	,469

a. Exact statistic
b. Design: Intercept + geneone + genetwo + genethree + genefour + genesixteen + geneseventeen + geneeighteen + genenineteen + genetwentyfour + genetwentyfive + genetwentysix + genetwentyseven + genethirtyone + genethirtytwo + genethirtythree + genethirtyfour + genethirtyseven + genethirtyeight + genethirtynine + geneforty + genefortyone + genefortytwo + genefortyfive + genefifty

Like manova, canonical analysis is based on multiple linear regression, used to find the best fit correlation coefficients for your data. However, because it works with Wilks'statistic and beta distributions rather than Pillai's statistic and normal distributions, it is able to more easily calculate overall correlation coefficients between sets of variables. Along this way, an overall canonical model can be further improved by removing unimportant variables. Canonical analysis may be arithmetically equivalent to factor-analysis/partial least squares analysis, but, conceptionally, it is very different. Unlike the latter, the former method does not produce new (latent) variables, but rather makes use of two sets of manifest variables. Also, unlike the latter, it complies with all of the requirements of traditional linear regression, and is, therefore, scientifically rigorous. A canonical analysis should start with a correlation matrix. Variables with small correlation coefficients must be removed from the model. If in canonical models the clusters of predictor and outcome variables have a significant relationship, then this finding can, just like with linear regression, be used for making predictions about individual patients. We will again use SPSS statistical software. The Menu does not offer canonical analysis, but the Syntax program does. Unlike manova, canonical regression is able to calculate overall correlation coefficients between sets of variables, and, in addition, it can assess, how sets of variables as a whole are related to separate variables. In order to assess the overall effect of clusters of genes on the cluster of drug efficacy scores, a canonical regression will be performed. Canonical regression is like collinearity-matrices available at SPSS' Syntax program.

Command:
click File....click New....click Syntax....the Syntax Editor dialog box is displayed....enter the following text: "manova" and subsequently enter all of the outcome variables....enter the text "WITH"....then enter all of the gene-names.... then enter the following text: /discrim all alpha(1)/print=sig(eigen dim)....click Run....mark All.

The output sheets have an overwhelmingly large output. It starts with a sample description, and then shows the general fit of the model reporting Pillai's, Hotellings', Wilk's and Roy's multivariate criteria. The commonly used test is Wilk's lambda, but we here find, that all of these tests were significant at $p < 0.05$.
Multivariate tests of Significance

Test Name	Value	Approx. F	Hypoth. DF	Error DF	Sig. of F
Pillai's	1,43646	2,33476	96,00	400,00	,000
Hotelling's	5,16950	5,14257	96,00	382,00	,000
Wilks'	,09216	3,32596	96,00	386,78	,000
Roys's	,81377				

The next section reports the canonical correlation coefficients and the eigenvalues of the canonical roots. The eigenvalues of the canonical roots are the squared canonical correlations (Sq.Cor). The first canonical correlation is .81108 with an explained variance of the canonical correlation of 96.87114 %.
Eigenvalues and Canonical Correlations

Root No.	Eigenvalue	Pct.	Cum. Pct.	Canon Cor.	Sq. Cor
1	4,36968	84,52819	84,52819	,90209	,81377
2	,35906	6,94580	91,47399	,51400	,26420
3	,26959	5,21495	96,68894	,46081	,21234
4	,17117	3,31106	100,0000	,38230	,14615

The significance of each root is tested next. The eigenvalues from the roots 1-4 get smaller and smaller as shown above. We find that of the four possible roots only the first one is significant at p < 0.05. The Wilks statistic for dimension reduction, in contrast, will get larger and larger, if you compare root 1 versus 4, 2 versus 4 etc.

Dimension Reduction Analysis

Roots	Wilks L.	F	Hypoth. DF	Error DF	Sig. of F
1 TO 4	,09216	3,32596	96,00	386,78	,000
2 TO 4	,49486	1,12989	69,00	293,63	,245
3 TO 4	,67254	,98723	44,00	198,00	,502
4 TO 4	,85385	,81507	21,00	100,00	,696

Subsequently, results are presented separately for each of the two sets of variables. With each set (1) raw canonical coefficients dependent variables are given, then (2) standardized coefficients for dependent variables, then (3) correlations between dependent and canonical variates, and, (4), variances in dependent variables explained by the canonical variates.

Raw canonical coefficients for dependent variables

	Outcome No.			
Variable	1	2	3	4
outcomeone	-,20723	,23307	,60362	,59071
outcometwo	-,27143	,42078	-,77071	-,45204
outcomethree	-,04568	-,73588	-,18231	,36818
outcomefour	-,06014	-,09791	,31408	-,64729

Easier to interpret are the underneath standardized coefficients (mean = 0, standard deviation = 1). Only the overall model (first root) is relevant, because the other three are not significant. The strongest influence on the first root is given by the variable outcomeone.

Standardized canonical coefficients for dependent variables

	Outcome No.			
Variable	1	2	3	4
outcomeone	-,41924	,47151	1,22114	1,19503
outcometwo	-,48743	,75563	-1,38405	-,81178
outcomethree	-,08294	-1,33615	-,33101	,66851
outcomefour	-,11447	-,18635	,59782	-1,23204

Correlations between dependent and canonical variables

Outcome No.

Variable	1	2	3	4
outcomeone	-,93876	,09353	,26375	,20105
outcometwo	-,94806	,09704	-,29481	-,06964
outcomethree	-,76934	-,61754	-,12682	,10335
outcomefour	-,70334	-,30830	,38126	-,51469

Variance in dependent variables explained by canonical variables

CAN. VAR.	Pct Var DEP	Cum Pct DEP	Pct Var COV	Cum Pct COV
1	71,66655	71,66655	58,32003	58,32003
2	12,36423	84,03077	3,26661	61,58664
3	7,94783	91,97860	1,68766	63,27430
4	8,02140	100,0000	1,17232	64,44662

In practice, what we are most interested in, is the performance of the separate highly expressed genes. They are given by SPSS statistical software in two forms:

(1) raw canonical coefficients, and standardized canonical coefficients for the predictor variables (the covariates), and linear correlations between the predictor variables and the outcomes,
(2) multiple linear regressions between predictor variables and the outcomes.

Raw canonical coefficients for covariates

Outcome No.

COVARIATE	1	2	3	4
geneone	-,03015	,09123	-,06991	-,08351
genetwo	-,02490	-,09397	,15328	,00762
genethre	,01910	-,14362	-,13615	-,52709
genefour	,00863	,05182	,09987	,29043
genesixt	-,14834	,15976	,15857	,06347
geneseve	-,20628	-,35309	-,40433	,08853
geneeigh	-,05451	,18389	-,06243	-,03310
genenine	-,04075	,19228	-,15727	,21956
genetwen	-,06646	,02569	,35721	,09540
genetw_1	-,00881	,00112	,17449	-,01782
genetw_2	-,05875	-,00499	-,12299	-,05858
genetw_3	,06759	-,13239	,05305	-,15234
genethir	,01611	-,27397	,13172	,28156
geneth_1	,00088	,12573	-,08922	-,13862
geneth_2	-,02028	,01976	-,01340	,10703
geneth_3	,03267	,16245	,29664	-,05683
geneth_4	,01327	-,14575	,04381	-,10288
geneth_5	,00301	-,13328	-,21525	-,01882
geneth_6	-,01311	,27249	-,02058	-,11066
genefort	-,02162	,07212	-,00217	-,03129
genefo_1	-,08956	-,23357	-,02860	,26859
genefo_2	,06994	,11247	-,03157	-,08540
genefo_3	,02742	,15429	-,29585	-,12984
genefift	-,06579	-,13692	,00516	-,01756

Standardized canonical coefficients for covariate and outcomes 1-4

COVARIATE	1	2	3	4
geneone	-,05655	,17111	-,13112	-,15663
genetwo	-,04915	-,18550	,30259	,01504
genethre	,03462	-,26033	-,24679	-,95539
genefour	,01352	,08117	,15645	,45496
genesixt	-,33592	,36179	,35909	,14373
geneseve	-,41555	-,71128	-,81452	,17834
geneeigh	-,13037	,43977	-,14931	-,07915
genenine	-,09191	,43367	-,35471	,49518
genetwen	-,17351	,06707	,93260	,24906
genetw_1	-,01751	,00223	,34659	-,03539
genetw_2	-,15574	-,01323	-,32601	-,15528
genetw_3	,16414	-,32152	,12883	-,36997
genethir	,03295	-,56033	,26939	,57585
geneth_1	,00137	,19584	-,13898	-,21592
geneth_2	-,03546	,03456	-,02344	,18718
geneth_3	,07173	,35671	,65136	-,12479
geneth_4	,03465	-,38058	,11440	-,26863
geneth_5	,00636	-,28159	-,45480	-,03976
geneth_6	-,03524	,73216	-,05531	-,29732
genefort	-,04529	,15107	-,00455	-,06555
genefo_1	-,18093	-,47184	-,05777	,54260
genefo_2	,14740	,23704	-,06654	-,17999
genefo_3	,05330	,29993	-,57511	-,25239
genefift	-,13274	-,27625	,01042	-,03543

Correlations between covariates and outcomes 1–4

COVARIATE	1	2	3	4
geneone	-,42963	,06489	,04088	-,21349
genetwo	-,65539	-,09186	,14701	-,24731
genethre	-,70159	-,05005	,11020	-,44672
genefour	-,36673	,01323	,12275	,09791
genesixt	-,85787	,12883	,04881	,01551
geneseve	-,86852	-,22677	-,13245	,00323
geneeigh	-,60993	,17115	-,05772	-,05115
genenine	-,71660	,21535	-,00575	,16148
genetwen	-,79848	-,02434	,34534	-,12986
genetw_1	-,38351	-,10275	,38253	-,11397
genetw_2	-,75715	-,05221	,15614	-,19667
genetw_3	-,44085	-,26696	,30990	-,26853
genethir	-,00761	-,24227	-,03885	,17757
geneth_1	,02468	,01556	-,20785	,08371
geneth_2	-,05846	-,00992	-,07491	,07089
geneth_3	-,05272	,05096	,06076	-,12567
geneth_4	,09481	-,19547	-,15096	-,19031
geneth_5	,02052	-,07988	-,40702	-,15116
geneth_6	,01697	,19782	-,11331	-,22161
genefort	,12588	-,03432	-,10264	-,25134
genefo_1	-,05583	-,14843	-,10735	,02311
genefo_2	-,08181	-,07991	-,17714	-,03680
genefo_3	,00270	,02229	-,23933	-,14829
genefift	,04453	-,16500	-,07991	-,03764

The covariates, the highly expressed genes, were pretty good predictors of outcomes with correlation coefficients particularly with outcome 1 up to 0.868 and better than 0.3 in 12 of the 24 predictors. The outcomes 3 and 4 were less well predicted.

Multiple linear regression between covariates and dependent variable outcome 1

COVARIATE	B	Beta	Std. Err.	t-Value	Sig. of t	Lower -95%	CL- Upper
geneone	,0303491521	,0281366586	,08784	,34551	,730	-,14392	,20462
genetwo	,0723868183	,0706357307	,10988	,65880	,512	-,14561	,29038
genethre	-,1621286537	-,1452623734	,12136	-1,33588	,185	-,40291	,07866
genefour	,0599668514	,0464344997	,09535	,62892	,531	-,12920	,24914
genesixt	,3185314549	,3565531580	,08329	3,82420	,000	,15328	,48378
geneseve	,2334174059	,2324291884	,09291	2,51237	,014	,04909	,41774
geneeigh	,0907754331	,1073099035	,06305	1,43964	,153	-,03432	,21587
genenine	,0839831839	,0936286507	,06909	1,21557	,227	-,05309	,22105
genetwen	,2190201868	,2826513087	,08138	2,69139	,008	,05757	,38047
genetw_1	,0553427849	,0543364605	,06606	,83771	,404	-,07573	,18641
genetw_2	,0608220516	,0796906025	,07534	,80725	,421	-,08866	,21030
genetw_3	-,1393087908	-,1672329053	,06237	-2,23344	,028	,26306	,01556
genethir	,0219227755	,0221633675	,08793	,24931	,804	-,15253	,19638
geneth_1	-,0327719235	-,0252326351	,10287	-,31856	,751	-,23687	,17133
geneth_2	,0500085551	,0432298677	,09841	,50818	,612	-,14523	,24525
geneth_3	,0239330927	,0259774102	,08464	,28277	,778	-,14399	,19185
geneth_4	-,0421348984	-,0543849429	,06304	-,66841	,505	-,16720	,08293
geneth_5	-,0739707926	-,0772549998	,07287	-1,01516	,312	,21854	,07059
geneth_6	,0267006062	,0354624119	,06556	,40725	,685	-,10337	,15678
genefort	,0386566543	,0400278176	,06448	,59954	,550	-,08926	,16658
genefo_1	,1654607955	,1652258808	,12101	1,36736	,175	-,07462	,40554
genefo_2	-,1299219892	-,1353526423	,11451	-1,13459	,259	,35711	,09726
genefo_3	-,1248980934	-,1200163335	,08601	-1,45205	,150	,29555	,04575
genefift	,0979330145	,0976733104	, 08600	1,13875	,258	-,07269	,26856

Multiple linear regression between covariates and dependent variable outcome 2

COVARIATE	B	Beta	Std. Err.	t-Value	Sig. of t	Lower -95%	CL- Upper
geneone	,0755245028	,0788782991	,07601	,99367	,323	-,07527	,22632
genetwo	-,0079380455	-,0087261413	,09508	-,08349	,934	-,19656	,18069
genethre	,0162122519	,0163636584	,10501	,15438	,878	-,19213	,22456
genefour	-,0468667156	-,0408825283	,08250	-,56805	,571	-,21055	,11682
genesixt	,2004174743	,2527267717	,07207	2,78077	,006	,05743	,34341
geneseve	,3795987542	,4258198560	,08039	4,72189	,000	,22010	,53909
geneeigh	,1170059372	,1558199560	,05456	2,14455	,034	,00876	,22525
genenine	,1076806899	,1352377578	,05978	1,80123	,075	-,01092	,22629
genetwen	,0126689609	,0184183853	,07042	,17992	,858	-,12703	,15237
genetw_1	-,0280795441	-,0310573282	,05716	-,49121	,624	,14149	,08533
genetw_2	,1225959005	,1809529616	,06519	1,88046	,063	,00675	,25194
genetw_3	-,1213187431	-,1640645746	,05397	-2,24784	,027	,22840	,01424
genethir	-,0948765102	-,1080544398	,07609	-1,24696	,215	-,24583	,05608
geneth_1	,0383051461	,0332247332	,08902	,43032	,668	-,13830	,21491
geneth_2	,0310646546	,0302517032	,08515	,36482	,716	-,13787	,20000
geneth_3	-,1052675173	-,1287167640	,07324	-1,43736	,154	,25057	,04003
geneth_4	-,0392059665	-,0570075783	,05455	-,71878	,474	-,14742	,06901
geneth_5	,0368492505	,0433549495	,06305	,58445	,560	-,08824	,16194
geneth_6	,0548619232	,0820846363	,05673	,96706	,336	-,05769	,16741
genefort	,0416952036	,0486370752	,05579	,74735	,457	-,06899	,15238
genefo_1	,1107701198	,1246089671	,10471	1,05792	,293	-,09696	,31850
genefo_2	-,0855557462	-,1004099991	,09908	-,86347	,390	-,28213	,11102
genefo_3	,0500902036	,0542226884	,07443	,67301	,502	-,09757	,19775
genefift	,0883561889	,0992721579	,07442	1,18734	,238	-,05928	,23599

Multiple linear regression between covariates and dependent variable outcome 3

COVARIATE	B	Beta	Std. Err.	t-Value	Sig. of t	Lower -95%	CL- Upper
geneone	-,0131624650	-,0135962968	,09934	-,13250	,895	-,21025	,18393
genetwo	,0698118567	,0759017148	,12427	,56179	,576	-,17673	,31635
genethre	,0353384092	,0352775000	,13726	,25746	,797	-,23698	,30765
genefour	-,0305057209	-,0263189320	,10784	-,28289	,778	-,24445	,18344
genesixt	,0825764606	,1029877740	,09420	,87660	,383	-,10432	,26947
geneseve	,5126924887	,5688160307	,10507	4,87935	,000	,30423	,72116
geneeigh	-,0330389041	-,0435165596	,07131	-,46331	,644	-,17452	,10844
genenine	-,0270309862	-,0335765265	,07814	-,34594	,730	-,18205	,12799
genetwen	,0378833605	,0544719343	,09203	,41162	,681	-,14471	,22048
genetw_1	-,0093328434	-,0102094362	,07472	-,12491	,901	,15757	,13890
genetw_2	,0857634815	,1252004507	,08521	1,00648	,317	,08329	,25482
genetw_3	-,0254224520	-,0340030672	,07054	-,36039	,719	,16538	,11453
genethir	,1438194336	,1620000807	,09945	1,44619	,151	-,05348	,34112
geneth_1	-,0740487274	-,0635236903	,11635	-,63645	,526	-,30488	,15678
geneth_2	,0232622496	,0224051965	,11129	,20901	,835	-,19754	,24407
geneth_3	-,1703400008	-,2060018497	,09572	-1,77952	,078	,36025	,01957
geneth_4	,0552478834	,0794529113	,07129	,77495	,440	-,08619	,19669
geneth_5	,0945078603	,1099744248	,08241	1,14683	,254	-,06899	,25800
geneth_6	-,1462750535	-,2164586068	,07415	-1,97273	,051	,29338	,00083
genefort	-,0163321870	-,0188425396	,07292	-,22397	,823	-,16100	,12834
genefo_1	,2697766313	,3001544180	,13685	1,97127	,051	-,00174	,54129
genefo_2	-,1557285246	-,1807630627	,12951	-1,20249	,232	,41266	,10121
genefo_3	-,1013948089	-,1085569699	,09728	-1,04231	,300	,29439	,09160
genefift	,1600040744	,1778014390	,09726	1,64507	,103	-,03296	,35297

Multiple linear regression between covariates and dependent variable outcome 4

COVARIATE	B	Beta	Std. Err.	t-Value	Sig. of t	Lower -95%	CL- Upper
geneone	,0167888327	,0165433709	,11495	,14605	,884	-,21127	,24485
genetwo	,1068125941	,1107809190	,14379	,74283	,459	-,17847	,39209
genethre	,1721235919	,1639122102	,15882	1,08373	,281	-,14298	,48723
genefour	-,1014265153	-,0834754127	,12478	-,81285	,418	-,34898	,14613
genesixt	,1602095770	,1906066209	,10900	1,46978	,145	-,05605	,37647
geneseve	,1872564333	,1981854290	,12158	1,54014	,127	-,05396	,42848
geneeigh	,0018837173	,0023668174	,08252	,02283	,982	-,16183	,16559
genenine	-,1436043097	-,1701615565	,09041	-1,58830	,115	,32298	,03577
genetwen	,1562354943	,2143009555	,10650	1,46706	,145	,05505	,36752
genetw_1	,0753287113	,0786083027	,08646	,87130	,386	-,09620	,24685
genetw_2	,0532717383	,0741857445	,09860	,54028	,590	-,14235	,24889
genetw_3	,0331055543	,0422397775	,08163	,40558	,686	-,12884	,19505
genethir	,0017801782	,0019128514	,11507	,01547	,988	-,22652	,23008
geneth_1	-,0169054862	-,0138345771	,13463	-,12557	,900	-,28400	,25019
geneth_2	-,0260399361	-,0239252817	,12878	-,20220	,840	-,28154	,22946
geneth_3	,0320295982	,0369509890	,11076	,28917	,773	-,18772	,25178
geneth_4	,0811135732	,1112776141	,08249	,98327	,328	-,08255	,24478
geneth_5	-,0283683548	-,0314903885	,09536	-,29750	,767	-,21755	,16082
geneth_6	-,0317945662	-,0448825577	,08580	-,37057	,712	-,20202	,13843
genefort	,0153521273	,0168959944	,08438	,18195	,856	-,15205	,18276
genefo_1	,0684579443	,0726581554	,15836	,43230	,666	-,24572	,38263
genefo_2	-,0969584663	-,1073612009	,14985	-,64702	,519	-,39426	,20035
genefo_3	-,1299547485	-,1327254620	,11256	-1,15450	,251	,35328	,09337
genefift	,1290501272	,1367989512	,11255	1,14665	,254	-,09424	,35234

In the regression analyses the genes 16, 17, 20 and 23 were frequently significantly predictors of outcomes 1, 2, 3 with p-values like 0.000, 0.014, 0.008. The outcome 4 was not well predicted by the highly expressed genes. The main conclusion from the above overwhelmingly large output is, thus, pretty limited. The genes 16, 17, 20, 23 were the main predictors of three of the four outcome variables. Nonetheless, a clinically relevant conclusion can be made from this analysis.

Canonical Networks, Big Data Model with Optimal Scaling

The term functional data analysis is sometimes used in connection with big data analysis. It was fist applied by Ramsay in a book entitled likewise and edited by Springer Heidelberg Germany in 2005. It particularly applied to analyses that include more than a single statistical method in one and the same analysis. Omics studies can easily include thousands of predictor variables but a "functional data analysis" combining a canonical data dimension reduction, and subsequent optimal scaling of the reduced dimensions is helpful. More information of "functional data analysis" is in the Chaps. 25 and 26 of Regression Analysis in Medical Research edited by Springer Heidelberg Germany, 2018, from the same authors. More information of Optimal Scaling is in the current edition Chap. 23.

Expression of genes is sometimes highly complex and often regulated by the expression of many other genes. A joint analysis will be needed, if such associations are expected. Multivariate techniques are based on models with multiple predictor and multiple outcome variables. Canonical regressions is better suitable for the purpose than traditional multivariate analyses of variance (manovas) (Chap. 22) or factor analyses (Chap. 22). The problems with traditional manovas as compared to canonical analysis is, that, with the former, statistical power is rapidly lost with increased numbers of variables, and with concealed negative correlations between the outcome variables. The problems with factor analyses as compared to canonical analysis is, that the former involves subjective decisions about the choice of the principle components, while the latter does not. The joint analysis with canonical regression and optimal scaling is called sparse canonical regression. It is a pretty novel methodology and will be addressed more broadly in the next chapter. For now, an important advantage of sparse canonical regressions is, that it can handle more oredictor variables, and, at the same time, leaves little room for subjective decisions about the choice of the principle components of the latent factors. In addition, an optimal scaling procedure is part of the analysis, and so is a penalization with ridge or lasso penalties, further reducing the numbers of predictor variables, that, with omics research, not rarely exceeds the number of subjects. A real data example will be given in the next chapter.

Conclusion

Canonical variates are variables like the latent factor of a factor analysis. However, canonical variates are linearly determined by all of the predictor and all of the outcome variables in a network, rather than by a subjectively selected subgroup of them. This makes canonical correlations scientifically more rigorous than factor analysis is. We should add, that, although computationally similar to canonical variates, they are conceptually very different, because of the subjectively selected variables to constitute latent variables. Of the latent variables models, multivariate discriminant analysis is most similar to canonical correlation analysis.

The benefit of penalization procedures using ridge, lasso and/or elastic web penalties is, that it enables to include thousands of predictors in a single canonical analysis. Therefore, particularly penalized canonical correlation analysis is like no other current methodology suitable for big data and multidimensional data like in omics research. This may be exciting, but, at this time, still in a very preliminary stage of development. In the next chapter penalized canonical regression will be addressed more broadly.

Note

Big data analysis is increasingly the subject of machine learning methodologies, and is often performed with canonical correlation analysis, particularly sparse canonical correlation is capable of analyzing thousands of predictor variable, and suitable for genome-wide diagnostic testing. Methodologies are reviewed in the Chaps. 27, 53, and the current chapter. The Chap. 20, in the 2019 edition "Efficacy Analysis in Clinical Trials an Update", Springer Heidelberg Germany, from the same authors, addresses validation procedures of big data prior to analyses.

Chapter 53
Sparse Canonical Correlation Analysis

General Purpose

In clinical research big data are particularly observed with genetic studies of the relationships between the genome and clinical outcomes like metabolics and more. With genome wide research we have to take into account the presence of 250.0000 genes in every human cell, and 2000 nucleic acids in every gene. This chapter is to address whether sparse canonical correlation analysis performs better in identifying predictor-outcome relationships than other analytic methods so far.

Background

Canonical-correlation analysis (CCA), also called canonical variates analysis, is a way of inferring information from cross-covariance matrices. If we have two vectors $X = (X_1, \ldots, X_n)$ and $Y = (Y_1, \ldots, Y_m)$ of random variables, and there are correlations among the variables, then canonical-correlation analysis will find linear combinations of X and Y which have maximum correlation with one another. It was discussed already in the Chaps. 27 and 52 of this edition. It is adequate for assessing the level of correlation between multiple predictors on multiple outcomes, and does better so than does traditional multivariate analysis, because it accounts the relative importance of separate variables. Underneath the model of a simple canonical analysis is described.

A simple example of a canonical network with two datasets of respectively three predictor (x) variables and two outcome (y) variables is given underneath. The ovals are variables with left from CVx1 the dataset 1 with three predictor variables (variable 1, 2, 3) and right from CVx1 in dataset 2 two outcome variables (variable 4, 5). The arrows are positive linear correlations.

CVx1 is the left canonical variate of the first root.

© Springer Nature Switzerland AG 2020
T. J. Cleophas, A. H. Zwinderman, *Machine Learning in Medicine – A Complete Overview*, https://doi.org/10.1007/978-3-030-33970-8_53

CVy1 is the right canonical variate of the first root.
CVx2 is the left canonical variate of the second root.
CVy2 is the right canonical variate of the second root.

Root is the name of a pair of canonical variates. A canonical variate is the weighted sum of variables in a canonical analysis. Multiple x and y variables can be used to construct a canonical model using CVs. The underneath terms a_1 to a_6 and b_1 to b_4 are best fit linear regression coefficients.

$CVx_1 = a_1 x_1 + a_2 x_2 + a_3 x_3$
$CVy_1 = b_1 y_1 + b_2 y_2$
$CVx_2 = a_4 x_1 + a_5 x_2 + a_6 x_3$
$CVy_1 = b_3 y_1 + b_4 y_2$

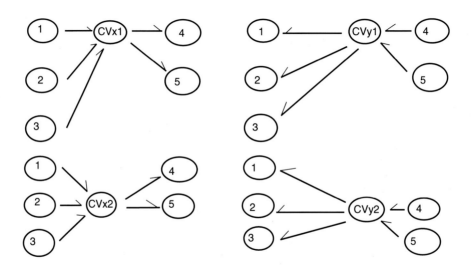

Canonical variates (CVs) are variables like the latent factor of a factor analysis. However, canonical variates are linearly determined by all of the predictor and all of the outcome variables in a network, rather than by a subjectively selected subgroup of them. This does make canonical correlations more rigorous than factor analysis does. The linear correlation between the x and y variables in the first root is called the *first-root* canonical correlation. It covers much of the variability in the data from five variables. However, as observable from the above graphs, all variables work simultaneously, and some variability is left in the model. In the *second-root* CVx2 is tested against CVy2. This does not produce as strong a canonical correlation as did the first root, but often some rest variability is present, and this can be estimated from the eigenvalues of the canonical correlation of the roots. Eigenvalues are squared correlation coefficients that can be interpreted as amounts of certainty in the data explained by CVx variables about CVy variables. Additional information of eigenvalues is given in the Chap. 54.

Canonical regression analysis is available in SPSS statistical software. In the past few years it is being extended by another methodology entitled sparse canonical, otherwise called penalized canonical correlation analysis. It is not yet available in SPSS, but PMA package in R statistical software is helpful for the purpose.

Waaijenborg and Zwinderman and others (Stat Applic in Gen Mol Biol 2008; 7:1, and Parhomenko et al 2007; 1: s 19) contributed to its development, and showed that, with shrinking factors (λ-factors) included, regression coefficients reduced from b to $b/(1+\lambda)$, enabling dimension reductions in data models with very many variables, and that this method will be particularly suitable, if you are searching for a limited number of strong predictors. A simple example of various shrinkings suitable for univariate prediction models is given in the Chap. 23. With sparse canonical regressions the shrinkings are similar, but the computation are more complex because of multiple outcome variables in the multivariate models here applied.

In order for a predictive model to make reliable, otherwise called reproducible, predictions a validation procedure of the variables is required. For the purpose various methods are available, one more complex but usually better than the other examples of basic validations is given in the Chap. 58, where decision trees with either continuous or binary outcomes are applied for making predictions. However, this method is not entirely appropriate, because a decision tree is built from a data file, and, subsequently, the same data file is applied once more for computing the health risk probabilities from the built tree. Obviously, the accuracy must be close to 100%, because the test sample is 100% identical to the sample used for building the tree, and, therefore, this accuracy does not mean too much. With neural networks this problem of duplicate usage of the same data is solved by randomly splitting the data into two samples, a training sample and a test sample (Chap. 12 in Machine learning in medicine part one, pp 145–156, Artificial intelligence, multilayer perceptron modeling, Springer Heidelberg Germany, 2013, from the same authors). The Chap. 8 shows, that the splitting methodology, otherwise called partitioning, is also feasible for assessing diagnostic accuracy, and that it performed pretty well with a sensitivity of 90–100 % and an overall accuracy of 94%. However, measures of error of predictive models like the above one are based on residual methods, assuming a-priori defined data distributions, particularly normal distributions. Big data and other machine learning data file may not meet such assumptions, and distribution free methods of validation, like cross-validations may be more safe. For the purpose cross-validation splitting the data into a k-fold scale and comparing it with a k-1 fold scale is a common method. The principle methods of it are in the Chap. 79.

Specific Scientific Question

Is sparse canonical correlation analysis capable of analyzing thousands of predictor variables and is it, therefore, suitable for genome-wide diagnostic testing.

Example

As example, a study of the group of Zwinderman from Amsterdam University was taken. In 12209 genes, as measured in 45 genetic carriers of glioblastoma, Waaijenborg and Zwinderman (BMC Bioinformatics 2009; 10: 315) tried and identified 25 genes with a correlation of over 0.9 with genes known to be in the glioblastoma pathway of genes. The authors performed a sparse canonical analysis of the over 12000 genes in 45 patients with the aggressive genetic brain tumor glioblastoma. So far known metabolic pathways are in the database KEGG (Kanehisa et al: Nucleic Acids Research 2008; 36: D 480)). No less than 12.209 genes were identified by the authors from genome-wide gene-expression microarray data. A prior pilot study showed, that genes are correctly identified, if the correlation with the pathway genes for glioblastoma was 0.3 or more. Sparse canonical regression is "functional data analysis" combining canonical dimension reduction with optimal scaling of the reduced dimensions with spline smoothing, and subsequent ridge, lasso, or elastic net regularization for increased precision in a single analysis with a final analysis result with better precision than that of the traditional canonical regression of the same data. For their best result they combined ridge and lasso penalties. Information of the penalties are in the Chap. 23, albeit in a univariate rather than multivariate version.

The univariate version is available in SPSS and for multivariate penalizing the authors applied R statistics, a free software with a very limited menu, but for those, who have the time to learn the syntax, a reliable program ahead of many expensive alternatives. Both cross correlations between pathway genes and canonical variates of the remaining genes, and those between remaining genes and canonical variates of the pathway genes were computed by the software. In the underneath tables the results are summarized. No less than 32 genes had a cross correlation over 90%.

Shrinking Factor
In their sparse canonical model they applied ridge regression for the purpose of adjusting multicollinearities and overdispersion in the data. The regression coefficient b is minimized by a shrinking factor λ such that $b_{ridge} = b/(1+\lambda)$, and that, with $\lambda = 0$, $b_{ridge} = b$, and, with $\lambda = \infty$, $b_{ridge} = 0$. Calculations are based on likelihood statistics adjusted for degrees of freedom, and it seems true, that there always exists a value for λ such, that it provides a better scale model than does the traditional linear model. Knowing this, one elegant approach is the Monte Carlo approach, i.e. perform multiple tests in order to find the best fit scale.

Permutation Analysis
If the number of variables is very large, as in the data example given, there is a high probability that a random pair of variables has a high correlation just by chance at least 5% of the times. To identify a canonical correlation that is large by chance, a permutation analysis was performed. In the permuted validation dataset the correlation coefficient will be zero, unlike in the non-permuted comparisons.

Example 403

Cross-validation

The optimal level of the shrinkage factor for each canonical variate pair, i.e., the level with producing the best fit correlation coefficient, was determined by p-fold cross-validations with the data divided into p subgroups of patients, p-1 subgroups as training set and 1 subgroup as validation set.

Simulated Data

Simulated data from 50 individuals consistent of 50 standard normally distributed x-variables whose covariances were determined from weakly correlated components ($r = 0.1$). We should add, that simulated data may not be as good as real data, but real data are in practice frequently unavailable.

Results of Simulated Data Analysis

Cross-validations with 10 training sets and the validation-sets showed, that, in the event of a correlation over 0.3, the existence of a glioblastoma pathway was correctly identified.

Root 1	2	3	4	5	6	7	8	9
1 -0.15	-0.06	0.30	0.72	0.21	0.06	-0.12	0.00	0.16
2 -0.03	-0.18	0.08	0.46	0.25	-0.24	-0.05	-0.24	0.17
3 -0.53	0.28	0.23	-0.01	0.12	-0.07	0.32	-0.14	0.05
4 -0.16	-0.28	0.14	-0.15	0.20	0.05	-0.05	-0.36	-0.18
5 0.10	0.15	0.14	0.02	0.01	-0.22	-0.13	0.17	-0.25
6 0.89	0.00	0.08	-0.09	-0.02	0.02	0.04	0.03	0.07
7 -0.16	0.23	0.26	-0.01	0.39	0.05	-0.08	-0.04	0.26
8 0.44	-0.16	-0.27	0.12	-0.18	0.05	-0.20	0.12	-0.12
9 -0.28	-0.09	0.31	0.06	0.51	0.12	-0.18	-0.19	0.14
10 -0.10	0.63	0.04	0.03	0.52	0.13	0.13	0.09	-0.10
11 -0.21	0.74	0.29	-0.22	0.11	0.04	-0.03	0.02	-0.10
12 -0.11	-0.24	0.87	0.01	-0.11	0.01	-0.03	-0.01	-0.02
13 -0.21	-0.16	0.61	0.22	-0.18	-0.02	0.23	0.04	-0.12
14 -0.16	0.38	-0.31	-0.16	0.06	-0.04	0.06	0.07	-0.13
15 -0.17	-0.38	0.06	0.04	0.11	-0.16	0.02	0.43	0.32
16 -0.06	0.15	-0.09	0.71	0.03	0.08	0.11	0.18	-0.01
17 0.33	-0.13	0.05	0.07	-0.28	0.05	0.10	0.51	-0.14
18 0.01	0.10	-0.02	0.30	0.17	-0.12	0.04	-0.14	0.63
19 0.28	0.22	0.03	-0.40	0.26	-0.25	-0.06	0.28	0.04
20 -0.01	0.73	-0.17	-0.14	-0.05	0.11	-0.07	0.30	0.14

The above table gives the first 20 of 50 correlation assessments between gene expressions of Glioblastoma pathway genes and those of the 45 patient genes remaining after removal of their Glioblastoma pathway genes. The data from nine root canonical correlations are given. Correlation > 0.3 or < -0.3 were, thus, correctly identified.

Results of Real Data Analysis

The underneath table shows the correlation assessments between the gene expressions of the 45 patient genes after removal of their Glioblastoma pathway genes and those of Glioblastoma pathway genes. Cross-correlations (Cs) between the gene expressions of Glioblastoma pathway genes and those of nine root canonical variates (Root 1 to 9) of the patients studied are shown.

Root	1	2	3	4	5	6	7	8	9
C2	-0.11	0.93	-0.03	-0.01	-0.03	0.08	-0.08	0.07	-0.02
CD68	-0.26	0.92	-0.03	0.05	-0.13	0.00	-0.04	-0.11	-0.03
CENPF	-0.26	-0.12	0.92	0.02	-0.02	0.06	0.00	0.05	-0.03
CLTB	0.91	0.01	-0.02	0.17	0.09	0.01	-0.06	-0.10	-0.08
SERPIN	-0.11	0.91	0.02	-0.01	0.14	0.04	0.05	-0.16	-0.07
EPB49	0.90	0.06	-0.09	-0.02	0.01	0.14	0.04	0.09	0.08
FCGR2A	-0.28	0.92	-0.01	-0.09	0.00	0.00	0.01	-0.04	-0.06
FCGR2B	-0.27	0.93	-0.03	-0.02	0.01	-0.01	-0.04	0.03	0.03
FCGR3A	-0.26	0.91	0.10	0.04	-0.09	0.06	-0.01	0.02	-0.01
CXCL2	0.09	0.91	0.03	0.22	-0.03	-0.16	-0.03	0.08	-0.01
LYN	-0.20	0.93	0.04	0.11	0.05	0.03	-0.01	0.02	0.04
NEF3	0.93	0.14	-0.03	-0.15	0.01	0.02	0.01	-0.08	0.01
NEFL	0.94	-0.01	0.01	0.01	0.00	0.03	0.08	-0.10	-0.01
NRGN	0.93	0.00	0.16	-0.02	-0.02	0.01	0.01	0.02	0.00
RAB3A	0.92	-0.20	0.07	0.11	0.04	-0.08	-0.04	-0.06	0.03
SNCG	0.91	0.03	-0.12	-0.15	-0.06	0.17	0.07	0.04	0.05
STK6	-0.21	0.01	0.93	0.01	0.00	-0.01	0.04	0.16	-0.03
TNFAIP	-0.08	0.95	-0.04	0.00	0.10	-0.03	-0.02	-0.01	-0.02
VSNL1	0.96	0.04	0.03	0.03	0.01	0.02	-0.04	-0.02	-0.02
VAMP8	-0.20	0.94	0.01	0.04	-0.07	-0.03	0.09	-0.06	-0.02
CCNB2	-0.26	-0.18	0.90	0.04	0.03	-0.08	0.07	-0.04	0.01
PHYHIP	0.94	-0.04	-0.07	-0.03	0.01	-0.02	-0.06	0.02	-0.10
TACC3	-0.30	0.04	0.90	-0.11	-0.07	-0.10	-0.06	0.00	0.01
NPC2	-0.30	0.92	-0.11	-0.01	-0.01	-0.01	-0.01	0.01	-0.03
UBE2C	-0.25	-0.20	0.93	0.01	-0.01	0.05	-0.05	0.04	-0.01
SULT4A1	0.95	0.06	0.03	-0.05	-0.05	-0.02	-0.05	0.04	-0.02
OSTF1	0.16	0.91	0.03	0.02	0.02	-0.10	-0.05	0.09	0.03
MS4A4A	-0.20	0.90	-0.06	0.06	-0.23	0.00	-0.03	0.00	-0.06
SLC17A7	0.92	-0.03	0.14	-0.02	-0.09	0.10	0.10	0.06	-0.02
NAPB	0.95	0.02	0.00	0.04	0.04	-0.02	0.02	0.15	0.01
FLJ145	0.93	-0.01	-0.04	0.10	0.07	-0.03	0.05	-0.10	0.06
LOC441	-0.17	0.91	-0.01	-0.01	-0.02	0.01	0.03	-0.04	0.15

The above 32 path Gliobastoma pathway genes, according to Babelonics in Nucleic Acid Research 2006; W 4742-7, were significantly involved in immunoglobin binding like observed in brain cancers (Ueda et al, Int J Cancer 2007; 120: 1704). Obviously, the cross-correlations of the roots 1-3 provided the best sensitivity with correlation coefficients over 0.9 in respectively 13, 14, and 5 of the 32 path way genes. In the remainder of the canonical variates cross-correlations with the pathway genes were very low and negligible.

Conclusion

In the Hadoop framework 2014 for processing and storing big data (www. tutorialspoint.com), multiple standard computers with multiple relatively simple programs are advisedly applied for accomplishing big data validations. With cross-validations the data are divided into a subgroup, a training set and a remaining subgroup entitled the validation set.

In the current chapter a sparse canonical regression of a 9 root canonical model with 12209 predictor variables, all of them gene expression levels, was successfully performed. In order for the overall analysis to be successful, the sparse canonical model was supported by additional methodologies including optimal penalization of the regression coefficients, simulation studies, permutations and cross-validations. Obviously, the effort was not without pain, but the result was excellent. In a micoarray data set of 12209 genes 25 novel genes ready for incorporation into the currently already existing Glioma pathway network, were detected by the analysis. Canonical like any other analytic tool only works with validated data. This may be hard to obtain with big data, and it is a lot of work. What is validation ? Validation may be a semantic term. Yet validation is the most important part of big data studies, and, currently, demands more than half of the time spent on big data analysis (Xie C, Big data validation case study. Published by IEEE (Institute for Electrical Electronic Engineers) Computer Society, 2017, Doi 10.1109 BigDataService). In clinical research the term validation refers, according to the American Food Drug Administration (Process Validation Document 2016), to process design, process qualification, continuous process verification, and different types are implicated, like retrospective, prospective, concurrent validation, and re-validation. With diagnostic tests, which are commonly called the basis of clinical research, validation consists of accuracy, reproducibility, precision assessments (Chap 51: in Statistics applied to clinical studies 5th edition, from the same authors, Springer Heidelberg Germany, 2012). With clinical trial protocols validation consists of a clearly defined prior hypothesis, a valid design, explicit description of methods, and uniform data analysis. Validating big data can, theoretically, be accomplished using all of the rules applied with small data, but this is very laborious, if not hardly possible. If big data consists of a pool of multiple small data, special checks are required, like publication bias, heterogeneity, robustness checks. Tentative alternatives for big data validation are occasionally given. In the above reference from Xie it says: multiple teams are appointed to validate fractions of data analyses. In the Hadoop framework 2014, an open-source framework to process and store big data (www.tutorialspoint.com), multiple standard computers with multiple relatively simple programs are advisedly applied for accomplishing big data validations. The current chapter example did not apply the traditional method of validation based on null hypothesis testings but rather applied data driven training of validation sets based on cross-validations and permutations of simulated data. For the purpose data were divided into a subgroup, a training set and a remaining subgroup entitled the validation set. Big data analysis is increasingly the subject of machine learning methodologies, and is often performed with canonical correlation analysis. Particularly sparse canonical correlation is capable of analysing thousands of predictor variable, and suitable for genome-wide diagnostic testing. Methodologies are reviewed in the Chaps. 27, 52, and the current chapter. The Chap. 20, in: the 2019 edition Efficacy Analysis in Clinical Trials an Update, Springer Heidelberg Germany, from the same authors, also addresses validation procedures prior to big data analyses.

Note

Big data analysis is increasingly the subject of machine learning methodologies, and is often performed with canonical correlation analysis. Particularly sparse canonical correlation is capable of analysing thousands of predictor variable, and suitable for genome-wide diagnostic testing. Methodologies are reviewed in the Chaps. 27, 52, and the current chapter. The Chap. 20, in the 2019 edition "Efficacy Analysis in Clinical Trials an Update", Springer Heidelberg Germany, from the same authors, addresses validation procedures prior to big data analyses.

Chapter 54
Eigenvalues, Eigenvectors and Eigenfunctions (45 and 250 Patients)

General Purpose

This chapter will, with the help of patient data, explain, how eigenvalues can be efficiently used to estimate proportions of uncertainty in multidimensional datasets. Data examples previously applied in this edition will be applied again.

Background

David Hilbert died in 1943, Göttingen Germany. He was an important contributor to formalistic foundations of current mathematics. He was the first to use the German word "eigen", which means "own" or "proper", to denote "eigenvalues" and "eigenvectors" in 1904, though he may have been following a related usage 100 years earlier by the German mathematician Helmholtz. For some time, the term in English was "proper value", but the term "eigenvalue" is standard today. Defining eigenvalues is hard, and their meaning is not always consistently used. But they are sometimes described as the length and width of the best fit ellipse pattern that can be drawn around the data from two variables plotted along an orthogonal x- and y-axis. The division sum of length and width could be called eigenfunctions, and, with their place in a graph taken into account, they can be called eigenvectors. Dividing the length of their "eigen values" by that of their widths always gives a term >1, and is also called the condition index. The larger the condition index the stronger the correlation between the two variables, and the closer we will be to 100% collinearity. Eigenvalues and Eigenvectors and all of the terms, as we shall see, related to them are important in the study of covariance assessments of variables. More broadly,

Electronic Supplementary Material The online version of this chapter (https://doi.org/10.1007/978-3-030-33970-8_54) contains supplementary material, which is available to authorized users.

T. J. Cleophas, A. H. Zwinderman, *Machine Learning in Medicine – A Complete Overview*, https://doi.org/10.1007/978-3-030-33970-8_54

eigenvalues are sometimes defined as the proportion variance explained in a datamodel, and if that is an unpaired analysis of variance model, it will be obtained by computing between group sums divided by within group sums. Collinearity diagnostics is an important application of eigenvalues.

Principal component analysis is also based on eigenvalues of the components, that are used to produce a reduced noise in the data. Discriminant Analysis is another application: categorical outcomes and multiple linear predictor variables are used to constitute functions with eigenvalues, that will be stronger the larger they are.

Obviously, eigenvalues are currently recognized as a concept at the heart of data science. Like expressed by Fahrad Malik, mathematician at Harvard's FinTechExplained, it may even be considered the basis of computing and mathematics (2018).

Specific Scientific Question

This chapter will, with the help of data examples, explain, how eigenvalues can be efficiently used to estimate proportions of uncertainty in multidimensional datasets.

Collinearity Diagnostics and Eigenvalues

In statistics, multicollinearity (also collinearity) is a phenomenon in which one predictor variable in a multiple regression model can be linearly predicted from other predictors with a substantial degree of accuracy. In this situation the coefficient estimates of the multiple regression may change erratically in response to small changes in the model or the data. A 45 patient dataset was assessed for the predictive effect of all kinds of laboratory values on the erythocyte sedimentation rate (ESR), which was used as a surrogate endpoint for severity of disease. The datafile has already been used in the Chap. 24 of this edition. It is in extras/springer.com, and is entitled "discriminantanalysis". Start by opening the datafile in your computer mounted with SPSS statistical software.

Command:
Analyze. . . .Correlate. . . .click Bivariate. . . .click Bivariate Correlations. . . .enter: gammagt. . . .asat. . . .alat. . . .bili. . . .ureum. . . .creatinine. . . .creatinine clearance. . . . c-reactive proteine. . . .leucos. . . .mark Pearson. . . .click OK.

A correlation matrix of all of the supposedly predicting laboratory variables on severity of disease is given.

Correlations

		gammagt	asat	alat	bili	ureum	creatinine	creatinine clearance	c-reactive protein	leucos
gammagt	Pearson Correlation	1	,916**	,921**	,904**	,842**	,821**	-,739**	,467**	,765**
	Sig. (2-tailed)		,000	,000	,000	,000	,000	,000	,001	,000
	N	45	45	45	45	45	45	45	45	45
asat	Pearson Correlation	,916**	1	,819**	,836**	,761**	,809**	-,642**	,286	,702**
	Sig. (2-tailed)	,000		,000	,000	,000	,000	,000	,057	,000
	N	45	45	45	45	45	45	45	45	45
alat	Pearson Correlation	,921**	,819**	1	,919**	,888**	,884**	-,765**	,643**	,805**
	Sig. (2-tailed)	,000	,000		,000	,000	,000	,000	,000	,000
	N	45	45	45	45	45	45	45	45	45
bili	Pearson Correlation	,904**	,836**	,919**	1	,890**	,872**	-,814**	,583**	,847**
	Sig. (2-tailed)	,000	,000	,000		,000	,000	,000	,000	,000
	N	45	45	45	45	45	45	45	45	45
ureum	Pearson Correlation	,842**	,761**	,888**	,890**	1	,919**	-,795**	,668**	,865**
	Sig. (2-tailed)	,000	,000	,000	,000		,000	,000	,000	,000
	N	45	45	45	45	45	45	45	45	45
creatinine	Pearson Correlation	,821**	,809**	,884**	,872**	,919**	1	-,805**	,642**	,888**
	Sig. (2-tailed)	,000	,000	,000	,000	,000		,000	,000	,000
	N	45	45	45	45	45	45	45	45	45
creatinine clearance	Pearson Correlation	-,739**	-,642**	-,765**	-,814**	-,795**	-,805**	1	-,670**	-,932**
	Sig. (2-tailed)	,000	,000	,000	,000	,000	,000		,000	,000
	N	45	45	45	45	45	45	45	45	45
c-reactive protein	Pearson Correlation	,467**	,286	,643**	,583**	,668**	,642**	-,670**	1	,750**
	Sig. (2-tailed)	,001	,057	,000	,000	,000	,000	,000		,000
	N	45	45	45	45	45	45	45	45	45
leucos	Pearson Correlation	,765**	,702**	,805**	,847**	,865**	,888**	-,932**	,750**	1
	Sig. (2-tailed)	,000	,000	,000	,000	,000	,000	,000	,000	
	N	45	45	45	45	45	45	45	45	45

**. Correlation is significant at the 0.01 level (2-tailed).

The intercorrelations between most of the x-variables in the predictive model were statistically very significant. This could mean that a number of predictors were so much similar to one another that they were no longer independent predictor of the outcome "severity of disease" as estimated with the ESR values. This situation is called multicollinearity and needs to be assessed, because it will produce an invalid multiple regression analysis.

Command:

Analyze....Regression....Linear....Dependent; enter erythocyte sedimentation rate....Independent (s) : enter all of the predictors already used in the correlation matrix....Collinearity Statistics....click OK.

The underneath tables are in the output.

Coefficients[a]

Model		Collinearity Statistics	
		Tolerance	VIF
1	gammagt	,053	18,762
	asat	,075	13,349
	alat	,060	16,752
	bili	,095	10,491
	ureum	,103	9,708
	creatinine	,074	13,483
	creatinine clearance	,106	9,421
	c-reactive protein	,188	5,307
	leucos	,049	20,464

a. Dependent Variable: esr

A tolerance < 0.3 is often observed. It means that over 70% of the variability in the data is explained by other predictors than the ones included in the analysis. A VIF (variance inflating factor) over the amount of 2, generally, confirms a problem with collinearity. This is, obviously, observed all the time. Also in the output is the underneath table of eigenvalues and condition indices.

Collinearity Diagnostics[a]

Model	Dimension	Eigenvalue	Condition Index	Variance Proportions									
				(Constant)	gammagt	asat	alat	bili	ureum	creatinine	creatinine clearance	c-reactive protein	leucos
1	1	7,790	1,000	,00	,00	,00	,00	,00	,00	,00	,00	,00	,00
	2	1,493	2,284	,00	,00	,00	,00	,00	,00	,00	,02	,00	,00
	3	,402	4,400	,00	,01	,04	,00	,00	,00	,00	,01	,09	,00
	4	,094	9,093	,00	,05	,02	,09	,01	,04	,08	,02	,05	,00
	5	,073	10,303	,00	,01	,03	,03	,01	,29	,02	,09	,02	,01
	6	,060	11,422	,00	,00	,18	,00	,36	,05	,04	,01	,21	,00
	7	,039	14,082	,00	,20	,00	,10	,24	,34	,13	,01	,01	,00
	8	,032	15,540	,01	,03	,22	,24	,30	,03	,07	,07	,34	,00
	9	,013	24,211	,01	,69	,39	,46	,07	,21	,61	,05	,01	,01
	10	,002	62,053	,97	,01	,12	,09	,01	,02	,05	,72	,27	,97

a. Dependent Variable: esr

An eigenvalue close to zero confirms the presence of multicollinearity. Except for the one dimension and 2 dimension data model all of the eigenvalues were under 1.0 and close to zero. The condition indices furthermore support things. A condition index is obtained by taking the square root of the ratio of the largest eigenvalue and each successive eigenvalue. A value over 15 means a problem with multicollinearity. Values over 30 mean a serious problem of multicollinearity. The table is very obvious. Through the step down method insignificant predictors can be successively removed from the multiple regression model until a model has remained with maximal numbers of significant predictors.

Command:

Analyze....Regression....Linear....Dependent; enter erythocyte sedimentation rate....Independent (s) : enter all of the predictors already used in the correlation matrix....click OK.

The multiple linear regression of the complete model shows, that, overall, the predictor significantly predicts the outcome severity of disease.

ANOVA[b]

Model		Sum of Squares	df	Mean Square	F	Sig.
1	Regression	76964,094	9	8551,566	30,502	,000[a]
	Residual	9812,706	35	280,363		
	Total	86776,800	44			

a. Predictors: (Constant), leucos, asat, c-reactive protein, ureum, bili, creatinine clearance, creatinine, alat, gammagt
b. Dependent Variable: esr

Coefficients[a]

Model		Unstandardized Coefficients		Standardized Coefficients	t	Sig.
		B	Std. Error	Beta		
1	(Constant)	-15,031	38,657		-,389	,700
	gammagt	-,002	,030	-,018	-,074	,941
	asat	,019	,017	,228	1,099	,279
	alat	,008	,032	,056	,242	,810
	bili	-,019	,077	-,044	-,241	,811
	ureum	-,009	,366	-,004	-,025	,980
	creatinine	,069	,040	,357	1,712	,096
	creatinine clearance	-,077	,180	-,075	-,429	,671
	c-reactive protein	,032	,171	,024	,185	,854
	leucos	1,844	1,381	,343	1,336	,190

a. Dependent Variable: esr

None of the predictors were, however, significant predictors due to the multicollinearity in the model.

After removing the most insignificant predictors from the analysis. The underneath results were obtained.

Model Summary

Model	R	R Square	Adjusted R Square	Std. Error of the Estimate
1	,941[a]	,886	,877	15,55462

a. Predictors: (Constant), leucos, asat, creatinine

ANOVA[b]

Model		Sum of Squares	df	Mean Square	F	Sig.
1	Regression	76857,007	3	25619,002	105,887	,000[a]
	Residual	9919,793	41	241,946		
	Total	86776,800	44			

a. Predictors: (Constant), leucos, asat, creatinine
b. Dependent Variable: esr

Coefficients[a]

Model		Unstandardized Coefficients		Standardized Coefficients	t	Sig.
		B	Std. Error	Beta		
1	(Constant)	-30,018	11,817		-2,540	,015
	asat	,017	,008	,200	2,223	,032
	creatinine	,073	,027	,376	2,694	,010
	leucos	2,279	,619	,424	3,684	,001

a. Dependent Variable: esr

The model summary and analysis of variance (ANOVA) tables show, that the current model is much more precise than the first model with a F statistic of 105.8 versus one of only 30.5. In the final model three significant predictors were present with p-values between 0.01 and 0.03.

Discriminant Analysis and Eigenvalues

A discriminant analysis has a categorical rather than continuous or binary dependent variable. Discriminant analysis can be used to make a diagnosis from categorical outcomes. The data example already applied in the Chap. 24 and in the above section of this chapter will be used again. Laboratory screenings were performed in patients with different types of sepsis (urosepsis, bile duct sepsis, and airway sepsis) as outcomes. The 45 patients data file is in extras.springer.com, and is entitled "discriminantanalysis". The analysis of the Chap. 24 will be partly repeated, but now attention will be given to the magnitudes of the eigenvalues of the correlations between the pooled discriminating variables and the different outcome scores, called the functions one, two, and three. In the example applied laboratory screenings were performed in patients with different types of sepsis (urosepsis, bile duct sepsis, and airway sepsis). Can discriminant analysis of laboratory screenings improve reliability of diagnostic processes.

Var 1	Var 2	Var 3	Var 4	Var 5	Var 6	Var 7	Var 8	Var 9	Var 10	Var 11
8,00	5,00	28,00	4,00	2,50	79,00	108,00	19,00	18,00	16,00	2,00
11,00	10,00	29,00	7,00	2,10	94,00	89,00	18,00	15,00	15,00	2,00
7,00	8,00	30,00	7,00	2,20	79,00	96,00	20,00	16,00	14,00	2,00
4,00	6,00	16,00	6,00	2,60	80,00	120,00	17,00	17,00	19,00	2,00
1,00	6,00	15,00	6,00	2,20	84,00	108,00	21,00	18,00	20,00	2,00
23,00	5,00	14,00	6,00	2,10	78,00	120,00	18,00	17,00	21,00	3,00
12,00	10,00	17,00	5,00	3,20	85,00	100,00	17,00	20,00	18,00	3,00
31,00	8,00	27,00	5,00	,20	68,00	113,00	19,00	15,00	18,00	3,00
22,00	7,00	26,00	5,00	1,20	74,00	98,00	16,00	16,00	17,00	3,00
30,00	6,00	25,00	4,00	2,40	69,00	90,00	20,00	18,00	16,00	3,00
2,00	12,00	21,00	4,00	2,80	75,00	112,00	11,00	14,00	19,00	1,00
10,00	21,00	20,00	4,00	2,90	70,00	100,00	12,00	15,00	20,00	1,00

Var = variable
Var 1 gammagt
Var 2 asat
Var 3 alat
Var 4 bilirubine
Var 5 ureum
Var 6 creatinine
Var 7 creatinine clearance
Var 8 erythrocyte sedimentation rate
Var 9 c-reactive protein
Var 10 leucocyte count
Var 11 type of sepsis (1-3 as described above)

The first 12 patients are shown only, the entire data file is entitled "discriminantanalysis" and is in extras.springer.com. Start by opening again the datafile in your computer mounted with SPSS statistical software.

Command:
Analyze....Grouping Variable(s): enter diagnosisgroup....click Define Range....
Minimum 1....maximum 3....Continue....Independent(s): enter all of the predictors variables....click Statistics....mark All groups equal....mark Summary table....mark Within-groups....mark Combined groups....click Continue....
click OK.

In the output the underneath tables are given. In addition to measures for checking the contribution of individual predictors to your discriminant model, the discriminant analysis procedure has provided eigenvalues and Wilks' lambdas for seeing how well the discriminant model as a whole fits the data.

Eigenvalues

Function	Eigenvalue	% of Variance	Cumulative %	Canonical Correlation
1	1,045[a]	86,5	86,5	,715
2	,164[a]	13,5	100,0	,375

a. First 2 canonical discriminant functions were used in the analysis.

The above eigenvalues table provides information about the relative efficacy of each discriminant function. When there are two groups, the canonical correlation is the most useful measure in the table, and it is equivalent to Pearson's correlation between the discriminant scores and the groups. The magnitude of the eigenvalues with discriminant analysis is small as compared to those with collinearity statistics, but this is normally so, and no problem, as long as they are nonnegative values. The larger they are, the stronger predictions can be made from the models. Thus, here, virtually all of the variance explained by the model is due to the first two discriminant functions. The third function's eigenvalue was minuscule and has been skipped from the analysis by SPSS. The eigenvalue can be defined as an estimate of the proportion of the variance in the functions explained by the discriminant model.

Wilks' Lambda

Test of Function(s)	Wilks' Lambda	Chi-square	df	Sig.
1 through 2	,420	32,500	20	,038
2	,859	5,681	9	,771

The above Wilks' lambdas are measures of how well each function separates cases into groups. It is equal to the proportion of the total variance in the discriminant scores not explained by differences among the groups. Smaller values of Wilks' lambda indicate greater discriminatory ability of the function.

The associated chi-square statistic tests the hypothesis, that the means of the functions listed are equal across groups. A significance value at $p < 0.05$ indicates, that the discriminant function performs better than does chance at separating the groups.

Structure Matrix

	Function	
	1	2
asat	,574*	,184
gammagt	,460*	,203
c-reactive protein	-,034	,761*
leucos	,193	,537*
ureum	,461	,533*
creatinine	,462	,520*
alat	,411	,487*
bili	,356	,487*
esr	,360	,487*
creatinine clearance	-,083	-,374*

Pooled within-groups correlations between discriminating variables and standardized canonical discriminant functions
Variables ordered by absolute size of correlation within function.

*. Largest absolute correlation between each variable and any discriminant function

When there is more than one discriminant function (here two), an asterisk(*) marks each variable's largest absolute correlation with one of the functions. Within each function, these marked variables are then ordered by the size of the correlation. The asat and gammagt variables produced the largest correlations with the first canonical discriminate function, while the other predictor variables produced the best correlations for the second discriminate function. But as the second discriminate function is useless here, so are the asterisk-marked predictors here.

In conclusion, the eigenvalues are estimates of proportion of variance in the models explained by the models. Like the above collinearity statistics, discriminant analysis is based on eigenvalues of regression models between predictor variables and outcome categories, each of one is called a function here. Although we have three outcome categories only two functions produced virtually 100% of the variability in the model.

The Wilk's lambda is a multivariate test-statistic to assess whether a predictive model 's effect is significantly different from a zero effect. Obviously, only the first discriminant function produced a p-value statistically significant at 0.038, which needs not be adjusted for multiple testing, because everything is in a single test. And so, despite the low level of significance, it is not necessarily meaningless. More information on discriminant analyses is given in the Chap. 24 of this edition.

Principal Components and Eigenvalues

In the Chap. 22 of this edition latent variables models were assessed. A few unmeasured factors, otherwise called latent factors, are identified to explain a much larger number of measured factors, e.g., highly expressed chromosome-clustered genes. Unlike factor analysis, partial least squares (PLS) identifies not only exposure (x-value), but also outcome (y-value) variables. The measured factors are commonly called components and the latent factor analysis is commonly just called factor analysis. We will use the data example from the Chap. 22 once more. Twelve highly expressed genes are used to predict drug efficacy in 250 patients.

G1	G2	G3	G4	G16	G17	G18	G19	G24	G25	G26	G27	O1	O2	O3	O4
8	8	9	5	7	10	5	6	9	9	6	6	6	7	6	7
9	9	10	9	8	8	7	8	8	9	8	8	8	7	8	7
9	8	8	8	8	9	7	8	9	8	9	9	9	8	8	8
8	9	8	9	6	7	6	4	6	6	5	5	7	7	7	6
10	10	8	10	9	10	10	8	8	9	9	9	8	8	8	7
7	8	8	8	8	7	6	5	7	8	8	7	7	6	6	7
5	5	5	5	5	6	4	5	5	6	6	5	6	5	6	4
9	9	9	9	8	8	8	8	9	8	3	8	8	8	8	8
9	8	9	8	9	8	7	7	7	7	5	8	8	7	6	6
10	10	10	10	10	10	10	10	10	8	8	10	10	10	9	10
2	2	8	5	7	8	8	8	9	3	9	8	7	7	7	6
7	8	8	7	8	6	6	7	8	8	8	7	8	7	8	8
8	9	9	8	10	8	8	7	8	8	9	9	7	7	8	8

Var G1-27 highly expressed genes estimated from their arrays' normalized ratios
Var O1-4 drug efficacy scores (the variables 20-23 from the initial data file).

The data from the first 13 patients are shown above (see extras.springer.com for the entire data file entitled "optscalingfactorplscanonical"). Start by opening the datafile in your computer.

Command:

Analyze....Dimension Reduction....Factor....enter variables into Variables box....click Extraction....Method: click Principle Components....mark Correlation Matrix, Unrotated factor solution....mark Based on eigenvalues....Eigenvalues greater than; enter 0....Maximal Iterations plot Convergence: enter 25.... Continue....click Rotation....Method: click Varimax....mark Rotated solution....mark Loading Plots....Maximal Iterations: enter 25....Continue.... click Scores.... mark Save as variables....click Regression....mark Display factor score coefficient matrix ....click OK.

In the output many tables are given.

Communalities

	Initial	Extraction
geneone	1,000	,721
genetwo	1,000	,772
genethree	1,000	,770
genefour	1,000	,709
genesixteen	1,000	,768
geneseventeen	1,000	,584
geneeighteen	1,000	,466
genenineteen	1,000	,662
genetwentyfour	1,000	,732
genetwentyfive	1,000	,586
genetwentysix	1,000	,717
genetwentyseven	1,000	,741

Extraction Method: Principal
Component Analysis.

Extraction communalities are estimates of the variance in each variable accounted for by the components. The communalities in this table are all pretty high, which indicates that the extracted components represent the variables well. If any communalities are very low in a principal components extraction, you may need to extract another component.

Total Variance Explained

Component	Initial Eigenvalues			Extraction Sums of Squared Loadings			Rotation Sums of Squared Loadings		
	Total	% of Variance	Cumulative %	Total	% of Variance	Cumulative %	Total	% of Variance	Cumulative %
1	6,017	50,145	50,145	6,017	50,145	50,145	3,718	30,984	30,984
2	1,192	9,930	60,075	1,192	9,930	60,075	2,398	19,985	50,968
3	1,019	8,491	68,566	1,019	8,491	68,566	2,112	17,597	68,566
4	,888	7,402	75,968						
5	,529	4,409	80,377						
6	,463	3,856	84,233						
7	,416	3,465	87,697						
8	,406	3,385	91,082						
9	,368	3,067	94,149						
10	,268	2,236	96,385						
11	,243	2,029	98,414						
12	,190	1,586	100,000						

Extraction Method: Principal Component Analysis.

The total variance explained by the initial solution, extracted components, and rotated components is displayed. This first section of the table shows the initial eigenvalues. The "Totals" column gives the eigenvalues, or amount of variance in the original variables accounted for by each component.

The % of variance column gives the ratio, expressed as a percentage, of the variance accounted for by each component to the total variance in all of the variables.

The cumulative % column gives the percentage of variance accounted for by the first n components. For example, the cumulative percentage for the second component is the sum of the percentage of variance for the first and second components.

For the initial solution, there are as many components as variables, and in a correlations analysis, the sum of the eigenvalues equals the number of components. You appear to have requested, that eigenvalues greater than 1 be extracted, so 3 principal components form the extracted solution.

The second section of the table shows the extracted components. They explain nearly 70% of the variability in the original ten variables, so you can considerably reduce the complexity of the data set by using these components, although with a 30% loss of information.

Total Variance Explained

Component	Initial Eigenvalues			Extraction Sums of Squared Loadings			Rotation Sums of Squared Loadings		
	Total	% of Variance	Cumulative %	Total	% of Variance	Cumulative %	Total	% of Variance	Cumulative %
1	6,017	50,145	50,145	6,017	50,145	50,145	3,718	30,984	30,984
2	1,192	9,930	60,075	1,192	9,930	60,075	2,398	19,985	50,968
3	1,019	8,491	68,566	1,019	8,491	68,566	2,112	17,597	68,566

The underneath scree plot helps you to determine the optimal number of components. The eigenvalue of each component in the initial solution is plotted.

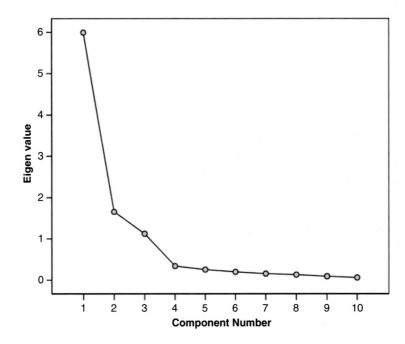

In conclusion, the three components model of the above principal components analysis shows a meaningful data dimension reduction model with three instead of

12 predictive variables, although 30% information has been lost. The best fit coefficients of the original variables constituting the 3 components and additional information are given in the Chap. 22 of this edition.

Conclusion

For some time, the term in English of eigenvalues was "proper value", but the term "eigenvalue" is standard today. Defining eigenvalues is hard, and their meaning is not always consistently used. But they are sometimes described as the length and width of the best fit ellipse pattern, that can be drawn around the data from two variables plotted along an orthogonal x- and y-axis. The division sum of length and place could be called eigenfunctions, and with their place in a graph taken into account they can be called eigenvectors. Dividing the length of their eigen values by that of their widths generally gives a term >1, and is called the condition index. The larger the condition index the stronger the correlation between the two variables, and the closer we will be to 100% collinearity. Eigenvalues and Eigenvectors are important and currently even often used as the basis in the study of covariance assessments of variables. More broadly, eigenvalues are sometimes defined as the proportion variance explained in a datamodel, and if that is an unpaired analysis of variance model, it will be obtained by computing between group sums divided by within group sums. Collinearity diagnostics, principal component analysis, and discriminant analysis are important applications based on eigenvalues. Eigenvalues are currently recognized as the heart of data science. It may even be considered the basis of computing and mathematics.

Note

This chapter focuses on eigenvalues, defined as the proportion of variance in a data model explained by the model itself. Understanding of the current chapter will be enhanced, if, simultaneously, studied with the Chaps. 22 and 24, as well as the Chaps. 52 and 53.

Part III
Rules Models

Chapter 55
Neural Networks for Assessing Relationships that are Typically Nonlinear (90 Patients)

General Purpose

Unlike regression analysis which uses algebraic functions for data fitting, neural networks uses a stepwise method called the steepest descent method for the purpose. This chapter is to asses whether typically nonlinear relationships can be adequately fit by this method.

Background

Artificial intelligence was first proposed by the group of the American neurophysiologist McCulloch in the fifties. Initially, it was merely to explore and simulate informational processing of the human brain. In the sixties Rosenblatt (Spartan, Washington DC) developed a three-layer perceptron model, that, with the help of a traditional digital computer system, was capable to process experimental data samples. A simple three-layer neural network: each layer of neurons after having received a signal beyond some threshold propagates it forward to the next layer as shown in the graph underneath. In the mid-seventies models were shown with more than three layers, and required to perform with the precision of current multiple regression models. Particularly, perceptrons with learning samples, otherwise called back propagation (BP) models, have been successful in the past two decades, and have been applied for various purposes including sales forecasting, process control, and target marketing. Also in clinical research it has been increasingly applied. In

---

This chapter was previously published in "Machine learning in medicine-cookbook 1" as Chap. 13, 2013.

Electronic Supplementary Material The online version of this chapter (https://doi.org/10.1007/978-3-030-33970-8_55) contains supplementary material, which is available to authorized users.

T. J. Cleophas, A. H. Zwinderman, *Machine Learning in Medicine – A Complete Overview*, https://doi.org/10.1007/978-3-030-33970-8_55

oncology research it has been used for diagnostic purposes and survival analysis, in critical care medicine for patient monitoring, and in cardiovascular medicine for making diagnoses, including the presence of myocardial infarction and coronary artery disease, and cardiovascular risk predictions.

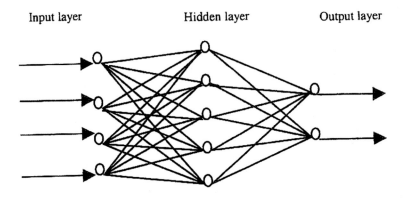

The BP neural networks software include one input layer, one or more hidden layers and one output layer. Each layer consists of various artificial neurons taking on two phases: activity or inactivity. The above graph gives a simple example with a single hidden layer. Each neuron in the input layer after having received a signal beyond some threshold propagates it forward to the next layer. This process will not stop until the signal reaches the output layer sending out the processed signal. The magnitude of the input values and output values is determined by the structure and functioning of the network. The network is also provided with previously observed outcome data, the learning sample. The computer will find, by modifying the weights for all signal-transfers, an outcome as close to the observed outcome as possible. In other words, the neural network tries to find the best-fit outcome for making predictions about the observed outcome data from the imputed data, in a way, similar to regression models. However, unlike regression models no Gaussian distribution models are required, but rather weighted signal-transfers from one layer to another. The underneath tables give examples of weights matrices of imputed signals in the first and second hidden layer of a real data example which will be used in the next section. For finding the best-fit weights the computer uses a technique called iteration or bootstrapping, which means it makes maximally 2000 guesses, depending on the setting when running the neural network, and then picks out the combination of guesses with the best-fit. The output activity is determined by all input activities times their weights, and, subsequently, the various hidden layer activities times their weights. The BP principle is, that all imput produces error. Error is assessed, in the usual way, by taking the sums of squared difference from the means of the observed variables. The result with the smallest error is the one with the best-fit. At present, there is no matured theory on how to select the numbers of artificial neurons and hidden layers. The precision of the neural network is improved by feedback signaling (negative weights in the matrices).

Part of weights matrix of transferred signals to the first hidden layer

-0.040	0.370	0.117	0.066	-0.082	-0.227	0.36	-0.321
-0.288	0.070	0.178	-0.190	-0.275	0.283	-0.467	0.032
-0.128	-0.052	-0.305	-0.237	0.442	0.350	0.077	-0.378
-0.585	-0.247	0.271	-0.045	-0.213	0.272	0.403	0.383
0.248	-0.221	-0.149	0.152	-0.012	0.204	-0.233	-0.007
-0.108	-0.338	0.523	-0.046	-0.321	0.309	0.433	-0.068
0.068	0.142	-0.346	0.014	-0.154	-0.052	-0.048	0.160

Part of weights matrix of transferred signals to the second hidden layer

-0.148	0.602	-0.571	-0.207	0.256	-0.495
0.098	0.684	-0.559	-0.731	1.364	0.097
0.336	-0.541	0.505	-0.241	0.632	-0.188
-0.287	-0.108	0.186	0.124	-0.458	-0.215
0.710	-0.002	-0.387	-0.301	0.735	-0.500

Specific Scientific Question

Body surface is a better indicator for drug dosage than body weight. The relationship between body weight, length and surface are typically nonlinear. Can a neural network be trained to predict body surface of individual patients.

Var 1	Var 2	Var 3
30,50	138,50	10072,90
15,00	101,00	6189,00
2,50	51,50	1906,20
30,00	141,00	10290,60
40,50	154,00	13221,60
27,00	136,00	9654,50
15,00	106,00	6768,20
15,00	103,00	6194,10
13,50	96,00	5830,20
36,00	150,00	11759,00
12,00	92,00	5299,40
2,50	51,00	2094,50
19,00	121,00	7490,80
28,00	130,50	9521,70

Var = variable

Var 1 weight (kg)

Var 2 height (m)

Var 3 body surface measured photometrically (cm^2)

The first 14 patients are shown only, the entire data file is entitled "neuralnetworks" and is in extras.springer.com.

The Computer Teaches Itself to Make Predictions

SPSS 19.0 and up can be used for training and outcome prediction. It uses XML (eXtended Markup Language) files to store data. MLP stands for multilayer perceptron, and indicates the neural network methodology used.

Command:

Click Transform....click Random Number Generators....click Set Starting Point....click Fixed Value (2000000)....click OK....click Analyze....Neural Networks.... Multilayer Perceptron....Dependent Variable: select body surface ....Factors: select weight and height....click Partitioning: set the training sample (7), test sample (3), hold out sample (0)....click Architecture: click Custom Architecture....set the numbers of hidden layers (2)....click Activation Function: click hyperbolic tangens....click Save: click Save predicted values or category for each dependent variable....click Export: click Export synaptic weight estimates to XML file....click Browse....File name: enter "exportnn"....click Save.... Options: click Maximum training time Minutes (15)....click OK.

The output warns that in the testing sample some cases have been excluded from analysis because of values not occurring in the training sample. Minimizing the output sheets shows the data file with predicted values (MLP_PredictedValue).

They are pretty much similar to the measured body surface values. We will use linear regression to estimate the association between the two.

Command:

Analyze....Regresssion....Linear....Dependent: bodysurface ....Independent: MLP_PredictedValue....click OK.

The output sheets show that the r-value is 0.998, r-square 0.995, p < 0.0001. The saved XML file will now be used to compute the body surface in five individual patients.

patient no	weight	height
1	36,00	130,50
2	28,00	150,00
3	12,00	121,00
4	19,00	92,00
5	2,50	51,00

Enter the above data in a new SPSS data file.

Command:

Utilities....click Scoring Wizard....click Browse....click Select....Folder: enter the exportnn.xml file....click Select....in Scoring Wizard click Next....click Use value substitution....click Next....click Finish.

The above data file now gives the body surfaces computed by the neural network with the help of the XML file.

Patient no	weight	height	computed body surfaces
1	36,00	130,50	10290,23
2	28,00	150,00	11754,33
3	12,00	121,00	7635,97
4	19,00	92,00	4733,40
5	2,50	51,00	2109,32

Conclusion

Multilayer perceptron neural networks can be readily trained to provide accurate body surface values of individual patients, and other nonlinear clinical outcomes. Instead of multilayer perceptron neural networks, radial basis function neural networks is possible (see Neural networks for efficacy analysis, Chap. 16, in: Efficacy analysis in clinical trials an update, Springer Heidelberg Germany, 2019, from the same authors). It is equivalent to Gaussian kernel regression, and may, better than multilayer perceptrons, predict medical data, because it uses a Gaussian activation function, although, to date, it is rarely used.

Note

More background, theoretical and mathematical information of neural networks is available in Machine learning in medicine part one, the Chaps. 12 and 13, entitled "Artificial intelligence, multilayer perceptron" and "Artificial intelligence, radial basis functions", pp 145–156 and 157–166, Springer Heidelberg Germany 2013., and the Chap. 63.

Chapter 56
Complex Samples Methodologies
for Unbiased Sampling (9678 Persons)

General Purpose

The research of entire populations is costly and obtaining information from selected samples instead is generally biased by selection bias. Complex sampling produces weighted, and, therefore, unbiased population estimates. This chapter is to assess, whether this method can be trained for predicting health outcomes.

Background

A real data example of the problems with the analysis of big data is in the 2000 National Institute of Health study of health parameters of the USA citizens including smoking habits, vitamin and mineral supplies, multivitamin consumption, body weight, daily exercise information, and herbal supplies. The study included about 0.3 billion of inhabitants, and census information was used to obtain most of the values of different states, city districts, and even townships and neighborhoods. However, little was known about the health parameters. It was decided to randomly sample 30,000 inhabitants throughout the country as a representative sample of the entire population, and these data could be used for comparisons between states, cities and other subgroups. However, it was recognized that different parts of the country would have different probabilities of being included in the sample. First, the states were not equally sized, and, thus, larger states had a larger chance of including individuals. Second, the sampled individuals were taken from different cities and

This chapter was previously published in "Machine learning in medicine-cookbook 1" as Chap.14, 2013.

Electronic Supplementary Material The online version of this chapter (https://doi.org/10.1007/ 978-3-030-33970-8_56) contains supplementary material, which is available to authorized users.

© Springer Nature Switzerland AG 2020

T. J. Cleophas, A. H. Zwinderman, *Machine Learning in Medicine – A Complete Overview*, https://doi.org/10.1007/978-3-030-33970-8_56

429

city districts, and these were again different in probability of being included. For these differences probability corrections had to be performed and a correction factor, otherwise called weighting factor, had to be added to each individual in the sample prior to data analysis. Such a complex analysis is hard to accomplish without complex sampling procedures.

Health scores, including measures of physical, mental and social health are increasingly considered important to estimate public health. If in one territorial division 40% has a low health score, and in another equally large territorial divisions 60%, then on average 50% has a low health score. If the first territorial division is larger than the second, e.g. 1.5 times larger (with similar population density), then we have 1.5 times larger chance that an individual from the 40% low scores is sampled. This would mean that, instead of an average of 50% low health scores for the two territorial divisions,

$$(1/2 \times 40 + 1/2 \times 60)/2 = 50\%,$$

the following average will be measured:

$$(3/5 \times 40 + 2/5 \times 60)/2 = 48\%.$$

This result is 2% smaller, and this is due to the difference in size of the two territorial divisions. Complex sample methodology adjusts these kinds of effects by adding appropriate weights to the individual data. However, with experimental data, uncertainty should be taken into account, and this is also true for the weights to be added as a multiplication factor to the individuals' data. This complicates statistical analyses. Different mathematical methods are available for adjusting the biased estimations. The replication method randomly selects a set of subsamples from the sampled data and overall estimates are computed from them. The Jack-knife method works similarly and calculates means and variances by repeatedly deleting one measured value. Both are Monte Carlo methods and can be applied without the need to take account of theoretical data distribution patterns. They are, respectively, used in SPSS with proportional and numeric data. Taylor series makes use of the algebraic phenomenon that any function $f(x)$ can be expressed as the sum of another function $f(a)$ and its derivative times $(x-a)^2$. It enables to account and compute the variances of ratio data and weighted ratios. We should add that computations are further complicated by the repeated nature of many observations in population studies, requiring paired analyses, and accounting, not only the variances but also the co-variances in the data.

In this chapter efficacy analyses of the effects of territorial divisions and of time on population health scores were assessed. Traditional efficacy analysis will be tested against a machine learning methodology entitled complex-samples methodology. The traditional efficacy analysis consists of confidence intervals, and simple linear regressions.

Specific Scientific Question

Can complex samples be trained to predict unbiased current health outcomes from previous health outcomes in individual members of an entire population.

Var 1	Var 2	Var 3	Var 4	Var 5	Var 6
1	1	1	9	19,26	3,00
1	1	1	7	21,11	6,00
1	1	1	9	22,42	9,00
1	1	1	7	20,13	12,00
1	1	1	5	16,37	15,00
1	1	1	8	20,49	18,00
1	1	1	7	20,79	21,00
1	1	1	7	17,52	24,00
1	1	1	7	18,12	27,00
1	1	1	6	18,60	30,00

Var 1 neighborhood
Var 2 town
Var 3 county
Var 4 time (years)
Var 5 last health score
Var 6 case identity number (defined as property ID)

Prior health scores of a 9,768 member population recorded some 5-10 years ago were available as well as topographical information (the data file is entitled "complexsamples" and is in extras.springer.com. We wish to obtain information of individual current health scores. For that purpose the information of the entire data plus additional information on the current health scores from a random sample of 1000 from this population were used. First, a *sampling plan* was designed with different counties, townships and neighborhoods weighted differently. A *random sample* of 1000 was taken, and additional information was obtained from this random sample, and included.

The latter data file plus the *sampling plan* were, then, used for analysis. The SPSS modules complex samples (cs) "general linear model" and "ratios" modules were applied for analyses. A *sampling plan* of the above population data was designed using SPSS. Open in extras.springer.com the database entitled "complexsamples".

Command:
click Analyze....Complex Samples.... Select a sample.... click Design a sample, click Browse: select a map and enter a name, e.g., complexsamplesplan....click Next....Stratify by: select county....Clusters: select township....click Next...Type: Simple Random Sampling....click Without replacement....click

Next. . . .Units: enter Counts. . . .click Value: enter 4. . . .click Next. . . .click Next. . . . click (Yes, add stage 2 now). . . .click Next. . .Stratify by: enter neighbourhood. . . . next. . .Type: Simple random sampling. . . .click Without replacement. . . .click Next. . . .Units: enter proportions. . . .click Value: enter 0,25. . . .click Next. . . .click Next. . . .click (No, do not add another stage now). . . .click Next. . .Do you want to draw a sample: click Yes. . . .Click Custom value. . . .enter 123. . . .click Next. . . . click External file, click Browse: select a map and enter a name, e.g., complexsamplessample . . . .click Save. . . .click Next. . . .click Finish.

In the original data file the weights of 1006 randomly sampled individuals are now given. In the maps selected above we find two new files,

(1) entitled "complexsamplesplan" (this map can not be opened, but it can in closed form be entered whenever needed during further complex samples analyses of these data), and
(2) entitled "complexsamplessample" containing 1006 randomly selected individuals from the main data file.

The latter data file is first completed with current health scores before the definitive analysis. Only of 974 individuals the current information could be obtained, and these data were added as a new variable (see "complexsamplessample" at extras.springer.com). Also "complexsamplesplan" has for convenience been made available at extras.springer.com.

The Computer Teaches Itself to Predict Current Health Scores from Previous Health Scores

We now use the above data files "complexsamplessample" and "complexsamplesplan" for predicting individual current health scores and odds ratios of current versus previous health scores. Also, an XML (eXtended Markup Language) file will be designed for analyzing future data. First, open "complexsamplessample".

Command:
Click Transform. . . .click Random Number Generators. . . .click Set Starting Point. . . .click Fixed Value (2000000). . . .click OK. . . .click Analyze. . . .Complex Samples. . . .General Linear Model. . . .click Browse: select the appropriate map and enter complexsamplesplan. . . .click Continue. . .Dependent variable: enter curhealthscore . . . .Covariates: enter last healthscores. . . .click Statistics: mark Estimates, 95% Confidence interval, t-test. . . .click Save. . . .mark Predicted Values. . . . in Export Model as XML click Browse. . . .in appropriate folder enter File name: "exportcslin". . . .click Save. . . .click Continue. . . .click OK.

The underneath table gives the correlation coefficient and the 95% confidence intervals. The lower part gives the data obtained through the usual commands

(Analyze, Regression, Linear, Dependent (curhealthscore), Independent (s) (last healthscore), OK). It is remarkable to observe the differences between the two analyses. The correlation coefficients are largely the same but their standard errors are respectively 0.158 and 0.044. The t-value of the complex sampling analysis equals 5.315, while that of the traditional analysis equals no less than 19.635. Nonetheless, the reduced precision of the complex sampling analysis did not produce a statistically insignificant result, and, in addition, it was, of course, again adjusted for inappropriate probability estimates.

Parameter Estimates[a]

Parameter	Estimate	Std. Error	95% Confidence Interval		Hypothesis Test		
			Lower	Upper	t	df	Sig.
(Intercept)	8,151	2,262	3,222	13,079	3,603	12,000	,004
lasthealthscore	,838	,158	,494	1,182	5,315	12,000	,000

a. Model: curhealthscore = (Intercept) + lasthealthscore

Coefficients[a]

Model		Unstandardized Coefficients		Standardized Coefficients	t	Sig.
		B	Std. Error	Beta		
1	(Constant)	7,353	,677		10,856	,000
	last healthscore	,864	,044	,533	19,635	,000

a. Dependent Variable: curhealthscore

The saved XML file will now be used to compute the predicted current health score in five individual patients from this population (Var = variable).

	Var 5
1	19,46
2	19,77
3	16,75
4	16,37
5	18,35

Var 5 Last health score.

Enter the above data in a new SPSS data file.

Command:
Utilities....click Scoring Wizard....click Browse....click Select....Folder: enter the exportcslin.xml file....click Select....in Scoring Wizard click Next....mark Predicted Value....click Next....click Finish.

The above data file now gives the predicted current health scores with the help of the XML file.

	Var 5	Var 6
1	19,46	24,46
2	19,77	24,72
3	16,75	22,19
4	16,37	21,87
5	18,35	23,53

Var 5 last health score.
Var 6 predicted value of current health score

The Computer Teaches Itself to Predict Individual Odds Ratios of Current Health Scores Versus Previous Health Scores

Open again the data file "complexsamplessample".

Command:
Click Transform....click Random Number Generators....click Set Starting Point.... click Fixed Value (2000000)....click OK....click Analyze....Complex Samples ....Ratios....click Browse: select the appropriate map and enter "complexsamplesplan"....click Continue...Numerators: enter curhealthscore.... Denominator: enter last healthscore ....Subpopulations: enter County....click Statistics: mark Standard error, Confidence interval (enter 95%), Design effect....click Continue....click OK.

The underneath table (upper part) gives the overall ratio and the ratios per county plus 95% confidence intervals. The design effects are the ratios of the variances of the complex sampling method versus that of the traditional, otherwise called simple random sampling (srs), method. In the given example the ratios are mostly 3-4, which means that the uncertainty of the complex samples methodology is 3-4 times larger than that of the traditional method. However, this reduction in precision is compensated for by the removal of biases due to the use of inappropriate probabilities used in the srs method.

The lower part of the table gives the srs data obtained through the usual commands (Analyze, Descriptive Statistics, Ratio, Numerator (curhealthscore), Denominator (lasthealthscore), Group Variable (County), Statistics (means, confidence intervals etc). Again the ratios of the complex samples and traditional analyses are rather similar, but the confidence intervals are very different. E.g., the 95% confidence intervals of the Northern County went from 1.172 to 1.914 in the complex samples, and from 1.525 to 1.702 in the traditional analysis, and was thus over 3 times wider.

Ratios 1

Numerator	Denominator	Ratio Estimate	Standard Error	95% Confidence Interval		Design Effect
				Lower	Upper	
curhealthscore	last healthscore	1,371	,059	1,244	1,499	17,566

Ratios 1

County	Numerator	Denominator	Ratio Estimate	Standard Error	95% Confidence Interval		Design Effect
					Lower	Upper	
Eastern	curhealthscore	last healthscore	1,273	,076	1,107	1,438	12,338
"Southern	curhealthscore	last healthscore	1,391	,100	1,174	1,608	21,895
"Western	curhealthscore	last healthscore	1,278	,039	1,194	1,362	1,518
Northern	curhealthscore	last healthscore	1,543	,170	1,172	1,914	15,806

Ratio Statistics for curhealthscore / last healthscore

Group	Mean	95% Confidence Interval for Mean		Price Related Differential	Coefficient of Dispersion	Coefficient of Variation
		Lower Bound	Upper Bound			Median Centered
Eastern	1,282	1,241	1,323	1,007	,184	24,3%
"Southern	1,436	1,380	1,492	1,031	,266	33,4%
"Western	1,342	1,279	1,406	1,051	,271	37,7%
Northern	1,613	1,525	1,702	1,044	,374	55,7%
Overall	1,429	1,395	1,463	1,047	,285	41,8%

The confidence intervals are constructed by assuming a Normal distribution for the ratios.

In addition to the statistics given above, other complex samples statistics are possible, and they can be equally well executed in SPSS, that is if the data are appropriate. If you have a binary outcome variable (dichotomous) available, then logistic regression modeling is possible, if an ordinal outcome variable is available, complex samples ordinal regression, if time to event information is in the data, complex samples Cox regression can be performed.

Conclusion

Complex samples is a cost-efficient method for analyzing target populations that are large and heterogeneously distributed. Also it is time-efficient, and offers greater scope and deeper insight, because specialized equipments are feasible.

Traditional analysis of limited samples from heterogeneous target populations is a biased methodology, because each individual selected is given the same probability, and the spread in the data is, therefore, generally underestimated. In complex sampling this bias is adjusted for by assigning appropriate weights to each individual included.

Note

More background, theoretical and mathematical information of complex samples methodologies is given in Machine learning in medicine part three, Chap. 12, Complex samples, pp 127–139, Springer Heidelberg Germany 2013.

Chapter 57
Correspondence Analysis for Identifying the Best of Multiple Treatments in Multiple Groups (217 Patients)

General Purpose

Multiple treatments for one condition are increasingly available, and a systematic assessment would serve optimal care. Research in this field to date is problematic.

This chapter is to propose a novel method based on cross-tables, correspondence analysis.

Background

Correspondence analysis or reciprocal averaging is a multivariate statistical technique proposed by Herman Otto Hartley from Cambridge UK (1935) and later developed by Jean-Paul Benzécri from Paris 1973. It is conceptually similar to principal component analysis, but applies to categorical rather than continuous data. Correspondence analysis (CA) is a technique for graphically displaying a two-way table by calculating coordinates representing its rows and columns. All data should be on the same scale for CA to be applicable, keeping in mind that the method treats rows and columns equivalently. It is traditionally applied to contingency tables. CA decomposes the chi-squared statistics associated with this table into orthogonal factors. Because CA is a descriptive technique, it can be applied to table whether or not the statistic is appropriate.

Like principal components analysis (Chap. 22), correspondence analysis creates orthogonal components and, for each item in a table, a set of scores (sometimes

This chapter was previously published in "Machine learning in medicine-cookbook 1" as Chap.15, 2013.

Electronic Supplementary Material The online version of this chapter (https://doi.org/10.1007/978-3-030-33970-8_57) contains supplementary material, which is available to authorized users.

called factor scores, see factor analysis (Chap. 22). Correspondence analysis is performed on a contingency table, C, of size m × n where m is the number of rows and n is the number of columns.

Specific Scientific Question

Can correspondence analysis avoid the bias of multiple testing, and identify the best of multiple treatments in multiple groups

Var 1   Var 2

1	1
1	1
1	1
1	1
1	1
1	1
1	1
1	1
1	1
1	1
1	1
1	1

Var 1 treatment modality (1 -3)
Var 2 response (1 = complete remission, 2 = partial remission, 3 = no response)
Only the first 12 patients are given, the entire data file entitled "correspondenceanalysis" is in extras.springer.com. 217 patients were randomly treated with one of three treatments (treat = treatment) and produced one of three responses (1 = complete remission, 2 = partial remission, 3 = no response). We will use SPSS statistical software 19.0.

Correspondence Analysis

First, a multiple groups chi-square test is performed. Start by opening the data file.

Command:
Analyze....Descriptive Statistics....Crosstabs....Row(s): enter treatment.... Column(s): enter remission, partial, no [Var 2]....click Statistics....mark Chi-square....click Continue....click Cell Display ....mark Observed....mark Expected ....click Continue....click OK.

treatment * remission, partial, no Crosstabulation

			remission, partial, no			
			1,00	2,00	3,00	Total
treatment	1,00	Count	19	21	18	58
		Expected Count	21,6	10,7	25,7	58,0
	2,00	Count	41	9	39	89
		Expected Count	33,2	16,4	39,4	89,0
	3,00	Count	21	10	39	70
		Expected Count	26,1	12,9	31,0	70,0
Total		Count	81	40	96	217
		Expected Count	81,0	40,0	96,0	217,0

The output file compares the observed counts (patients) per cell with the expected count, if no significant difference existed. Also, a chi-square value is given, 21.462 with 4 degrees of freedom, p-value < 0.0001. There is a significantly different pattern in numbers of responders between the different treatment groups. To find out what treatment is best a correspondence analysis is performed. For that purpose the individual chi-square values are calculated from the values of the above table according to the underneath equation.

$$\left[(\text{observed count} - \text{expected count})^2/\text{expected count}\right]$$

Then, the individual chi-square values are converted to similarity measures. With these values the software program creates a two-dimensional quantitative distance measure that is used to interpret the level of nearness between the treatment groups and response groups. We will use again SPSS 19.0 statistical software for the analysis.

Command:
Analyze....Dimension Reduction....Correspondence Analysis ....Row: enter treatment....click Define Range....Minimum value: enter1....Maximum value: enter 3....click Update....Column: enter remission, partial, no [Var 2] ....click Define Range....Minimum value: enter1....Maximum value: enter 3....click Update....click Continue ....click Model....Distance Measure: click Chi square....click Continue....click Plots....mark Biplot....click OK.

Treatment		Remission yes	partial	no
1	residual	-2,6	10,3	-7,7
	$(o-e)^2 / e$	0,31	9,91	2,31
	similarity	-0,31	9,91	-2,31
2	residual	7,9	-7,4	-0,4
	$(o-e)^2 / e$	1,88	3,34	0,004
	similarity	1,88	-3,34	-0.004
3	residual	-4,1	-2,9	8,0
	$(o-e)^2 / e$	0,64	0.65	2,65
	similarity	-0,64	-0,65	2,65

The above table of similarity values is given in the output. Also the underneath plot of the coordinates of both the treatment groups and the response groups in a two-dimensional plane is shown in the output. This plot is meaningful. As treatment group 2 and response group 1 tend to join, and treatment group 1 and response group 2 do, equally, so, we have reason to believe that treatment group 2 has the best treatment and treatment group 1 the second best. This is, because response group 1 has a complete remission, and response group 2 has a partial remission. If a 2 × 2 table of the treatment groups 1 and 2 versus the response groups 1 and 2 shows a significant difference between the treatments, then we can argue, that the best treatment is, indeed, significantly better than the second best treatment.

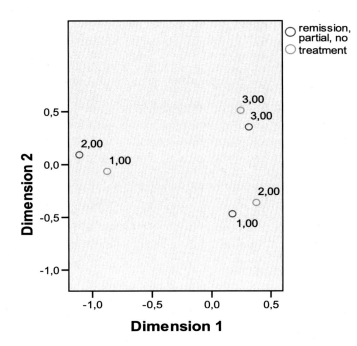

For statistical testing response 1 and 2 versus treatment 1 and 2 recoding of the variables is required, but a simpler solution is to use a pocket calculator method for computing the chi-square value.

	response		
treatment	1	2	total
1	19	21	40
2	41	9	50
	60	30	90

Chi-square $= \frac{[(9 \times 19)-(21 \times 41)]^2 \times 90}{60 \times 30 \times 50 \times 40} = 11.9$ with 1 degree of freedom, $p < 0.0001$

Treatment 2, indeed, produced significantly more complete remissions than did treatment 1, as compared to the partial remissions.

Conclusion

In our example correspondence analysis was able to demonstrate which one of three treatments was best, and it needed, instead of *multiple* 2 × 2 tables, only a single 2 × 2 table for that purpose. The advantage of this procedure will be even more obvious, if larger sets of categorical data have to be assessed. A nine cells data file would require only nine 2 × 2 tables to be tested, a sixteen cells data file would require thirty-six of them. This procedure will almost certainly produce significant effects by chance rather than true effects, and is, therefore, rather meaningless. In contrast, very few tests are needed, when a correspondence analysis is used to identify the proximities in the data, and the risk of type I errors is virtually negligible.

Note

We should add that, instead of a two-dimensional analysis as used in the current chapter, correspondence analysis can also be applied for multidimensional analyses. More background, theoretical and mathematical information of correspondence analysis is given in Machine learning in medicine part two, Chap. 13, Correspondence analysis, pp 129–137, Springer Heidelberg Germany 2013.

Chapter 58
Decision Trees for Decision Analysis (1004 and 953 Patients)

General Purpose

Decision trees are, so-called, non-metric or non-algorithmic methods adequate for fitting nominal and interval data (the latter either categorical or continuous). Better accuracy from decision trees is sometimes obtained by the use of a training sample (Chap. 8). This chapter is to assess whether decision trees can be appropriately applied to predict health risks and improvements.

Background

A decision tree is a decision support tool, that uses a tree-like model of decisions and their possible consequences, including chance event outcomes, resource costs, and utility. It is one way to display an algorithm that only contains conditional control statements. One model for performing decision tree analysis was created by J. Ross Quinlan at the University of Sydney and presented in his book Machine Learning, vol.1, no. 1, 1975. His first algorithm for decision tree creation was called the Iterative Dichotomiser 3 (ID3).

This chapter was previously published in "Machine learning in medicine-cookbook 1" as Chap.16, 2013.

Electronic Supplementary Material The online version of this chapter (https://doi.org/10.1007/978-3-030-33970-8_58) contains supplementary material, which is available to authorized users.

T. J. Cleophas, A. H. Zwinderman, *Machine Learning in Medicine – A Complete Overview*, https://doi.org/10.1007/978-3-030-33970-8_58

Specific Scientific Question

Can decision trees be trained to predict in individual future patients risk of infarction and ldl (low density lipoprotein) cholesterol decrease.

Decision Trees with a Binary Outcome

Var 1	Var 2	Var 3	Var 4	Var 5	Var 6
,00	44,86	1,00	,00	1,00	2,00
,00	42,71	2,00	,00	1,00	2,00
,00	43,34	3,00	,00	2,00	2,00
,00	44,02	3,00	,00	1,00	2,00
,00	67,97	1,00	,00	2,00	2,00
,00	40,31	2,00	,00	2,00	2,00
,00	66,56	1,00	,00	2,00	2,00
,00	45,95	1,00	,00	2,00	2,00
,00	52,27	1,00	,00	1,00	2,00
,00	43,86	1,00	,00	1,00	2,00
,00	46,58	3,00	,00	2,00	1,00
,00	53,83	2,00	,00	2,00	2,00
,00	49,48	1,00	,00	2,00	1,00

Var = variable
Var 1 infarct_rating (,00 no, 1,00 yes)
Var 2 age (years)
Var 3 cholesterol_level (1,00-3,00)
Var 4 smoking (,00 no, 1,00 yes)
Var 5 education (levels 1,00 and 2,00)
Var 6 weight_level (levels 1,00 and 2,00)

The data from the first 13 patients are shown only. See extra.springer.com for the entire data file entitled "decisiontreebinary": in a 1004 patient data file of risk factors for myocardial infarct a so-called chi-squared automatic interaction (CHAID) model is used for analysis. Also an XML (eXtended Markup Language) will be exported for the analysis of future data. Start by opening the data file.

Command:
Click Transform....click Random Number Generators....click Set Starting Point.... click Fixed Value (2000000)....click OK....click Classify....Tree.... Dependent Variable: enter infarct rating....Independent Variables: enter age, cholesterol level, smoking, education, weight level....Growing Method: select CHAID....click Categories: Target mark yes....Continue....click Output: mark Tree in table format....Criteria: Parent Node type 200, Child Node type 100.... click Continue.... click Save: mark Terminal node number, Predicted

probabilities. . . . in Export Tree Model as XML mark Training sample. . . .click Browse. . . . . . . .in File name enter "exportdecisiontreebinary" . . . .in Look in: enter the appropriate map in your computer for storage. . . .click Save. . . .click OK.

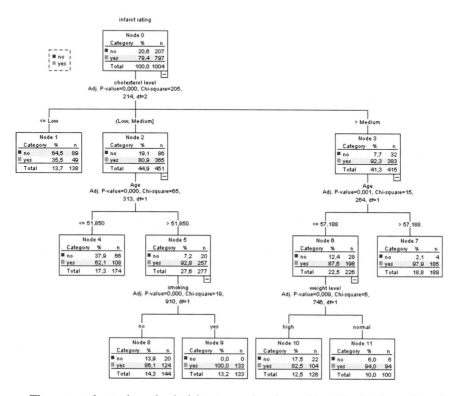

The output sheets show the decision tree and various tables. The Cholesterol level is the best predictor of the infarct rating. For low cholesterol the cholesterol level is the only significant predictor of infarction: only 35.5% will have an infarction. In the medium and high cholesterol groups age is the next best predictor. In the elderly with medium cholesterol smoking contributes considerably to the risk of infarction. In contrast, in the younger with high cholesterol those with normal weight are slightly more at risk of infarction than those with high weights. For each node (subgroup) the number of cases, the chi-square value, and level of significance is given. A p-value < 0.05 indicates that the difference between the 2×2 or 3×2 tables of the paired nodes are significantly different from one another. All of the p-values were very significant.

The risk and classification tables indicate that the category infarction predicted by the model is wrong in $0.166 = 16.6\%$ of the cases (underneath table). A correct prediction of 83.4% is fine. However, in those without an infarction no infarction is predicted in only 43.0% of the cases (underneath table).

Risk

Estimate	Std. Error
,166	,012

Growing Method:
CHAID
Dependent Variable:
infarct rating

Classification

Observed	Predicted		
	no	yes	Percent Correct
no	89	118	43,0%
yes	49	748	93,9%
Overall Percentage	13,7%	86,3%	83,4%

Growing Method: CHAID
Dependent Variable: infarct rating

When returning to the original data file we will observe 3 new variables, (1) the terminal node number, (2) the predicted probabilities of no infarction for each case, (3) the predicted probabilities of yes infarction for each case. In a binary logistic regression it can be tested that the later variables are much better predictors of the probability of infarction than each of the original variables are. The saved XML file will now be used to compute the predicted PAF rate in 6 novel patients with the following characteristics. For convenience the XML file is given in extras.springer.com.

Var 2	Var 3	Var 4	Var 5	Var 6
59,16	2,00	,00	1,00	2,00
53,42	1,00	,00	2,00	2,00
43,02	2,00	,00	2,00	2,00
76,91	3,00	1,00	1,00	1,00
70,53	2,00	,00	1,00	2,00
47,02	3,00	1,00	1,00	1,00

Var 2 age (years)
Var 3 cholesterol_level (1,00-3,00)
Var 4 smoking (,00 no, 1,00 yes)
Var 5 education (level 1,00 and 2,00)
Var 6 weight_level (1,00 and 2,00)

Enter the above data in a new SPSS data file.

Command:
Utilities....click Scoring Wizard....click Browse....click Select....Folder: enter
the exportdecisiontreebinary.xml file....click Select....in Scoring Wizard click
Next....mark Node Number....mark Probability of Predicted Category....click
Next....click Finish.

The above data file now gives the individual predicted nodes numbers and
probabilities of infarct for the six novel patients as computed by the linear model
with the help of the XML file. Enter the above data in a new SPSS data file.

Var 2	Var 3	Var 4	Var 5	Var 6	Var 7	Var 8
59,16	2,00	,00	1,00	2,00	8,00	,86
53,42	1,00	,00	2,00	2,00	1,00	,64
43,02	2,00	,00	2,00	2,00	4,00	,62
76,91	3,00	1,00	1,00	1,00	7,00	,98
70,53	2,00	,00	1,00	2,00	8,00	,86
47,02	3,00	1,00	1,00	1,00	11,00	,94

Var 2 age
Var 3 cholesterol_level
Var 4 smoking
Var 5 education
Var 6 weight_level
Var 7 predicted node number
Var 8 predicted probability of infarct

Decision Trees with a Continuous Outcome

Var 1	Var 2	Var 3	Var 4	Var 5	Var 6
3,41	0	1	3,00	3	0
1,86	-1	1	2,00	3	1
,85	-2	1	1,00	4	1
1,63	-1	1	2,00	3	1
6,84	4	0	4,00	2	0
1,00	-2	0	1,00	3	0
1,14	-2	1	1,00	3	1
2,97	0	1	3,00	4	0
1,05	-2	1	1,00	4	1
,63	-2	0	1,00	3	0
1,18	-2	0	1,00	2	0
,96	-2	1	1,00	2	0
8,28	5	0	4,00	2	1

Var 1 ldl_reduction
Var 2 weight_reduction
Var 3 gender
Var 4 sport
Var 5 treatment_level
Var 6 diet

For the decision tree with continuous outcome the classification and regression tree (CRT or CART) model is applied, otherwise called recursive partitioning (= the partitioning with the largest difference is chosen after multiple partitionings). A 953 patient data file is used of various predictors of ldl (low-density-lipoprotein)-cholesterol reduction including weight reduction, gender, sport, treatment level, diet. The file is in extras.springer.com and is entitled "decisiontreecontinuous". The file is opened.

Command:
Click Transform....click Random Number Generators....click Set Starting Point.... click Fixed Value (2000000)....click OK....click Analyze.... Classify...Tree.... Dependent Variable: enter ldl_reduction.... Independent Variables: enter weight reduction, gender, sport, treatment level, diet....Growing Methods: select CRT ....click Criteria: enter Parent Node 300, Child Node 100....click Output: Tree mark Tree in table format....click Continue....click Save....mark Terminal node number....mark Predicted value....in Export Tree Model as XML mark Training sample....click Browse........in File name enter "exportdecisiontreecontinuous" ....in Look in: enter the appropriate map in your computer for storage....click Save....click OK.

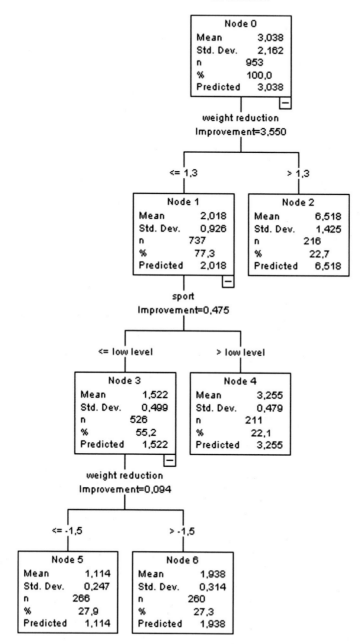

The output sheets show the classification tree. Only weight reduction and sport significantly contributed to the model, with the overall mean and standard deviation dependent variable ldl cholesterol in the parent (root) node. Weight reduction with a cut-off level of 1.3 units is the best predictor of ldl reduction. In the little weight reduction group sport is the best predictor. In the low sport level subgroup again weight reduction is a predictor, but here there is a large difference between weight gain (<-1.5 units) and weight loss (>-1.5 units). Minimizing the output shows the original data file. It now contains two novel variables, the npde classification and the predicted value of ldl cholesterol reduction. They are entitled NodeId and PredictedValue. The saved XML (eXtended Markup Language) file will now be used to compute the predicted node classification and value of ldl cholesterol reduction in five novel patients with the following characteristics. For convenience the XML file is given in extras.springer.com.

Var 2	Var 3	Var 4	Var 5	Var 6
-,63	1,00	2,00	1,00	,00
2,10	,00	4,00	4,00	1,00
-1,16	1,00	2,00	1,00	1,00
4,22	,00	4,00	1,00	,00
-,59	,00	3,00	4,00	1,00

Var 2 weight_reduction
Var 3 gender
Var 4 sport
Var 5 treatment_level
Var 6 diet

Enter the above data in a new SPSS data file.

Command:
Utilities....click Scoring Wizard....click Browse....click Select....Folder: enter the exportdecisiontreecontinuous.xml file....click Select....in Scoring Wizard click Next....mark Node Number....mark Predicted Value....click Next....click Finish.

The above data file now gives individually predicted node classifications and predicted ldl cholesterol reductions as computed by the linear model with the help of the XML file.

Var 2	Var 3	Var 4	Var 5	Var 6	Var 7	Var 8
-,63	1,00	2,00	1,00	,00	6,00	1,94
2,10	,00	4,00	4,00	1,00	2,00	6,52
-1,16	1,00	2,00	1,00	1,00	6,00	1,94
4,22	,00	4,00	1,00	,00	2,00	6,52
-,59	,00	3,00	4,00	1,00	4,00	3,25

Var 2 weight_reduction
Var 3 gender
Var 4 sport
Var 5 treatment_level
Var 6 diet
Var 7 predicted node classification
Var 8 predicted ldl cholesterol reduction

Conclusion

The module decision trees can be readily trained to predict in individual future patients risk of infarction and ldl (low density lipoprotein) cholesterol decrease. Instead of trained XML files for predicting about future patients, also syntax files are possible for the purpose. They perform better if predictions from multiple instead of single future patients are requested.

Note

More background, theoretical and mathematical information of decision trees as well as the steps for utilizing syntax files is available in Machine learning in medicine part three, Chap. 14, entitled "Decision trees", pp 153–168, Springer Heidelberg, Germany 2013. Better accuracy from decision trees is sometimes obtained by the use of a training sample (Chap. 8).

Decision trees works with either chi-square tests or, for continuous outcomes, with the CART (classification and regression trees) method. Y- axis are transformed into log y -values.

Decision trees applies two models: (1) outcomes are scores or rates, predictors are category levels, (2) outcomes are continuous, predictors are again category levels.

Chapter 59
Multidimensional Scaling for Visualizing Experienced Drug Efficacies (14 Pain-killers and 42 Patients)

General Purpose

To individual patients, objective criteria of drug efficacy, like pharmaco-dynamic / -kinetic and safety measures may not mean too much, and patients' personal opinions are important too. This chapter is to assess whether multidimensional scaling can visualize subgroup differences in experienced drug efficacies, and whether data-based dimensions can be used to match dimensions as expected from pharmacological properties.

Background

JB Kruskal, a mathematician and computer scientist from Chicago, wrote the book entitled "Multidimensional scaling, Springer Heidelberg Germany", in 1978. Although based on principles dating back to the classical Greek geometry of Euclides, and provided with algebraic methods by Rene Descartes in the seventeenth century, the work of Kruskal and others in the 70s were important contributions to currently important methodology of multidimensional scaling. Multidimensional scaling (MDS) is a means of visualizing the level of similarity of individual cases of a dataset. MDS is used to translate "information about the pairwise 'distances' among a set of n objects or individuals" into a configuration of n points mapped into an abstract Cartesian space. A Cartesian coordinate system is a coordinate system that specifies each point uniquely in a plane by a set of numerical coordinates, which

This chapter was previously published in "Machine learning in medicine-cookbook 1" as Chap.17, 2013.

Electronic Supplementary Material The online version of this chapter (https://doi.org/10.1007/978-3-030-33970-8_59) contains supplementary material, which is available to authorized users.

are the signed distances to the point from two fixed perpendicular oriented lines, measured in the same unit of length. Each reference line is called a coordinate axis or just axis (plural axes) of the system, and the point where they meet is its origin, at ordered pair (0, 0). The coordinates can also be defined as the positions of the perpendicular projections of the point onto the two axes, expressed as signed distances from the origin. One can use the same principle to specify the position of any point in three-dimensional space by three Cartesian coordinates, its signed distances to three mutually perpendicular planes (or, equivalently, by its perpendicular projection onto three perpendicular lines). In general, n Cartesian coordinates specify the point in an n-dimensional Euclidean space for any dimension n.

Specific Scientific Question

Can proximity and preference scores of pain-killers as judged by patient samples be used for obtaining insight in the real priorities both in populations and in individual patients. Can the data-based dimensions as obtained by this procedure be used to match dimensions as expected from pharmacological properties.

Proximity Scaling

Var == variable

Var	Var 1	Var 2	Var 3	Var 4	Var 5	Var 6	Var 7	Var 8	Var 9	Var 10	Var 11	Var 12	Var 13	Var 14
1	0													
2	8	0												
3	7	2	0											
4	5	4	5	0										
5	8	5	4	6	0									
6	7	5	6	6	8	0								
7	4	5	6	3	7	4	0							
8	8	5	4	6	3	8	7	0						
9	3	7	9	4	8	7	5	8	0					
10	5	6	7	6	9	4	4	9	6	0				
11	9	5	4	6	3	8	7	3	8	9	0			
12	9	4	3	7	5	7	7	5	8	9	5	0		
13	4	6	6	3	7	5	4	8	4	5	7	7	0	
14	6	6	7	6	8	2	4	9	7	3	9	7	5	0

Var 1–14 one by one distance scores of the pain-killers 1–14, mean estimates of 20 patients (scale 0–10). The 14 pain-killers are also given in the first column. The data file is entitled "proxscal" and is in extras.springer.com.

The above matrix mean scores can be considered as one by one distances between all of the medicines connected with one another by straight lines in 14 different ways. Along an x- and y-axis they are subsequently modeled using the equation: the distance between drug i and drug $j = \sqrt{[(x_i - x_j)^2 + (y_i - y_j)^2]}$. SPSS statistical software 19.0 will be used for analysis. Start by opening the data file.

Command:
Analyze....Scale....Multidimensional scaling (PROXSCAL)....Data Format: click The data are proximities....Number of Sources: click One matrix source.... One Source: click The proximities are in a matrix across columns....click Define.... enter all variables (medicines) into "Proximities"....Model: Shape: click Lower-triangular matrix....Proximity Transformation: click Interval.... Dimensions: Minimum: enter 2....Maximum: enter 2....click Continue....click Plots....mark Common space....mark Transformed proximities vs distances.... click Continue ....click: Output....mark Common space coordinates....mark Multiple stress measures....click Continue....click OK.

Stress and Fit Measures

Normalized Raw Stress	,00819
Stress-I	,09051[a]
Stress-II	,21640[a]
S-Stress	,02301[b]
Dispersion Accounted For (D.A.F.)	,99181
Tucker's Coefficient of Congruence	,99590

PROXSCAL minimizes Normalized Raw Stress.

a. Optimal scaling factor = 1,008.

b. Optimal scaling factor = ,995.

The output sheets gives the uncertainty of the model (stress = standard error) and dispersion values. The model is assumed to appropriately describe the data if they are respectively < 0.20 and approximately 1.0.

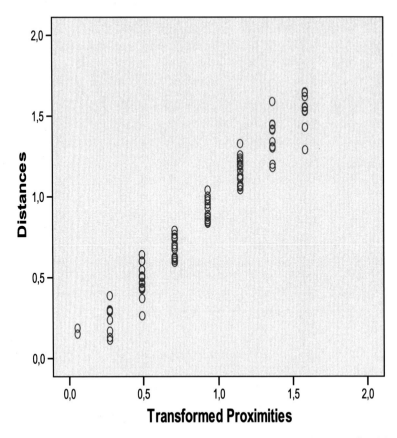

Also, a plot of the actual distances as observed versus the distances fitted by the statistical program is given. A perfect fit should produce a straight line, a poor fit produces a lot of spread around a line or even no line at all. The figure is not perfect but it shows a very good fit as expected from the stress and fit measures.

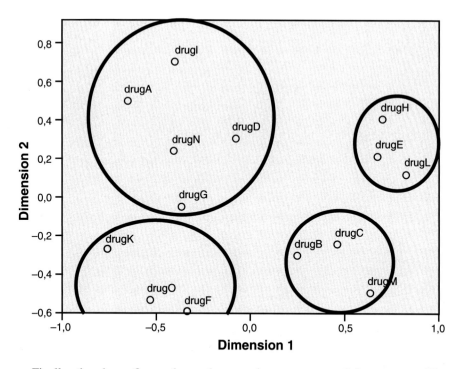

Finally, the above figure shows the most important part of the outcome. The standardized x- and y-axes values give some insight in the relative position of the medicines according to perception of our study population. Four clusters are identified. Using Microsoft's drawing commands we can encircle the clusters as identified. The cluster at the upper right quadrant comprises high priorities of the patients along both the x- an the y-axis. The cluster at the lower left quadrant comprises low priorities of the patients along both axes. If, pharmacologically, the drugs in the right upper quadrant were highly potent with little side effects, then the patients' priorities would fairly match the pharmacological properties of the medicines.

Preference Scaling

Var 1	2	3	4	5	6	7	8	9	10	11	12	13	14	15
12	13	7	4	5	2	8	10	11	14	3	1	6	9	15
14	11	6	3	10	4	15	8	9	12	7	1	5	2	13
13	10	12	14	3	2	9	8	7	11	1	6	4	5	15
7	14	11	3	6	8	12	10	9	15	4	1	2	5	13
14	9	6	15	13	2	11	8	7	10	12	1	3	4	5
9	11	15	4	7	6	14	10	8	12	5	2	3	1	13
9	14	5	6	8	4	13	11	12	15	7	2	1	3	10
15	10	12	6	8	2	13	9	7	11	3	1	5	4	14
13	12	2	4	5	8	10	11	3	15	7	9	6	1	14
15	13	10	7	6	4	9	11	12	14	5	2	8	1	3
9	2	4	13	8	5	1	10	6	7	11	15	14	12	3

Var 1–15 preference scores (1 = most prefered, 15 = least prefered)

Only the first 11 patients are given. The entire data file is entitled "prefscal" and is in extras.springer.com.

To 42 patients 15 different pain-killers are administered, and the patients are requested to rank them in order of preference from 1 "most prefered" to 15 "least prefered". First will try and draw a three dimensional view of the individually assigned preferences. We will use SPSS 19.0. Start by opening the data file.

Command:
Graphs....Legacy Dialogs....3-D Bar....X-axis represents: click Separate variables....Z-axis represents: click Individual cases....Define....Bars Represent: enter pain-killers 1–15....Show Cases on: click Y-axis....Show Cases with: click Case number....click OK.

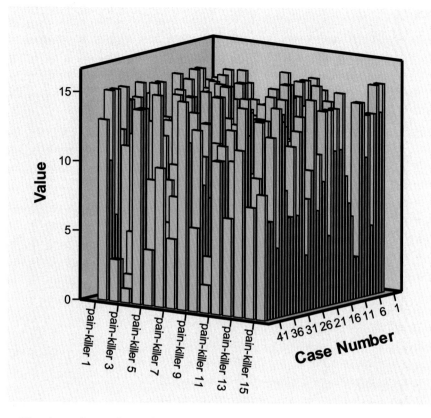

The above figure shows the result: a very irregular pattern consisting of multiple areas with either high or low preference is observed. We will now perform a preference scaling analysis. Like with proximity scaling, preference assessments is mapped in a 2 dimensional plane with the rank orders of the medicines as measures of distance between the medicines. Two types of maps are constructed: an aggregate map giving average distances of the entire population or individual maps

of single patients, and an ideal point map where ideal points have to be interpreted as a map with ideal medicines, one for each patient. SPSS 19.0 is used once more.

Command:

Analyze....Scale....Multidimensional Unfolding (PREFSCAL)....enter all variables (medicines) into "Proximities"....click Model....click Dissimilarities.... Dimensions: Minimum enter 2 ....Maximum enter 2....Proximity Transformations: click Ordinal ....click Within each row separately....click Continue.... click Options: imputation by: enter Spearman....click Continue....click Plots: mark Final common space....click Continue....click Output: mark Fit measures ....mark Final common space....click Continue....click OK.

Measures

Iterations		115
Final Function Value		,7104127
Function Value Parts	Stress Part	,2563298
	Penalty Part	1,9688939
Badness of Fit	Normalized Stress	,0651568
	Kruskal's Stress-I	,2552582
	Kruskal's Stress-II	,6430926
	Young's S-Stress-I	,3653360
	Young's S-Stress-II	,5405226
Goodness of Fit	Dispersion Accounted For	,9348432
	Variance Accounted For	,7375011
	Recovered Preference Orders	,7804989
	Spearman's Rho	,8109694
	Kendall's Tau-b	,6816390
Variation Coefficients	Variation Proximities	,5690984
	Variation Transformed Proximities	,5995274
	Variation Distances	,4674236
Degeneracy Indices	Sum-of-Squares of DeSarbo's Intermixedness Indices	,2677061
	Shepard's Rough Nondegeneracy Index	,7859410

The above table gives the stress (standard error) and fit measures. The best fit distances as estimated by the model are adequate: measures of stress including normalized stress and Kruskal's stress-I are close to 0.20 or less, the value of dispersion measures (Dispersion Accounted For) is close to 1.0. The table also shows whether there is a risk of a *degenerate* solution, otherwise called loss function. The individual proximities have a tendency to form circles, and when averaged for obtaining average proximities, there is a tendency for the average treatment places to center in the middle of the map. The solution is a penalty term, but in our example we need not worry. The DeSarbo's and Shepard criteria are close to respectively 0 and 80%, and no penalty adjustment is required.

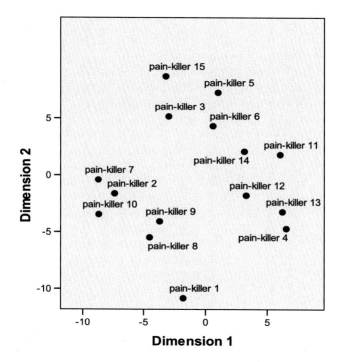

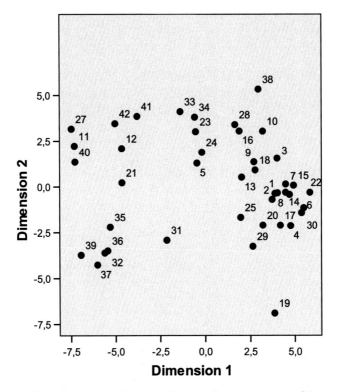

The above figure (upper graph) gives the most important part of the output. The standardized x- and y-axes values of the upper graph give some insight in the relative position of the medicines according to our study population. The results can be understood as the relative position of the medicines according to the perception of our study population. Both the horizontal and the vertical dimension appears to discriminate between different preferences. The lower graph gives the patients' *ideal points*. The patients seem to be split into two clusters with different preferences, although with much variation along the y-axis. The dense cluster in the right lower quadrant represented patients with preferences both along the x- and y-axis. Instead of two-dimensions, multidimensional scaling enables to assess multiple dimensions each of which can be assigned to one particular cause for proximity. This may sound speculative, but if the pharmacological properties of the drugs match the place of the medicines in a particular dimension, then we will be more convinced that the multi-dimensional display gives, indeed, an important insight in the real priorities of the patients. In order to address this issue, we will now perform a multidimensional scaling procedure of the above data including three dimensions.

Command:

Analyze....Scale....Multidimensional Unfolding (PREFSCAL)....enter all variables (medicines) into "Proximities"....click Model....click Dissimilarities....
Dimensions: Minimum enter 3 ....Maximum enter 3....Proximity Transformations: click Ordinal ....click Within each row separately....click Continue....
click Options: imputation by: enter Spearman....click Continue....click Plots: mark Final common space....click Continue....click Output: mark Fit measures ....mark Final common space....click Continue....click OK.

Final Column Coordinates

Painkiller no.	Dimension 1	2	3
1	-2.49	-9.08	-4.55
2	-7.08	-1.81	1.43
3	-3.46	3.46	-2.81
4	5.41	-4.24	1.67
5	-.36	6.21	5.25
6	.17	1.88	-3.27
7	-7.80	-2.07	-1.59
8	-5.17	-4.18	2.91
9	4.75	-.59	4.33
10	-6.80	-4.83	.27
11	6.22	2.50	.88
12	3.71	-1.27	-.49
13	5.30	-2.95	1.51
14	2.82	1.66	-2.09
15	-4.35	2.76	-6.72

The output sheets shows the standardized mean preference values of the different pain-killers as x- y-, and z-axis coordinates. The best fit outcome of the three-dimensional (3-D) model can be visualized in a 3-D figure. SPSS 19.0 is used. First cut and paste the data from the above table to the preference scaling file or another file. Then proceed.

Command:

Graphs....Legacy Dialogs....Scatter/Dot....click 3-D Scatter....click Define....
Y-Axis: enter dimension 1....X-Axis: enter dimension 2....Z-Axis: enter dimension 3....click OK.

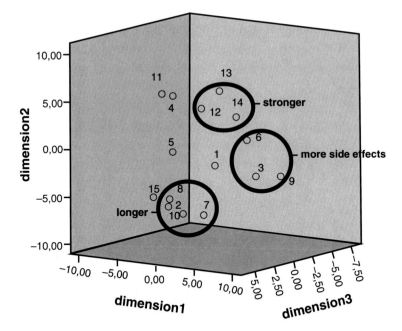

The above figure is in the output, and gives the best fit outcome of a 3-dimensional scaling model. Three clusters were identified, consistent with patients' preferences along an x-, y-, and z-axis. Using Microsoft's drawing commands we can encircle the clusters as identified. In the figure an example is given of how pharmacological properties could be used to explain the cluster pattern.

Conclusion

Multidimensional scaling is helpful both to underscore the pharmacological properties of the medicines under studies, and to identify what effects are really important to patients, and uses for these purposes estimated proximities as surrogates for counted estimates of patients' opinions. Multidimensional scaling can, like regression analysis, be used two ways, (1) for estimating preferences of treatment modalities in a population, (2) for assessing the preferred treatment modalities in individual patients.

Note

More background, theoretical and mathematical information of multidimensional scaling is given in Machine learning in medicine part two, Chap. 12, Multidimensional scaling, pp 115–127, Springer Heidelberg Germany 2013.

Chapter 60
Stochastic Processes for Long Term Predictions from Short Term Observations

General Purpose

Markov modeling, otherwise called stochastic processes, assumes that per time unit the same % of a population will have an event, and it is used for long term predictions from short term observations. This chapter is to assess whether the method can be applied by non-mathematicians using an online matrix-calculator.

Background

In probability theory, a Markov model is a stochastic model used to model
  randomly changing systems where it is assumed that future states depend only on the current state not on the events that occurred before it (that is, it assumes the Markov property).

  Markov is a pretty brilliant mathematician from Saint Petersburg who died in 1922.

  One of the most frequently used methods for modeling and understanding human internet actions are Markov chains.

This chapter was previously published in "Machine learning in medicine-cookbook 1" as Chap.18, 2013.

Electronic Supplementary Material The online version of this chapter (https://doi.org/10.1007/978-3-030-33970-8_60) contains supplementary material, which is available to authorized users.

© Springer Nature Switzerland AG 2020
T. J. Cleophas, A. H. Zwinderman, *Machine Learning in Medicine – A Complete Overview*, https://doi.org/10.1007/978-3-030-33970-8_60

Specific Scientific Questions

If per time unit the same % of patients will have an event like surgery, medical treatment, a complication like a co-morbidity or death, what will be the average time before such events take place.

Example 1

Patients with three states of treatment for a disease are checked every 4 months. The underneath matrix is a so-called transition matrix. The states 1–3 indicate the chances of treatment: 1 = no treatment, 2 = surgery, 3 = medicine. If you are in state 1 today, there will be a 0.3 = 30% chance that you will receive no treatment in the next 4 months, a 0.2 = 20% chance of surgery, and a 0.5 = 50% chance of medicine treatment. If you are still in state 1 (no treatment) after 4 months, there will again be a 0.3 chance that this will be the same in the second 4 month period etc. So, after 5 periods the chance of being in state 1 equals $0.3 \times 0.3 \times 0.3 \times 0.3 \times 0.3 = 0.00243$. The chance that you will be in the states 2 or 3 is much larger, and there is something special about these states. Once you are in these states you will never leave them anymore, because the patients who were treated with either surgery or medicine are no longer followed in this study. That this happens can be observed from the matrix: if you are in state 2, you will have a chance of 1 = 100% to stay in state 2 and a chance of 0 = 0% not to do so. The same is true for the state 3.

	State in next period (4 months)		
State in current time	1	2	3
1	0.3	0.2	0.5
2	0	1	0
3	0	0	1

Now we will compute what will happen with the chances of a patient in the state 1 after several 4 month periods.

	chances of being in state:		
	state 1	state 2	state 3
4 month period			
1st	30%	20%	50%
2nd	30x0.3= 9%	20+0.3x20= 26%	50+0.3x50= 65%
3rd	9x0.3= 3%	26+9x0.2= 27.8%	65+9x0.5= 69.5%
4th	3x0.3= 0.9%	27.8+3x0.2= 28.4%	69.5+3x0.5= 71.0%
5th	0.9x0.3= 0.27%	28.4+0.9x0.2= 28.6%	71.0+0.9x0.5= 71.5..

Example 1   467

Obviously, the chances of being in the states 2 or 3 will increase, though increasingly slowly, and the chance of being in state 1 is, ultimately, going to approximate zero. In clinical terms: postponing the treatment does not make much sense, because everyone in the no treatment group will eventually receive a treatment and the ultimate chances of surgery and medicine treatment are approximately 29 and 71%. With larger matrices this method for calculating the ultimate chances is rather laborious. Matrix algebra offers a rapid method.

	State in next period (4 months)			
	1	2 3		
State in current time				
1	[0.3]	[0.2 0.5]	matrix Q	matrix R
2	[0]	[1 0]	matrix O	matrix I
3	[0]	[0 1]		

The states are called transient, if they can change (the state 1), and absorbing if not (the states 2 and 3). The original matrix is partitioned into four submatrices, otherwise called the canonical form:

[0.3]   Upper left corner:
                     This square matrix Q can be sometimes very large with rows and
                     columns respectively presenting the transient states.

[0.2 0.5]   Upper right corner:
                     This R matrix presents in rows the chance of being absorbed
                     from the transient state.

[1   0]   Lower right corner:
[0   1]   This identity matrix I presents rows and columns with chances of
                     being in the absorbing states, the I matrix must be adjusted to the
                     size of the Q matrix (here it will look like [1] instead of [1 0]
                                                                                    [0 1]

[0]   Lower left corner.
[0]   This is a matrix of zeros (0 matrix).

From the above matrices a fundamental matrix (F) is constructed.

$$[(\text{matrix I}) - (\text{matrix R})]^{-1} = [0.7]^{-1} = 10/7$$

With larger matrices a matrix calculator, like the Bluebit Online Matrix Calculator can be used to compute the matrix to the -1 power by clicking "Inverse".

The fundamental matrix F equals 10/7. It can be interpreted as the average time, before someone goes into the absorbing state ($10/7 \times 4$ months $= 5.714$ months).

The product of the fundamental matrix F and the R matrix gives more exact chances of a person in state 1 ending up in the states 2 and 3.

$$F \times R = (10/7) \times [0.2 \ 0.5] = [2/75/7] = [0.2857140.714286]$$

The two latter values add up to 1.00, which indicates a combined chance of ending up in an absorbing state equal to 100%.

Example 2

Patients with three states of treatment for a chronic disease are checked every 4 months.

	State in next period (4 months)		
	1	2	3
State in current time			
1	0.3	0.6	0.1
2	0.45	0.5	0.05
3	0	0	1

The above matrix of three states and second periods of time gives again the chances of different treatment for a particular disease, but it is slightly different from the first example. Here state 1 = no treatment state, state 2 = medicine treatment, state 3 = surgery state. We assume that medicine can be stopped while surgery is irretrievable, and, thus, an absorbing state. We first partition the matrix.

	State in next period (4 months)				
	1	2	3		
State in current time					
1	[0.3	0.6]	[0.1]	matrix Q	matrix R
2	[0.45	0.5]	[0.05]		
3	[0	0]	[1]	matrix O	matrix I

Example 3   469

The R matrix $\begin{bmatrix} 0.1 \\ 0.05 \end{bmatrix}$ is in the upper right corner.

The Q matrix $\begin{bmatrix} 0.3 & 0.6 \\ 0.45 & 0.5 \end{bmatrix}$ is in the left upper corner.

The I matrix $[\,1\,]$ is in the lower right corner, and must be adjusted, before it can be subtracted from the Q matrix according

The 0 matrix $[\,0\ 0\,]$ is in the lower left corner.

$$I - Q = \begin{bmatrix} 1 & 0 \\ 0 & 1 \end{bmatrix} - \begin{bmatrix} 0.3 & 0.6 \\ 0.45 & 0.5 \end{bmatrix} = \begin{bmatrix} 0.7 & -0.6 \\ 0.45 & -0.5 \end{bmatrix}$$

The inverse of $[I - Q]$ is obtained by marking "Inverse" at the online Bluebit Matrix Calculator and equals

$$[I - Q]^{-1} = \begin{bmatrix} 6.25 & 7.5 \\ 5.625 & 8.75 \end{bmatrix}$$

$$= \text{fundamental matrix F.}$$

It is interpreted as the average periods of time before some transient state goes into the absorbing state:

$(6.25 + 7.5 = 13.75) \times 4$ months for the patients in state 1 first and state 2 second, $(5.625 + 8.75 = 14.375) \times 4$ months for the patients in state 2 first and state 1 second).

Finally, the product of matrix F times matrix R is calculated. It gives the chances of ending up in the absorbing state for those starting in the states 1 and 2.

$$\begin{bmatrix} 6.25 & 7.5 \\ 5.625 & 8.75 \end{bmatrix} \times \begin{bmatrix} 0.1 \\ 0.05 \end{bmatrix} = \begin{bmatrix} 1.00 \\ 1.00 \end{bmatrix}$$

Obviously the chance of both the transient states for ending up in the absorbing state is $1.00 = 100\%$.

Example 3

State 1 = stable coronary artery disease (CAD),
state 2 = complications,
state 3 = recovery state,
state 4 = death state).

	State in next period (4 months)			
	1	2	3	4
State in current time				
1	0.95	0.04	0	0.01
2	0	0	0.9	0.1
3	0	0.3	0.3	0.4
4	0	0	0	1

If you take higher powers of this transition matrix (P), you will observe long-term trends of this model. For that purpose use the matrix calculator and square the transition matrix (P^2 gives the chances in the 2nd 4 month period etc) and compute also higher powers (P^3, P^4, P^5, etc).

P^2
0.903 0.038 0.036 0.024
0.000 0.270 0.270 0.460
0.000 0.090 0.360 0.550
0.000 0.000 0.000 1.000

P^6
0.698 0.048 0.063 0.191
0.000 0.026 0.064 0.910
0.000 0.021 0.047 0.931
0.000 0.000 0.000 1.000

The above higher order transition matrices suggest that with rising powers, and, thus, after multiple 4 month periods, there is a general trend towards the absorbing state: in each row the state 4 value continually rises. In the end we all will die, but in order to be more specific about the time, a special matrix like the one described in the previous examples is required. In order to calculate the precise time before the transient states go into the absorbing state, we need to partition the initial transition matrix.

	State in next period (4 months)			
	1	2	3	4
State in current time				
1	$\begin{bmatrix} 0.95 & 0.04 & 0.0 \\ 0.0 & 0.0 & 0.9 \\ 0.0 & 0.3 & 0.3 \end{bmatrix}$	$\begin{bmatrix} 0.01 \\ 0.1 \\ 0.4 \end{bmatrix}$	matrix Q	matrix R
2				
3				
4	$[0 \ 0 \ 0]$	$[1]$	matrix O	matrix I

Example 3   471

$$F = (I - Q)^{-1}$$

$$I - Q = \begin{bmatrix} 1 & 0 & 0 \\ 0 & 1 & 0 \\ 0 & 0 & 1 \end{bmatrix} - \begin{bmatrix} 0.95 & 0.04 & 0.0 \\ 0.0 & 0.0 & 0.9 \\ 0.0 & 0.3 & 0.3 \end{bmatrix}$$

$$F = \begin{bmatrix} 0.5 & -0.04 & 0 \\ 0.0 & 1.0 & -0.9 \\ 0.0 & -0.3 & 0.7 \end{bmatrix}^{-1}$$

The online Bluebit Matrix calculator (mark inverse) produces the underneath result.

$$F = \begin{bmatrix} 20.0 & 1.3202 & 1.674 \\ 0.0 & 1.628 & 2.093 \\ 0.0 & 0.698 & 2.326 \end{bmatrix}$$

The average time before various transient states turn into the absorbing state (dying in this example) is given.

State 1: $(20 + 1.302 + 1.674) \times 4$ months $= 91.904$ months.
State 2: $(0.0 + 1.628 + 2.093) \times 4$ months $= 14.884$ months.
State 3: $(0.0 + 0.698 + 2.326) \times 4$ months $= 12.098$ months.

The chance of dying for each state is computed from matrix F times matrix R (click multiplication, enter the data in the appropriate fields and click calculate.

$$F.R = \begin{bmatrix} 20.0 & 1.3202 & 1.674 \\ 0.0 & 1.628 & 2.093 \\ 0.0 & 0.698 & 2.326 \end{bmatrix} \times \begin{bmatrix} 0.01 \\ 0.1 \\ 0.4 \end{bmatrix} = \begin{bmatrix} 1.0 \\ 1.0 \\ 1.0 \end{bmatrix}$$

Like in the previous examples again the products of the matrices F and R show that all of the states end up with death. However, in the state 1 this takes more time than it does in the other states.

Conclusion

Markov chains are used to analyze the long-term risks of reversible and irreversible complications including death. The future is not shown, but it is shown, what will happen, if everything remains the same. Markov chains assume, that the chance of an event is not independent, but depends on events in the past.

Note

More background, theoretical and mathematical information of Markov chains (stochastic modeling) is given in Machine learning in medicine part three, Chaps. 17 and 18, "Stochastic processes: stationary Markov chains" and "Stochastic processes: absorbing Markov chains", pp 195–204 and 205–216, Springer Heidelberg Germany 2013.

Chapter 61
Optimal Binning for Finding High Risk Cut-offs (1445 Families)

General Purpose

Optimal binning is a so-called non-metric method for describing a continuous predictor variable in the form of best fit categories for making predictions. Like binary partitioning (Machine Learning in Medicine Part One, Chap. 7, Binary partitioning, pp 79–86, Springer Heidelberg Germany, 2013) it uses an exact test called the entropy method, which is based on log likelihoods. It may, therefore, produce better statistics than traditional tests. In addition, unnecessary noise due to continuous scaling is deleted, and categories for identifying patients at high risk of particular outcomes can be identified. This chapter is to assess its efficiency in medical research.

Background

Optimal Binning was introduced by SPSS 15 and its forerunner, the Clementine data mining workbench (2006). It is a supervised method for discretizing a scale numeric variable (numeric and treated as continuous), i.e. grouping the values of that variable into a relatively small set of discrete values (bins), each of which represent a range of values on the original variable. The discretization may be performed to allow analysis that is restricted to categorical variables. The Optimal binning procedure discretizes one or more scale variables (referred to henceforth as binning input variables) by distributing the values of each variable into bins. Bin formation is

This chapter was previously published in "Machine learning in medicine-cookbook 1" as Chap.19, 2013.

Electronic Supplementary Material The online version of this chapter (https://doi.org/10.1007/978-3-030-33970-8_61) contains supplementary material, which is available to authorized users.

optimal with respect to a categorical guide variable that "supervises" the binning process. Bins can then be used instead of the original data values for further analysis. Bins are, thus, equally-spaced intervals that are used to sort data. If on graphs, it will usually be called histograms. By default, the number of values in each bin is represented by bars on histograms or by stacks of dots on dotplots. For example, on the underneath histogram, the height of each bar represents the frequency of observations within the corresponding range of values. On the underneath dotplot, the height of each stack of dots represents the frequency of observations within the corresponding range of values.

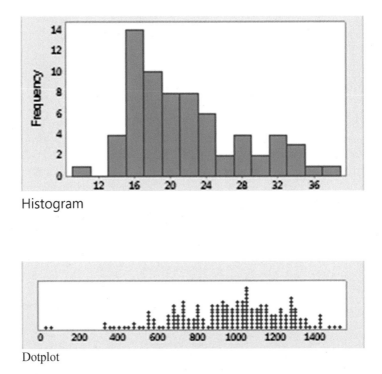

Histogram

Dotplot

The optimal binning procedure discretizes a scale variable, such that bin formation will be optimal. Bin formation will be optimal, if it is according to a categorical variable that "supervises" the binning process. Bins can then be used as consecutive intervals of one (or more) variables. Examples include (1) categorical variables of crosstabs, (2) binned values instead of actual values safeguarding the privacy of your data sources, (3) reduced bin numbers instead of distinct values for improved process efficiencies. Histograms are an example of a method using binning. To construct a histogram, the first step is to "bin" (or "bucket") the range of values, that is, divide the entire range of values into a series of intervals, and, then, count how many values fall into different intervals.

Specific Scientific Question

The data example of the Chap.5 will be used once more. Increasingly unhealthy lifestyles cause increasingly high risks of overweight children. We are, particularly, interested in the best fit cut-off values of unhealthy lifestyle estimators to maximize the difference between low and high risk.

Var 1	Var 2	Var 3	Var 4	Var 5
0	11	1	8	0
0	7	1	9	0
1	25	7	0	1
0	11	4	5	0
1	5	1	8	1
0	10	2	8	0
0	11	1	6	0
0	7	1	8	0
0	7	0	9	0
0	15	3	0	0

Var 1fruitvegetables (0 = no, 1 = yes)
Var 2 unhealthysnacks (times per week)
Var 3 fastfoodmeal (times per week)
Var 4 physicalactivities (times per week)
Var 5 overweightchildren (0 = no, 1 = yes)
Only the first 10 families are given, the entire data file is entitled "optimalbinning" and is in extras.springer.com.

Optimal Binning

SPSS 19.0 is used for analysis. Start by opening the data file.

Command:
Transform....Optimal Binning....Variables into Bins: enter fruitvegetables, unhealthysnacks, fastfoodmeal, physicalactivities....Optimize Bins with Respect to: enter "overweightchildren"....click Output....Display: mark Endpoints.... mark Descriptive statistics....mark Model Entropy....click Save: mark Create variables that contain binned data....click OK.

Descriptive Statistics

	N	Minimum	Maximum	Number of Distinct Values	Number of Bins
fruitvegetables/wk	1445	0	34	33	2
unhealthysnacks/wk	1445	0	42	1050	3
fastfoodmeal/wk	1445	0	21	1445	2
physicalactivities/wk	1445	0	10	1385	2

In the output the above table is given. N = the number of adults in the analysis, Minimum/Maximum = the range of the original continuous variables, Number of Distinct Values = the separate values of the continuous variables as used in the binning process, Number of Bins = the number of bins (= categories) generated and is smaller than the initials separate values of the same variables.

Model Entropy

	Model Entropy
fruitvegetables/wk	,790
unhealthysnacks/wk	,720
fastfoodmeal/wk	,786
physicalactivities/wk	,805

Smaller model entropy indicates higher predictive accuracy of the binned variable on guide variable overweight children.

Model Entropy gives estimates of the usefulness of the bin models as predictor models for probability of overweight: the smaller the entropy, the better the model. Values under 0,820 indicate adequate usefulness.

fruitvegetables/wk

	End Point		Number of Cases by Level of overweight children		
Bin	Lower	Upper	No	Yes	Total
1	a	14	802	340	1142
2	14	a	274	29	303
Total			1076	369	1445

unhealthysnacks/wk

Bin	End Point		Number of Cases by Level of overweight children		
	Lower	Upper	No	Yes	Total
1	a	12	830	143	973
2	12	19	188	126	314
3	19	a	58	100	158
Total			1076	369	1445

fastfoodmeal/wk

Bin	End Point		Number of Cases by Level of overweight children		
	Lower	Upper	No	Yes	Total
1	a	2	896	229	1125
2	2	a	180	140	320
Total			1076	369	1445

physicalactivities/wk

Bin	End Point		Number of Cases by Level of overweight children		
	Lower	Upper	No	Yes	Total
1	a	8	469	221	690
2	8	a	607	148	755
Total			1076	369	1445

Each bin is computed as Lower <= physicalactivities/wk < Upper.

a. Unbounded

The above tables show the high risk cut-offs for overweight children of the four predicting factors. E.g., in 1142 adults scoring under 14 units of fruit/vegetable per week, are put into bin 1 and 303 scoring over 14 units per week, are put into bin 2. The proportion of overweight children in bin 1 is much larger than it is in bin 2: $340/1142 = 0.298$ (30%) and $29/303 = 0.096$ (10%). Similarly high risk cut-offs are found for

unhealthy snacks less than 12, 12–19, and over 19 per week
fastfood meals less than 2, and over 2 per week
physical activities less than 8 and over 8 per week.

These cut-offs can be used as meaningful recommendation limits to future families.

When we return to the dataview page, we will observe that the four variables have been added in the form of bin variables (with suffix _bin). They can be used as outcome variables for making predictions from other variables like personal characteristics of parents. Also they can be used, instead of the original variable, as predictors in regression modeling. A binary logistic regression with overweight children as dependent variable will be performed to assess their predictive strength as compared to that of the original variables. SPSS 19.0 will again be used.

Command:

Analyze....Regression....Binary Logistic....Dependent: enter overweight children ....Covariates: enter fruitvegetables, unhealthysnack, fastfoodmeal, physicalactivities....click OK.

Variables in the Equation

		B	S.E.	Wald	df	Sig.	Exp(B)
Step 1[a]	fruitvegetables	-,092	,012	58,775	1	,000	,912
	unhealthysnacks	,161	,014	127,319	1	,000	1,175
	fastfoodmeal	,194	,041	22,632	1	,000	1,214
	physicalactivities	,199	,041	23,361	1	,000	1,221
	Constant	-4,008	,446	80,734	1	,000	,018

a. Variable(s) entered on step 1: fruitvegetables, unhealthysnacks, fastfoodmeal, physicalactivities.

The output shows that the predictors are very significant independent predictors of overweight children. Next the bin variable will be used.

Command:

Analyze....Regression....Binary Logistic....Dependent: enter overweight children ....Covariates: enter fruitvegetables_bin, unhealthysnack_bin, fastfoodmeal_bin, physicalactivities_bin....click OK.

Variables in the Equation

		B	S.E.	Wald	df	Sig.	Exp(B)
Step 1[a]	fruitvegetables_bin	-1,694	,228	55,240	1	,000	,184
	unhealthysnacks_bin	1,264	,118	113,886	1	,000	3,540
	fastfoodmeal_bin	,530	,169	9,827	1	,002	1,698
	physicalactivities_bin	,294	,167	3,086	1	,079	1,341
	Constant	-2,176	,489	19,803	1	,000	,114

a. Variable(s) entered on step 1: fruitvegetables_bin, unhealthysnacks_bin, fastfoodmeal_bin, physicalactivities_bin.

If p < 0.10 is used to indicate statistical significance, all of the bin variables are independent predictors, though at a somewhat lower level of significance than the original variables. Obviously, in the current example some precision is lost by the binning procedure. This is, because information may be lost if you replace a continuous variable with a binary or nominal one. Nonetheless, the method is precious for identifying high risk cut-offs for recommendation purposes.

Conclusion

Optimal binning variables instead of the original continuous variables may either produce (1) better statistics, because unnecessary noise due to the continuous scaling may be deleted, (2) worse statistics, because information may be lost if your replace a continuous variable with a binary one. It is more adequate than traditional analyses, if categories are considered clinically more relevant

Note

More background, theoretical and mathematical information of optimal binning
   is given in Machine learning in medicine part three, Chap. 5, Optimal binning, pp 37–48, Springer Heidelberg Germany 2013. See also the Chap. 5 of this book for bin membership assessment in future families.

Chapter 62
Conjoint Analysis for Determining the Most Appreciated Properties of Medicines to Be Developed (15 Physicians)

General Purpose

Products like articles of use, food products, or medicines have multiple characteristics. Each characteristic can be measured in several levels, and too many combinations are possible for a single person to distinguish. Conjoint analysis models a limited, but representative and meaningful subset of combinations, which can, subsequently, be presented to persons for preference scaling. The chapter is to assess whether this method is efficient for the development of new medicines.

Background

Conjoint analysis is a survey-based statistical technique used in market research that helps determine how people value different attributes (feature, function, benefits) that make up an individual product or service. Conjoint analysis is sometimes called mathematical psychology and was developed by marketing professor Paul E. Green at the Wharton School of the University of Pennsylvania in the early 80s.

Depending on the type of model, different econometric and statistical methods can be used to estimate utility functions. These utility functions indicate the perceived value of the feature and how sensitive consumer perceptions and preferences are to changes in product features. The actual estimation procedure will depend on the design of the task and profiles for respondents, in the type of specification, and the scale of measure for preferences (it can be ratio, ranking, choice) which can have

This chapter was previously published in "Machine learning in medicine-cookbook 1" as Chap. 20, 2013.

Electronic Supplementary Material The online version of this chapter (https://doi.org/10.1007/978-3-030-33970-8_62) contains supplementary material, which is available to authorized users.

© Springer Nature Switzerland AG 2020
T. J. Cleophas, A. H. Zwinderman, *Machine Learning in Medicine – A Complete Overview*, https://doi.org/10.1007/978-3-030-33970-8_62

a limited range or not. For rated full profile tasks, linear regression may be appropriate, for choice based tasks, maximum likelihood estimation, usually with logistic regression are typically used. The original methods were monotonic analysis of variance or linear programming techniques, but contemporary marketing research practice has shifted towards choice-based models using multinomial logit, mixed versions of this model, and other refinements. Bayesian estimators are also very popular. Hierarchical Bayesian procedures are nowadays relatively popular as well.

Specific Scientific Question

Can conjoint analysis be helpful to pharmaceutical institutions for determining the most appreciated properties of medicines they will develop.

Constructing an Analysis Plan

A novel medicine is judged by 5 characteristics:

(1) safety expressed in 3 levels,
(2) efficacy in 3,
(3) price in 3,
(4) pill size in 2,
(5) prolonged activity in 2 levels.

From the levels $3 \times 3 \times 3 \times 2 \times 2 = 108$ combinations can be formed, which is too large a number for physicians to distinguish. In addition, some combinations, e.g., high price and low efficacy will never be prefered and could be skipped from the listing. Instead, a limited but representative number of profiles is selected. SPSS statistical software 19.0 is used for the purpose.

Command:
Data....Orthogonal Design....Generate....Factor Name: enter safety....Factor Label: enter safety design....click Add....click ?....click Define Values: enter 1,2,3 on the left, and A,B,C on the right side....Do the same for all of the characteristics (here called factors)....click Create a new dataset....Dataset name: enter medicine_plan....click Options: Minimum number of cases: enter 18....mark Number of holdout cases: enter 4....Continue....OK.

The output sheets show a listing of 22, instead of 108, combinations with two new variables (status_ and card_) added. The variable Status_ gives a "0" to the first 18 combinations used for subsequent analyses, and "1" to holdout combinations to be used by the computer for checking the validity of the program. The variable

Card_ gives identification numbers to each combination. For further use of the model designed so far, we will first need to perform the Display Design commands.

Command:
Data. . . .Orthogonal Design. . . .Display. . . .Factors: transfer all of the characteristics to this window. . . .click Listing for experimenter. . . .click OK.

The output sheet now shows a plan card, which looks virtually identical to the above 22 profile listing. It must be saved. We will use the name medicine_plan for the file. For convenience the design file is given on the internet at extras.springer. com. The next thing is to use SPSS' syntax program to complete the preparation for real data analysis.

Command:
click File. . . .move to Open. . . .move to Syntax. . . .enter the following text. . . .
CONJOINT PLAN='g:medicine_plan.sav'
/DATA='g:medicine_prefs.sav'
/SEQUENCE=PREF1 TO PREF22
/SUBJECT=ID
/FACTORS=SAFETY EFFICACY (DISCRETE)
PRICE (LINEAR LESS)
PILLSIZE PROLONGEDACTIVITY (LINEAR MORE)
/PRINT=SUMMARYONLY.

Save this syntax file at the directory of your choice. Note: the conjoint file entitled "conjoint" only works, if both the plan file and the data file to be analyzed are correctly entered in the above text. In our example we saved both files at a USB stick (recognised by our computer under the directory "g:"). For convenience the conjoint file entitled "conjoint" is also given at extras.springer.com. Prior to use it should also be saved at the USB-stick.

The 22 combinations including the 4 holdouts, can now be used to perform a conjoint analysis with real data. For that purpose 15 physicians are requested to express their preferences of the 22 different combinations.

The preference scores are entered in the data file with the IDs of the physicians as a separate variable in addition to the 22 combinations (the columns). For convenience the data file entitled "medicine_prefs" is given at extras.springer.com, but, if you want to use it, it should first be saved at the USB stick. The conjoint analysis can now be successfully performed.

Performing the Final Analysis

Command:
Open the USB stick. . . .click conjoint. . . .the above syntax text is shown. . . .click Run. . .select All.

Model Description

	N of Levels	Relation to Ranks or Scores
safety	3	Linear (more)
efficacy	3	Linear (more)
price	3	Linear (less)
pillsize	2	Discrete
prolongedactivity	2	Discrete

All factors are orthogonal.

The above table gives an overview of the different characteristics (here called factors), and their levels used to construct an analysis plan of the data from our data file.

Utilities

		Utility Estimate	Std. Error
pillsize	large	-1,250	,426
	small	1,250	,426
prolongedactivity	no	-,733	,426
	yes	,733	,426
safety	A*	1,283	,491
	B*	2,567	,983
	C*	3,850	1,474
efficacy	high	-,178	,491
	medium	-,356	,983
	low	-,533	1,474
price	$4	-1,189	,491
	$6	-2,378	,983
	$8	-3,567	1,474
(Constant)		10,328	1,761

The above table gives the utility scores, which are the overall levels of the preferences expressed by the physicians. The meaning of the levels are given:

safety level C: best safety
efficacy level high: best efficacy
pill size 2: smallest pill
prolonged activity 2: prolonged activity present
price $8: most expensive pill.

Generally, higher scores mean greater preference. There is an inverse relationship between pill size and preference, and between pill costs and preference. The safest pill and the most efficaceous pill were given the best preferences.

However, the regression coefficients for efficacy were, statistically, not very significant. Nonetheless, they were included in the overall analysis by the software program. As the utility scores are simply linear regression coefficients, the scores can be used to compute total utilities (add-up preference scores) for a medicine with known characteristic levels. An interesting thing about the methodology is that, like with linear regression modeling, the characteristic levels can be used to calculate an individual add-up utility score (preference score) for a pill with e.g., the underneath characteristics:

(1) pill size (small) + (2) prolonged activity (yes) + safety (C) + efficacy (high) + price ($4) = 1.250 + 0.733 + 3.850 − 0.178 − 1.189 + constant (10.328) = 14.974.

For the underneath pill the add-up utility score is, as expected, considerably lower.

(1) pill size (large) + (2) prolonged activity (no) + safety (A) + efficacy (low) + price ($8) = −1.250 − 0.733 + 1.283 − 0.533 − 3.567 + constant (10.328) = 5.528.

The above procedure is the real power of conjoint analysis. It enables to predict preferences for combinations that were not rated by the physicians. In this way you will obtain an idea about the preference to be received by a medicine with known characteristics.

Importance Values

pillsize	15,675
prolongedactivity	12,541
safety	28,338
efficacy	12,852
price	30,594

Averaged Importance
Score

The range of the utility (preference) scores for each characteristic is an indication of how important the characteristic is. Characteristics with greater ranges play a larger role than the others. As observed the safety and price are the most important preference producing characteristics, while prolonged activity, efficacy, and pill size appear to play a minor role according to the respondents' judgments. The ranges are computed such that they add-up to 100 (%).

Coefficients

	B Coefficient
	Estimate
safety	1,283
efficacy	-,178
price	-1,189

The above table gives the linear regression coefficients for the factors that are specified as linear. The interpretation of the utility (preference) score for the cheapest pill equals $4 \times (-1.189) = -4.756$

Correlations[a]

	Value	Sig.
Pearson's R	,819	,000
Kendall's tau	,643	,000
Kendall's tau for Holdouts	,333	,248

a. Correlations between observed and estimated preferences

The correlation coefficients between the observed preferences and the preferences calculated from conjoint model shows that the correlations by Pearson and Kendall's method are pretty good, indicating that the conjoint methodology produced a sensitive prediction model. The regression analysis of the holdout cases is intended as a validity check, and produced a pretty large p-value of 24.8%. Still it means that we have about 75% to find no type I error in this procedure.

Number of Reversals

Factor	efficacy		9
	price		5
	safety		4
	prolongedactivity		0
	pillsize		0
Subject	1	Subject 1	1
	2	Subject 2	0
	3	Subject 3	0
	4	Subject 4	1
	5	Subject 5	3
	6	Subject 6	1
	7	Subject 7	3
	8	Subject 8	2
	9	Subject 9	1
	10	Subject 10	0
	11	Subject 11	1
	12	Subject 12	1
	13	Subject 13	0
	14	Subject 14	1
	15	Subject 15	3

Finally, the conjoint program reports the number of physicians whose preference was different from what was expected. Particularly in the efficacy characteristic there were 9 of the 15 physicians who chose differently from expected, underlining the limited role of this characteristic.

Conclusion

Conjoint analysis is helpful to pharmaceutical institutions for determining the most appreciated properties of medicines they will develop. Disadvantages include: (1) it is pretty complex; (2) it may be hard to respondents to express preferences; (3) other characteristics not selected may be important too, e.g., physical and pharmacological factors.

Note

More background, theoretical and mathematical information of conjoint modeling is given in Machine learning in medicine part three, Chap. 19, Conjoint analysis, pp 217–230, Springer Heidelberg Germany 2013.

Chapter 63
Item Response Modeling for Analyzing Quality of Life with Better Precision (1000 Patients)

General Purpose

Item response tests are goodness of fit tests for analyzing the item scores of intelligence tests, and they perform better for the purpose than traditional tests, based on reproducibility measures, do. Like intelligence, quality of life is a multidimensional construct, and may, therefore, be equally suitable for item response modeling.

Background

Item response models are applied for analyzing item scores of psychological and intelligence tests, and they are based on exponential relationships between the psychological traits and the item responses. Items are usually questions with "yes" or "no" answers. Item response models were invented by Georg Rasch, a mathematician from Copenhagen who was unable to find work in his discipline in the 30ths and turned to work as a psychometrician. These models are, currently, the basis for modern psychological testing including computer-assisted adaptive testing. Advantages compared to classical linear testing include first that item response models do not use reliability as a measure of their applicability, but instead use formal goodness of fit tests. Second, the scale does not need to be of an interval nature. As a consequence the effects of covariates can be analyzed and reported with odds ratios,

This chapter was previously published in "Machine learning in medicine-cookbook 2" as Chap. 12, 2014.

Electronic Supplementary Material The online version of this chapter (https://doi.org/10.1007/978-3-030-33970-8_63) contains supplementary material, which is available to authorized users.

© Springer Nature Switzerland AG 2020
T. J. Cleophas, A. H. Zwinderman, *Machine Learning in Medicine – A Complete Overview*, https://doi.org/10.1007/978-3-030-33970-8_63

independently of the item format and population averages. Ceiling effects are, therefore, much less of a problem than they are with classical linear methods.

Our group was the first to apply item response modeling to quality of life assessments. Like psychometric properties quality of life is a multidimensional construct and is often investigated in homogeneous populations. Both aspects are a direct threat to the reliability, because reliability is a direct function of the dimensionality of the item pool and of the variance of the true score in the population. Indeed, item response modeling may be suitable for quality of life analyses, although not widely used so far. But this may be a matter of time. Quality of life (QOL) research is still in its infancy, and modern QOL batteries provide better validity and reliability, making it better suitable for methods like item response modeling.

Not only quality of life, but also current clinical diagnostic batteries are increasingly multidimensional, particularly, in clinical research like diagnostic test batteries in the vascular laboratory or catheterization laboratory: multiple tests are often used to assess the presence of a single disease or disease severity. To date item response modeling has not yet been applied in this field. The current chapter is the first effort for that purpose, and was also written to explain the principles of item response modeling to the readership of clinical investigators. Data examples are given of both a quality of life assessment and a diagnostic test battery in the vascular laboratory.

With psychometric item response modeling the data of a test sample are exponentially modeled according to:

$$\text{Probability of responding to an item (yes/no)}$$
$$= e^{(\text{ability level of patient}) - (\text{difficulty level of item})}.$$

This equation can also be described as:

$$\text{Log odds of responding to an item (yes/no)}$$
$$= (\text{ability level of patient}) - (\text{difficulty level of item}).$$

Multiple items in a single test can be simply added up:

$$\text{Probability of responding to a set of items (yes/no)}$$
$$= \Sigma \, e^{(\text{ability levels of patients}) - (\text{difficulty levels of items})}.$$

$$\text{Log odds of responding to a set of items (yes/no)}$$
$$= \Sigma \, (\text{ability levels of patients}) - (\text{difficulty levels of items}).$$

Software is used to calculate the best fit ability parameters, otherwise called latent traits, and the best fit difficulty parameters for the data given. Then, based on these parameters, just like with logistic models for making predictions from risk factor profiles, predictions can be made about individual levels of intellectual and psychological abilities. Similarly, predictions about levels of quality of life and, maybe also, severity of clinical diseases can respectively be made with quality of life data and diagnostic laboratory data.

For analysis the data are fitted within the standard Gaussian distribution. A problem is that item response modeling is not available in standard statistical software. However, for dichotomous items plenty software is commercially and freely available, and for polytomous items such software is rapidly being developed. All of the software can handle large data files, the numbers of items to be scored are now only limited by the memory capacities of the hardware. In the current paper, we will use the Free Software LTA-2 (latent trait analysis-2) (with binary items) of John Uebersax, 2006. The interesting things about item response modeling are

(1) that they are more realistic than classical methods: e.g., with a classical model the data would produce a quality of life between 0 and 100% while patients with a quality of life of 0 and 100% in reality do not exist; in contrast, with item response modeling quality of life levels are expressed as distances from an average level;

(2) that they are more flexible and precise, and, therefore, more suitable for making predictions about individual patients, for example, a set of 5 items will give 5 levels of quality of life or severity of disease in the usual classical model, with item response modeling it will give 32 levels.

The following type of data are suitable for item response modeling. A sub-domain of mental depression after a myocardial event is assessed with five items (answer yes/no): (1) not hopeful, (2) blue feeling, (3) tired in the morning, (4) worrier, (5) not talking. If we review the answers, we may observe that, for example, the items (4) and (5) are less often confirmed by our test sample subjects than the other three items. They may, therefore, be expressions of a more severe level of depression. Item response models, unlike the classical models for psychometric assessments, account for and make use of the different levels of severity of items in a test battery. By doing so they change largely qualitative data into fairly accurate quantitative data. They use for that purpose the (slight) differences between individual patients in response pattern to a set of items.

The results of the item response model are fitted to a standard normal Gaussian curve. Both the chi-square goodness of fit and Kolmogorov-Smirnov (KS) goodness of fit tests can be used to assess how closely the results actually follow the Gaussian curve, respectively using a significant chi-square value and using the largest cumulative difference between observed and expected frequencies according to the KS table, as criteria for adequacy of the model for making predictions.

Primary Scientific Question

Can quality of life data be analyzed through item response modeling, and provide more sensitivity than classical linear models do?

Example

As an example we will analyze the 5-items of a mobility-domain of a quality of life (QOL) battery for patients with coronary artery disease in a group of 1000 patients. Instead of 5 many more items can be included. However, for the purpose of simplicity we will use only 5 items: the domain mobility in a quality of life battery was assessed by answering "yes or no" to experienced difficulty (1) while climbing stair, (2) on short distances, (3) on long distances, (4) on light household work, (5) on heavy household work. In the underneath table the data of 1000 patients are summarized. These data can be fitted into a standard normal Gaussian frequency distribution curve (see underneath figure). From it, it can be seen that the items used here are more adequate for demonstrating low quality of life than they are for demonstrating high quality of life, but, nonetheless, an entire Gaussian distribution can be extrapolated from the data given. The lack of histogram bars on the right side of the Gaussian curve suggests that more high quality of life items in the questionnaire would be welcome in order to improve the fit of the histogram into the Gaussian curve. Yet it is interesting to observe that, even with a limited set of items, already a fairly accurate frequency distribution pattern of all quality of life levels of the population is obtained.

Example 493

No. response pattern	Response pattern (1 = yes, 2 = no) to items 1 to 5	Observed Frequencies
1	11111	4
2	11112	7
3	11121	3
4	11122	12
5	11211	2
6	11212	2
7	11221	4
8	11222	5
9	12111	2
10	12112	9
11	12121	1
12	12122	17
13	12211	1
14	12212	4
15	12221	3
16	12222	16
17	21111	11
18	21112	30
19	21121	15
20	21122	21
21	21211	4
22	21212	29
23	21221	16
24	21222	81
25	22111	17
26	22112	57
27	22121	22
28	22122	174
29	22211	12
30	22212	62
31	22221	29
32	22222	263

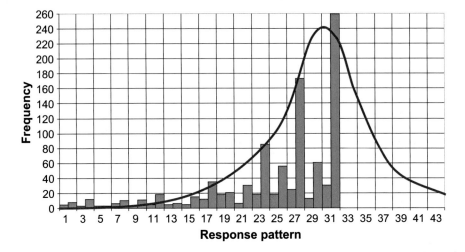

The LTA-2 (Latent Trait Analysis −2) free software program is used (Uebersax J. Free Software LTA (latent trait analysis) −2 (with binary items), 2006, www.john-uebersax.com/stat/ltal.htm). The data file entitled "itemresponsemodeling" is available in extras.springer.com. We enter the data file by the traditional copy and paste commands.

Command

Gaussian error model for IRF (Instrument Response Function) shape....chi-square goodness of fit for Fit Statistics.... Frequency table....EAP score table.

The software program calculates the quality of life scores of the different response patterns as EAP (Expected Ability a Posteriori) scores. These scores can be considered as the z-values of a normal Gaussian curve, meaning that the associated area under curve (AUC) of the Gaussian curve is an estimate of the level of quality of life.

There is, approximately,

> a 50% quality of life level with an EAP score of 0,
> a 35 % QOL level with an EAP score of -1 (standard deviations),
> a 2.5 %   "   "   "   of -2
> a 85 %   "   "   of +1
> a 97.5 %   "   "   of +2

Example   495

No.response Pattern	Response pattern (1 = yes, 2 = no) to items 1 to 5	EAP scores (SDs)	AUCs (QOL levels) (%)	Classical Scores (0-5)
1.	11111	-1.8315	3.4	0
2.	11112	-1.4425	7.5	1
3.	11121	-1.4153	7.8	1
4.	11122	-1.0916	15.4	2
5.	11211	-1.2578	10.4	1
6.	11212	-0.8784	18.9	2
7.	11221	-0.8600	19.4	2
8.	11222	-0.4596	32.3	3
9.	12111	-1.3872	8.2	1
10.	12112	-0.9946	16.1	2
11.	12121	-0.9740	16.6	2
12.	12122	-0.5642	28.8	3
13.	12211	-0.8377	20.1	2
14.	12212	-0.4389	33.0	3
15.	12221	-0.4247	33.4	3
16.	12222	0.0074	50.4	4
17.	21111	-1.3501	8.9	1
18.	21112	-0.9381	17.4	2
19.	21121	-0.9172	17.9	2
20.	21122	-0.4866	31.2	3
21.	21211	-0.7771	21.8	2
22.	21212	-0.3581	35.9	3
23.	21221	-0.3439	36.7	3
24.	21222	0.1120	54.4	4
25.	22111	-0.8925	18.7	2
26.	22112	-0.4641	32.3	3
27.	22121	-0.4484	32.6	3
28.	22122	0.0122	50.4	4
29.	22211	-0.3231	37.5	3
30.	22212	0.1322	55.2	4
31.	22221	0.1433	55.6	4
32.	22222	0.6568	74.5	5

EAP = expected ability a posteriori; QOL = quality of life.

In the above table the EAP scores per response pattern is given as well as the AUC (= quality of life level) values as calculated by the software program are given. In the fourth column the classical score is given ranging from 0 (no yes answers) to five (five yes answers). Unlike the classical scores, running from 0 to 100%, the item scores are more precise and vary from 3.4 to 74.5% with an overall mean score, by definition, of 50%. The item response model produce an adequate fit for the data as demonstrated by chi-square goodness of fit values/ degrees of freedom of 0.86. What is even more important, is, that we have 32 different QOL scores instead of no more than 5 as observed with the classical score method. With 6 items the numbers of scores would even rise to 64. The interpretation is: the higher score, the better the quality of life.

Conclusion

Quality of life assessments can be analyzed through item response modeling, and item response models provide more sensitivity than classical linear models do.

Note

More background theoretical and mathematical information of item response modeling is given in Machine learning in medicine part one, Chap. 8, Item response modeling, pp. 87–98, edited by Springer Heidelberg Germany, 2012, from the same authors. In the current chapter the LTA-2 the free software program is used (Uebersax J. Free Software LTA (latent trait analysis) −2 (with binary items), 2006, www.john-uebersax.com/stat/ltal.htm).

Chapter 64
Survival Studies with Varying Risks of Dying (50 and 60 Patients)

General Purpose

Patients' predictors of survival may change across time, because people may change their lifestyles. Standard statistical methods do not allow adjustments for time-dependent predictors. Time-dependent Cox regression has been introduced as a method adequate for the purpose.

Background

The Cox proportional-hazards regression model has achieved widespread use in the analysis of time-to-event data with censoring and covariates. The covariates may change their values over time. In 1999 Lloyd Fisher, statistician from the University of Washington discussed the use of such time-dependent covariates, which offer additional opportunities but must be used with caution. The interrelationships between the outcome and variable over time can lead to bias unless the relationships are well understood. The form of a time-dependent covariate is much more complex than in Cox models with fixed (non-time-dependent) covariates. It involves constructing a function of time. Further, the model does not have some of the properties of the fixed-covariate model; it cannot usually be used to predict the survival (time-to-event) curve over time. The estimated probability of an event over time is not related to the hazard function in the usual fashion.

This chapter was previously published in "Machine learning in medicine-cookbook 2" as Chap. 13, 2014.

Electronic Supplementary Material The online version of this chapter (https://doi.org/10.1007/978-3-030-33970-8_64) contains supplementary material, which is available to authorized users.

Primary Scientific Question

Predictors of survival may change across time, e.g., the effect of smoking, cholesterol, and increased blood pressure on cardiovascular disease, and patients' frailty in oncology research.

Examples

Cox Regression with a Time-Dependent Predictor

The level of LDL cholesterol is a strong predictor of cardiovascular survival. However, in a survival study virtually no one will die from elevated values in the first decade of observation. LDL cholesterol may be, particularly, a killer in the second decade of observation. The Cox regression model is not appropriate for analyzing the effect of LDL cholesterol on survival, because it assumes that the relative hazard of dying is the same in the first, second and third decade. If you want to analyze such data, an extended Cox regression model allowing for non-proportional hazards can be applied, and is available in SPSS statistical software. In the underneath example the first 10 of 60 patients are given. They were followed for 30 years for the occurrence of a cardiovascular event. Each row represents a patient, the columns are the patient characteristics, otherwise called the variables.

Variable (Var)					
1	2	3	4	5	6
1,00	1	0	65,00	0,00	2,00
1,00	1	0	66,00	0,00	2,00
2,00	1	0	73,00	0,00	2,00
2,00	1	0	54,00	0,00	2,00
2,00	1	0	46,00	0,00	2,00
2,00	1	0	37,00	0,00	2,00
2,00	1	0	54,00	0,00	2,00
2,00	1	0	66,00	0,00	2,00
2,00	1	0	44,00	0,00	2,00
3,00	0	0	62,00	0,00	2,00

Var 00001 = follow-up period (years) (Var = variable)
Var 00002 = event (0 or 1, event or lost for follow-up = censored)
Var 00003 = treatment modality (0 = treatment-1, 1 = treatment-2)
Var 00004 = age (years)
Var 00005 = gender (0 or 1, male or female)
Var 00006 = LDL-cholesterol (0 or 1, < 3.9 or > = 3.9 mmol/l)

The entire data file is in extras.springer.com, and is entitled "survivalvaryingrisks". Start by opening the file. First, a usual Cox regression is performed with LDL-cholesterol as predictor of survival (var = variable).

Command

Analyze....survival....Cox regression....time: follow months.... status: var. 2....define event (1)....Covariates....categorical: elevated LDL-cholesterol (Var 00006) = > categorical variables....continue....plots.... survival = > .... hazard....continue....OK.

Variables in the Equation

	B	SE	Wald	df	Sig.	Exp(B)
VAR00006	-,482	,307	2,462	1	,117	,618

Variables in the Equation

	B	SE	Wald	df	Sig.	Exp(B)
T_COV_	-,131	,033	15,904	1	,000	,877

The upper table shows that elevated LDL-cholesterol is not a significant predictor of survival with a p-value as large as 0.117 and a hazard ratio of 0.618. In order to assess, whether elevated LDL-cholesterol adjusted for time has an effect on survival, a time-dependent Cox regression will be performed as shown in the above lower table. For that purpose the time-dependent covariate is defined as a function of both the variable time (called "T_" in SPSS) and the LDL-cholesterol-variable, while using the product of the two. This product is applied as the "time-dependent predictor of survival, and a usual Cox model is, subsequently, performed (Cov = covariate).

Command

Analyze....survival....Cox w/Time-Dep Cov....Compute Time-Dep Cov.... Time (T_) = > in box Expression for T_Cov....add the sign * ....add the LDL-cholesterol variable....model....time: follow months....status: var. 00002....?: define event:1....continue....T_Cov = > in box covariates....OK.

The above lower table shows that elevated LDL-cholesterol after adjustment for differences in time is a highly significant predictor of survival. If we look at the actual data of the file, we will observe that, overall, the LDL-cholesterol variable is not an important factor. But, if we look at the blood pressures of the three decades separately, then it is observed that something very special is going on: in the first decade virtually no one with elevated LDL-cholesterol dies. In the second decade virtually everyone with an elevated LDL-cholesterol does: LDL cholesterol seems to be particularly a killer in the second decade. Then, in the third decade other reasons for dying seem to have occurred.

Cox Regression with a Segmented Time-Dependent Predictor

Some variables may have different values at different time periods. For example, elevated blood pressure may be, particularly, harmful not after decades but at the very time-point it is highest. The blood pressure is highest in the first and third decade of the study. However, in the second decade it is mostly low, because the patients were adequately treated at that time. For the analysis we have to use the socalled logical expressions. They take the value 1, if the time is true, and 0, if false. Using a series of logical expressions, we can create our time-dependent predictor, that can, then, be analyzed by the usual Cox model. In the underneath example 11 of 60 patients are given. The entire data file is in extras.springer.com, and is entitled "survivalvaryingrisks2" The patients were followed for 30 years for the occurrence of a cardiovascular event. Each row represents again a patient, the columns are the patient characteristics.

Var 1	2	3	4	5	6	7
7,00	1	76	,00	133,00	.	.
9,00	1	76	,00	134,00	.	.
9,00	1	65	,00	143,00	.	.
11,00	1	54	,00	134,00	110,00	.
12,00	1	34	,00	143,00	111,00	.
14,00	1	45	,00	135,00	110,00	.
16,00	1	56	1,00	123,00	103,00	.
17,00	1	67	1,00	133,00	107,00	.
18,00	1	86	1,00	134,00	108,00	.
30,00	1	75	1,00	134,00	102,00	134,00
30,00	1	65	1,00	132,00	121,00	126,00

Var 00001 = follow-up period years (Var = variable)
Var 00002 = event (0 or 1, event or lost for follow-up = censored)
Var 00003 = age (years)
Var 00004 = gender
Var 00005 = mean blood pressure in the first decade
Var 00006 = mean blood pressure in the second decade
Var 00007 = mean blood pressure in the third decade

In the second and third decade an increasing number of patients have been lost. The following time-dependent covariate must be constructed for the analysis of these data ($*$ = sign of multiplication) using the click Transform and click Compute Variable commands:

$$(T >= 1 \& T < 11) * \text{Var } 5 + (T >= 11 \& T < 21) * \text{Var } 6 + (T >= 21 \& T < 31)$$
$$* \text{Var } 7$$

This novel predictor variable is entered in the usual way with the commands (Cov = covariate):

Model....time: follow months....status: var. 00002....?: define event:1 - continue....T_Cov => in box covariates....OK.

The underneath table shows that, indeed, a mean blood pressure after adjustment for difference in decades is a significant predictor of survival at p = 0.040, and with a hazard ratio of 0.936 per mm Hg. In spite of the better blood pressures in the second decade, blood pressure is a significant killer in the overall analysis.

Variables in the Equation

	B	SE	Wald	df	Sig.	Exp(B)
T_COV_	-,066	,032	4,238	1	,040	,936

Conclusion

Many predictors of survival change across time, e.g., the effect of smoking, cholesterol, and increased blood pressure in cardiovascular research, and patients' frailty in oncology research.

Note

More background theoretical and mathematical information is given in Machine learning in medicine part one, Chap. 9, Time-dependent predictor modeling, pp. 99–111, Springer Heidelberg Germany, 2012, from the same authors.

Chapter 65
Fuzzy Logic for Improved Precision of Dose-Response Data (8 Induction Dosages)

General Purpose

Fuzzy logic can handle questions to which the answers may be "yes" at one time and "no" at the other, or may be partially true and untrue. Pharmacodynamic data deal with questions like "does a patient respond to a particular drug dose or not", or "does a drug cause the same effects at the same time in the same subject or not". Such questions are typically of a fuzzy nature, and might, therefore, benefit from an analysis based on fuzzy logic.

Background

Lofti Zadeh, professor of science at Berkeley, published in 1964 the concept of fuzzy truths, as answers that may be "yes" at one time and "no" at the other, or that may be partially true and partially untrue. He developed an analytical model based on this concept. When you think of real life, you can imagine many things that are not entirely certain, and it is remarkable, therefore, that it took over 20 years before this analytical model became successfully implemented in science. Nowadays Tokyo subway traffic uses fuzzy logic running and braking systems, and Maserati sportscars have a fuzzy logic automatic transmission with one position for forward instead of the usual three or four, and with much better performance.

In the field of medicine fuzzy logic is little used in spite of the, typically, uncertain character of this branch of science. When searching for published papers we found a few papers on diagnostic imaging and clinical decision analysis. In clinical pharmacology fuzzy logic has been applied for pharmacological treatment decision

This chapter was previously published in "Machine learning in medicine-cookbook 2" as Chap. 14, 2014.

T. J. Cleophas, A. H. Zwinderman, *Machine Learning in Medicine – A Complete Overview*, https://doi.org/10.1007/978-3-030-33970-8_65

analyses, and structure-activity modeling. However, we found no papers on fuzzy logic and pharmacodynamic modeling. Often the basic molecular mode of action of a drug is unknown, and pharmacodynamics is, then, used as a surrogate for studying the pharmacological response to a drug of the body. By its very nature pharmacodynamics can be argued to be particularly fuzzy. For example, the answer to the question "does a patient respond or not to a particular thiopental induction dose", or questions like "does propranolol cause the same effects at the same time in the same subject or not" are typically questions of a fuzzy nature, and might, thus, benefit from an analysis based on fuzzy logic.

In the present chapter we study whether fuzzy logic can improve the precision of predictive models for pharmacodynamic data, i.e., models that better fit the observed data, and, thus, better predict future data. We hope that the examples given will stimulate researchers analyzing pharmacodynamic data to more often apply fuzzy methodologies.

Specific Scientific Question

This chapter is to study whether fuzzy logic can improve the precision of predictive models for pharmacodynamic data.

Example

Input values	output values	fuzzy-modeled output
induction dosage of thiopental (mg/kg)	numbers of responders (n)	numbers of responders (n)
1	4	4
1.5	5	5
2	6	8
2.5	9	10
3	12	12
3.5	17	14
4	17	16
4.5	12	14
5	9	1

Example   505

We will use as an example the quantal pharmacodynamic effects of different induction dosages of thiopental on numbers of responding subjects. It is usually not possible to know what type of statistical distribution the experiment is likely to follow, sometimes Gaussian, sometimes very skewed. A pleasant aspect of fuzzy modeling is that it can be applied with any type of statistical distribution and that it is particularly suitable for uncommon and unexpected non linear relationships.

Quantal response data are often presented in the literature as S-shape dose-cumulative response curves with the dose plotted on a logarithmic scale, where the log transformation has an empirical basis. We will, therefore, use a logarithmic regression model. SPSS Statistical Software is used for analysis.

Command

Analyze...regression...curve estimation...dependent variable: data second column...independent variable: data first column...logarithmic...OK.

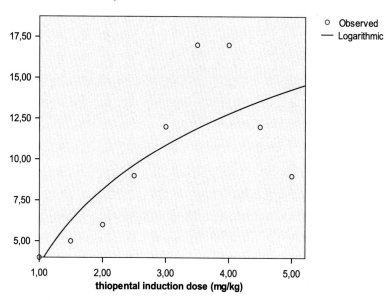

numbers of responders

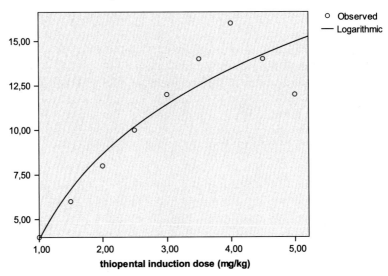

The analysis produces a moderate fit of the data (upper curve) with an r-square value of 0.555 (F-value 8.74, p-value 0.024).

We, subsequently, fuzzy-model the imput and output relationships (underneath figure). First of all, we create linguistic rules for the imput and output data.

For that purpose we divide the universal space of the imput variable into fuzzy memberships with linguistic membership names:

imput-*zero*, −*small*, −*medium*, −*big*, −*superbig*.

Then we do the same for the output variable:

output-*zero*, −*small*, −*medium*, −*big*.

Subsequently, we create linguistic rules.

Example   507

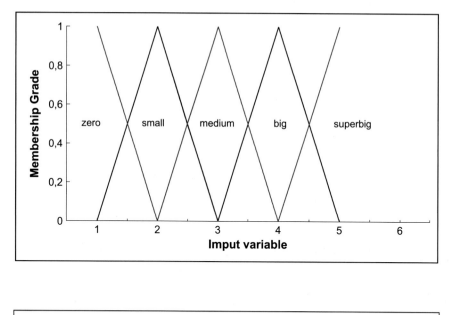

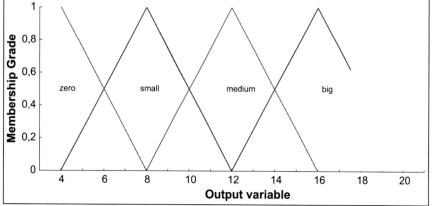

The above figure shows that imput-*zero* consists of the values 1 and 1.5.

> The value 1 (100% membership) has 4 as outcome value (100% membership of output-*zero*).
>
> The value 1.5 (50% membership) has 5 as outcome value (75% membership of output-*zero*, 25% of output-*small*).

The imput-*zero* produces 100% x 100% + 50% x 75% = 137.5% membership to output-*zero*, and 50% x 25% = 12.5% membership to output-*small*, and so, output-*zero* is the most important output contributor here, and we forget about the small contribution of output-*small*.

Imput-*small* is more complex, it consists of the values 1.5, and 2.0, and 2.5.

The value 1.5 (50% membership) has 5 as outcome value (75% membership of output-*zero*, 25% membership of output-*small*).

The value 2.0 (100% membership) has 6 as outcome value (50% membership of outcome-*zero*, and 50% membership of output-*small*).

The value 2.5 (50% membership) has 9 as outcome value (75% membership of output-*small* and 25% of output-*medium*).

The imput-*small* produces 50% x 75% + 100% x 50% = 87.5% membership to output-*zero*, 50% x 25% + 100% x 50% + 50%x75% = 100% membership to output-*small*, and 50% x 25% = 12.5% membership to output-*medium*. And so, the output-*small* is the most important contributor here, and we forget about the other two.

For the other imput memberships similar linguistic rules are determined:

Imput-*medium* → output-*medium*
Imput-*big* → output-*big*
Imput-*superbig* → output-*medium*

We are, particularly interested in the modeling capacity of fuzzy logic in order to improve the precision of pharmacodynamic modeling.

The modeled output value of imput value 1 is found as follows.

Value 1 is 100% member of imput-*zero*, meaning that according to the above linguistic rules it is also associated with a 100% membership of output-*zero* corresponding with a value of 4.

Value 1.5 is 50% member of imput-*zero* and 50% imput-*small*. This means it is 50% associated with the output-*zero* and –*small* corresponding with values of 50% x (4 + 8) = 6.

For all of the imput values modeled output values can be found in this way. The above table right column shows fuzzy-modeled results. We perform a logarithmic regression on the fuzzy-modeled outcome data similar to that for the un-modeled output values. The fuzzy-modeld output data provided a much better fit than did the un-modeled output values (lower curve) with an r-square value of 0.852 (F-value = 40.34) as compared to 0.555 (F-value 8.74) for the un-modeled output data.

Conclusion

Fuzzy logic can handle questions to which the answers may be "yes" at one time and "no" at the other, or may be partially true and untrue. Dose response data deal with questions like "does a patient respond to a particular drug dose or not", or "does a drug cause the same effects at the same time in the same subject or not". Such questions are typically of a fuzzy nature, and might, therefore, benefit from.

an analysis based on fuzzy logic.

Note

More background theoretical and mathematical information of analyses using fuzzy logic is given in Machine learning in medicine part one, Chap. 19, pp. 241–253, Springer Heidelberg Germany, 2012, from the same authors.

Chapter 66
Automatic Data Mining for the Best Treatment of a Disease (90 Patients)

General Purpose

SPSS modeler is a work bench for automatic data mining (current chapter) and data modeling (Chaps. 69 and 70). So far it is virtually unused in medicine, and mainly applied by econo−/sociometrists. We will assess whether it can also be used for multiple outcome analysis of clinical data.

Background

In interventional studies with multiple continuous outcomes, multiple one-way analyses of variances are possible, but these traditional analyses do not account interactions between the outcome variables. SPSS modeler is a work bench for automatic data mining and data modeling. So far it is virtually unused in medicine, and mainly applied by econo−/sociometrists. We will assess whether it can also be used for multiple outcome analysis of clinical data. In data mining the question "is a treatment a predictor of clinical improvement" is assessed by the question "is the outcome, clinical improvement, a predictor of the chance of having had a treatment". This approach may seem incorrect, but is also used with discriminant analysis, and it works fine, because it does not suffer from strong correlations between outcome variables. In this chapter a traditional efficacy analysis will be tested against a machine learning methodology entitled automatic data mining. The traditional

This chapter was previously published in "Machine learning in medicine-cookbook 2" as Chap. 15, 2014.

Electronic Supplementary Material The online version of this chapter (https://doi.org/10.1007/978-3-030-33970-8_66) contains supplementary material, which is available to authorized users.

© Springer Nature Switzerland AG 2020
T. J. Cleophas, A. H. Zwinderman, *Machine Learning in Medicine – A Complete Overview*, https://doi.org/10.1007/978-3-030-33970-8_66

efficacy analysis will consist of one-way analyses of variance, 3×2 crosstabs with 3×2 chi-square statistics, and 3-dimensional bars of treatment modalities versus outcomes.

Specific Scientific Question

Patients with sepsis have been given one of three treatments. Various outcome variables are used to assess which one of the treatments performs best.

Example

In data mining the question "is a treatment a predictor of clinical improvement" is assessed by the question "is the outcome, clinical improvement, a predictor of the chance of having had a treatment". This approach may seem incorrect, but is also used with discriminant analysis, and works fine, because it does not suffer from strong correlations between outcome variables (Machine Learning in Medicine Part One, Chap. 17, Discriminant analysis of supervised data, pp. 215–224, Springer Heidelberg Germany, 2013). In this example, 90 patients with sepsis are treated with three different treatments. Various outcome values are used as predictors of the output treatment.

asat	alat	ureum	creat	crp	leucos	treat	low bp	death
5,00	29,00	2,40	79,00	18,00	16,00	1,00	1	0
10,00	30,00	2,10	94,00	15,00	15,00	1,00	1	0
8,00	31,00	2,30	79,00	16,00	14,00	1,00	1	0
6,00	16,00	2,70	80,00	17,00	19,00	1,00	1	0
6,00	16,00	2,20	84,00	18,00	20,00	1,00	1	0
5,00	13,00	2,10	78,00	17,00	21,00	1,00	1	0
10,00	16,00	3,10	85,00	20,00	18,00	1,00	1	0
8,00	28,00	8,00	68,00	15,00	18,00	1,00	1	0
7,00	27,00	7,80	74,00	16,00	17,00	1,00	1	0
6,00	26,00	8,40	69,00	18,00	16,00	1,00	1	0
12,00	22,00	2,70	75,00	14,00	19,00	1,00	1	0
21,00	21,00	3,00	70,00	15,00	20,00	1,00	1	0
10,00	20,00	23,00	74,00	15,00	18,00	1,00	1	0
19,00	19,00	2,10	75,00	16,00	16,00	1,00	1	0
8,00	32,00	2,00	85,00	18,00	19,00	1,00	2	0
20,00	11,00	2,90	63,00	18,00	18,00	1,00	1	0
7,00	30,00	6,80	72,00	17,00	18,00	1,00	1	0
1973,00	846,00	73,80	563,00	18,00	38,00	3,00	2	0
1863,00	757,00	41,70	574,00	15,00	34,00	3,00	2	1
1973,00	646,00	38,90	861,00	16,00	38,00	3,00	2	1

asat = aspartate aminotransferase
alat = alanine aminotransferase
creat = creatinine
crp = c-reactive protein
treat = treatments 1-3
low bp = low blood pressure (1 no, 2 slight, 3 severe)
death = death (0 no, 1 yes)

Only the first 20 patients are above, the entire data file is in extra.springer.com and is entitled "spssmodeler.sav". SPSS modeler version 14.2 is used for the analysis. Start by opening SPSS modeler.

Step 1 Open SPSS Modeler

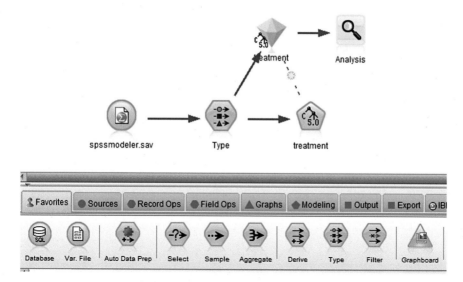

In the palettes at the bottom of the screen full of nodes, look and find the **Statistics File node**, and drag it to the canvas. Double-click on it....Import file: browse and enter the file "spssmodeler.sav"....click OK....in the palette find **Distribution node** and drag to canvas....right-click on the Statistics File node....a Connect symbol comes up....click on the Distribution node....an arrow is displayed.... double-click on the Distribution Node....after a second or two the underneath graph with information from the Distribution node is observed.

Step 2 the Distribution Node

Value /	Proportion	%	Count
1.00		38.89	35
2.00		40.0	36
3.00		21.11	19

It gives the frequency distribution of the three treatments in the 90 patient data file. All of the treatments are substantially present.

Next remove the Distribution node by clicking on it and press delete on the key board of your computer. Continue by dragging the Data audit node to the canvas. . . . perform the connecting manoeuvres as above. . . .double-click it again.

Step 3 the Data Audit Node

Field	Graph	Measurement	Min	Max	Mean	Std. Dev	Skewness	Unique	Valid
asat	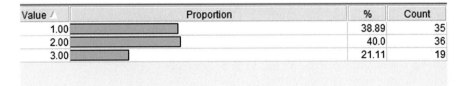	Continuous	5.000	2000.000	360.789	524.433	2.004	--	90
alat		Continuous	11.000	976.000	280.833	318.883	1.036	--	90
ureum		Continuous	2.000	83.000	20.310	19.381	1.338	--	90
creatinine		Continuous	59.000	861.000	272.767	231.551	0.967	--	90
creactiveprotein		Continuous	14.000	131.000	41.667	33.781	1.360	--	90
leucos		Continuous	14.000	42.000	26.822	8.222	0.151	--	90
treatment		Nominal	1.000	3.000	--	--	--	3	90
A lowbloodpress...		Nominal	--	--	--	--	--	3	90
A death		Nominal	--	--	--	--	--	2	90

The Data audit will be edited. Select "treatment" as target field (field is variable here). . . .click Run. The information from this node is now given in the form of a Data audit plot, showing that, as a beneficial effect from the best treaments low values are frequently more often observed than the high values. Particularly, the treatments 1 and 2 (light blue and red) are often associated with low values, these are probably the best treatments. Next remove the Data audit node by clicking on it and press delete on the key board of your computer. Continue by dragging the Plot node to the canvas....perform the connecting manoeuvres as above....double-click it again.

Step 4 the Plot Node

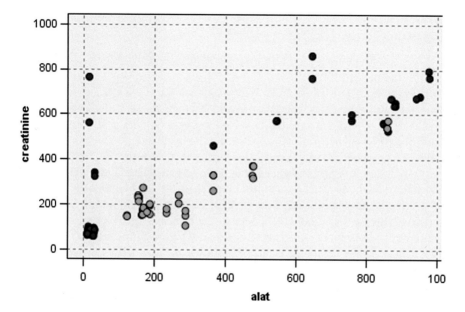

The Plot node will be edited. On the Plot tab select creatinine as y-variable and alat as x-variable, and treatment in the Overlay field at Color....click Run. The information from this node is now given in the form of a scatter plot of patients. This scatter plot of alat versus creatinine values shows that the three treatments are somewhat separately clustered. Treatment 1 (blue) in the left lower part, 2 (green) in the middle, and 3 in the right upper part. Low values means adequate effect of treatment. So treatment 1 (and also some patients with treatment 2) again perform pretty well. Next remove the Plot node by clicking on it and press delete on the key board of your computer. Continue by dragging the Web node to the canvas.... perform the connecting manoeuvres as above....double-click it again.

Step 5 the Web Node

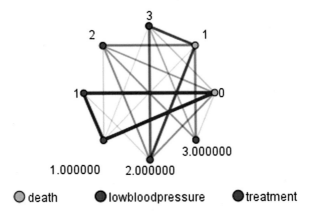

The Web node will be edited. In the Web node dialog box click Select All. . . .click Run. The web graph that comes up, shows that treatment 1 (indicated here as 1.000000) is strongly associated, based on regressions with path statistics very much like Bayesian networks (Chap. 70), with no death and no low blood pressure (thick line), which is very good. However, the treatments 2 (2.000000) and 3 (3.000000) are strongly associated with death and treatment 2 (2.000000) is also associated with the severest form of low blood pressure. Next remove the Web node by clicking on it and press delete on the key board of your computer. Continue by dragging both the Type and C5.0 nodes to the canvas. . . .perform the connecting manoeuvres respectively as indicated in the first graph of this chapter. . . .double-click it again. . . .a gold nugget is placed as shown above. . . .click the gold nugget.

Step 6 the Type and C5.0 Nodes

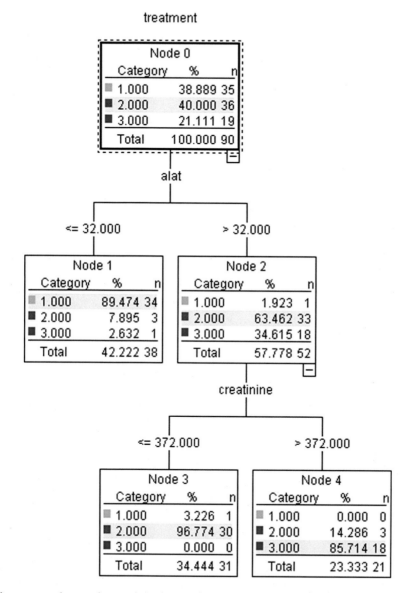

The output sheets give various interactive graphs and tables. One of them is the above C5.0 decision tree. C5.0 decision trees are an improved version of the traditional Quinlan decision trees with less, but more-relevant information.

The C5.0 classifier underscores the previous findings. The variable alat is the best classifier of the treatments with alat <32 over 89% of the patients having had treatment 1, and with alat >32 over 63% of the patients having had treatment 2. Furthermore, in the high alat class patients with a creatinine over 372 around 86% has treatment 3. And so all in all, the treatment 1 would seem the best treatment and treatment 3 the worst one.

Step 7 the Output Node

Results for output field treatment
Comparing $C-treatment with treatment

Correct	82	91,11%
Wrong	8	8,89%
Total	90	

In order to assess the accuracy of the C5.0 classifier output an Output node is attached to the gold nugget. Find Output node and drag it to the canvas. . . .perform connecting manoeuvres with the gold nugget. . . .double-click the Output node again. . . .click Run. The output sheet shows an accuracy (true positives and true negatives) of 91,11%, which is pretty good.

Conclusion

SPSS modeler can be adequately used for multiple outcomes analysis from multiple treatment groups. Finding the most appropriate treatment for a disease might be one of the goals of this kind of research.

Note

SPSS modeler is a software program entirely distinct from SPSS statistical software, though it uses most if not all of the calculus methods of it. It is a standard software package particularly used by market analysts, but, as shown, can perfectly well be applied for exploratory purposes in medical research. SPSS modeler is also applied in the Chaps. 69 and 70.

Chapter 67
Pareto Charts for Identifying the Main Factors of Multifactorial Outcomes (2000 Admissions to Hospital)

General Purpose

In 1906 the Italian economist Pareto observed that 20% of the Italian population possessed 80% of the land, and, looking at other countries, virtually the same seemed to be true. The Pareto principle is currently used to identify the main factors of multifactorial outcomes. Pareto charts is available in SPSS, and this chapter is to assess whether it is useful, not only in marketing science, but also in medicine.

Background

When analyzing observational studies with multifactorial effects, usually less than 20% of the factors determines over 80% of the effect. Vilfredo Pareto was a chief member of the school of elitism. In political science and sociology during the late nineteenth century, elite theory is a theory of the state that seeks to describe and explain power relationships in contemporary society. The theory posits that a small minority, consisting of members of the economic elite and policy-planning networks, holds the most power—and that this power is independent of democratic elections. Elite theory opposes pluralism, a tradition that assumes that all individuals, or at least the multitude of social groups, have equal power and balance each other out in contributing to democratic political outcomes representing the emergent, aggregate will of society. Elite theory argues either that democracy is a utopian

This chapter was previously published in "Machine learning in medicine-cookbook 2" as Chap. 16, 2014.

Electronic Supplementary Material The online version of this chapter (https://doi.org/10.1007/978-3-030-33970-8_67) contains supplementary material, which is available to authorized users.

© Springer Nature Switzerland AG 2020
T. J. Cleophas, A. H. Zwinderman, *Machine Learning in Medicine – A Complete Overview*, https://doi.org/10.1007/978-3-030-33970-8_67

folly, and not realizable within capitalism. Observations from pareto charts would be generally in agreement with the utopian folly, however injust.

Primary Scientific Question

To assess whether pareto charts can be applied to identify in a study of hospital admissions the main causes of iatrogenic admissions.

Example

2000 subsequent admissions to a general hospital in the Netherlands were classified.

Indications for admission	Numbers	%	confidence intervals (95%)
1. Cardiac condition and hypertension	810	40.5	38.0-42.1
2. Gastrointestinal condition	254	12.7	11.9-14.2
3. Infectious disease	200	10.0	9.2-12.0
4. Pulmonary disease	137	6.9	6.5-7.7
5. Hematological condition	109	5.5	4.0-6.2
6. Malignancy	74	3.7	2.7-4.9
7. Mental disease	54	2.7	1.9-3.8
8. Endocrine condition	49	2.5	1.7-3.5
9. Bleedings with acetyl salicyl / NSAIDS	47	2.4	1.6-3.4
10. Other	41	2.1	1.4-3.1
11. Unintentional overdose	31	1.6	1.0-2.5
12. Bleeding with acenocoumarol / dalteparin	28	1.4	0.8-2.2
13. Fever after chemotherapy	26	1.3	0.7-2.1
14. Electrolyte disturbance	26	1.3	0.7-2.1
15. Dehydration	23	1.2	0.7-2.0
16. Other problems after chemotherapy	20	1.0	0.5-1.8
17. Allergic reaction	17	0.9	0.4-1.7
18. Renal disease	16	0.8	0.3-1.5
19. Pain syndrome	8	0.4	0.1-1.0
20. Hypotension	8	0.4	0.1-1.0
21. Neurological disease	7	0.4	0.1-1.0
22. Vascular disease	6	0.3	0.06-0.7
23. Rheumatoid arthritis/arthrosis/osteoporosis	6	0.3	0.06-0.7
24. Dermatological condition	3	0.2	0.02-0.7
	2000	100	

NSAIDS = non-steroidal anti-inflammatory drugs

The data file is in extras.springer.com and is entitled "paretocharts.sav". Open it.

Example 521

Command

Analyze....Quality Control....Pareto Charts....click Simple....mark Value of individual cases....click Define....Values: enter "alladmissions"....mark Variable: enter "diagnosisgroups"....click OK.

The underneath graph shows that over 50% of the admissions is in the first two diagnosis groups. A general rule as postulated by Pareto says: when analyzing observational studies with multifactorial effects, usually less than 20% of the factors determines over 80% of the effect. This postulate seems to be true in this example. The graph shows that the first 5 diagnosis groups out of 21% determine around 80% of the effect (admission). When launching a program to reduce hospital admissions in general, it would make sense to prioritize these 5 diagnosis groups, and to neglect the other diagnosis groups.

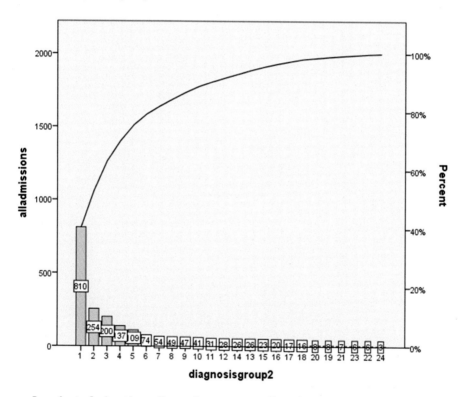

In order to find out how diagnosis groups contributed to the numbers of iatrogenic admissions, a pareto chart was constructed. The data are underneath, and are the variables 4 and 5 in "paretocharts.sav".

	Numbers	%	95% CIs
1. Cardiac condition and hypertension	202	35.1	31.1-38.9
2. Gastrointestinal condition	89	15.5	12.2-18.1
3. Bleedings with acetyl salicyl/NSAIDS	46	8.0	5.9-10.4
4. Infectious disease	31	5.4	3.6-7.4
5. Bleeding with acenocoumarol/dalteparin	28	4.9	3.1-6.8
6. Fever after chemotherapy	26	4.5	2.9-6.4
7. Hematological condition	24	4.2	2.7-6.1
8. Other problems after chemotherapy	20	3.5	2.1-5.3
9. Endocrine condition	19	3.3	2.0-5.1
10. Dehydration	18	3.1	1.9-4.9
11. Electrolyte disturbance	14	2.4	1.3-3.8
12. Pulmonary disease	9	1.6	0.8-3.0
13. Allergic reaction	8	1.4	0.6-2.8
14. Hypotension not due to antihypertensives	8	1.4	0.6-2.8
15. Other	7	1.2	0.5-2.4
16. Unintentional overdose	6	1.0	0.4-2.1
17. Malignancy	6	1.0	0.4-2.1
18. Neurological disease	4	0.7	0.2-1.7
19. Mental disease	4	0.7	0.2-1.7
20. Renal disease	2	0.3	0.04-1.2
21. Vascular disease	2	0.3	0.04-1.2
22. Dermatological condition	2	0.3	0.04-1.2
23. Rheumatoid arthritis/arthrosis/osteoporosis	1	0.2	0.0-0.9
Total	576	100	

NSAIDS = non-steroidal anti-inflammatory drugs; ns = not significant

Command

Analyze....Quality Control....Pareto Charts....click Simple....mark Value of individual cases....click Define....Values: enter "iatrogenicadmissions"....mark Variable: enter "diagnosisgroups"....click OK.

Example   523

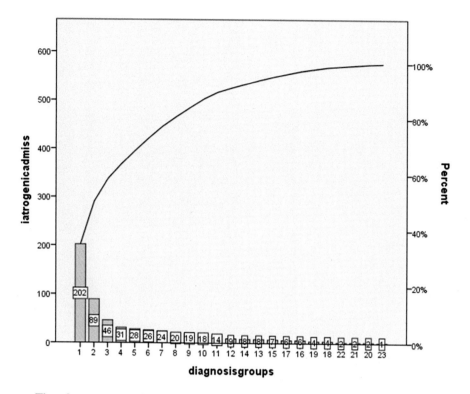

The above pareto chart has a breakpoint at 50%. Generally, a breakpoint is observed at around 50% of the effect with around 10% of the factors before the breakpoint. The breakpoint would be helpful for setting priorities, when addressing the problem of iatrogenic admissions. The diagnosis groups, cardiac condition and gastrointestinal condition, cause over 50% of all of the iatrogenic admissions.

In order to find which medicines were responsible for the iatrogenic admissions, again a pareto chart was constructed. The variables 1 and 2 of the data file "paretocharts.sav" will be used.

Command

Analyzed....Quality Control....Pareto Charts....click Simple....mark Value of individual cases....click Define....Values: enter "iatrogenicad"....mark Variable: enter "medicinecat"....click OK.

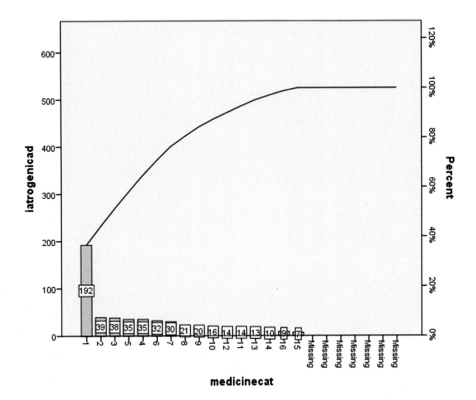

No breakpoint is observed, but the first two medicine categories were responsible for 50% of the entire number of iatrogenic admissions. We can conclude, that over 50% of the iatrogenic admissions were in two diagnosis groups, and over 50% of the medicines responsible were also in two main medicine categories.

Conclusion

Pareto charts are useful for identifying the main factors of multifactorial outcomes, not only in marketing science but also in medicine.

Note

In addition to flow charts, scattergrams, histograms, control charts, cause effects diagrams, and checklists, pareto charts are basic graphical tools of data analysis. All of them require little training in statistics. More information is given in "Machine learning in medicine-cookbook 2" as Chap. 16, 2014, Springer Heidelberg Germany, from the same authors.

Chapter 68
Radial Basis Neural Networks for Multidimensional Gaussian Data (90 Persons)

General Purpose

Radial basis functions may better than multilayer neural network (Chap. 55), predict medical data, because it uses a Gaussian activation function, but it is rarely used. This chapter is to assess its performance in clinical research.

Background

More information on neural networks is in the Chap. 55. Radial basis neural networks is more modern, and was first formulated in a 1988 paper by Broomhead at the Royal Signals and Radar Establishment, UK. Unlike multilayer perceptron it uses products between input and weight and a sigmoidal activation functions, and training is usually done through backpropagation for all layers (which can be as many as you want). This type of neural network is used in deep learning with the help of many techniques (such as dropout or batch normalization).

This chapter was previously published in "Machine learning in medicine-cookbook 2" as Chap.17, 2013.

Electronic Supplementary Material The online version of this chapter (https://doi.org/10.1007/978-3-030-33970-8_68) contains supplementary material, which is available to authorized users.

Specific Scientific Question

Body surface area is an indicator for metabolic body mass, and is used for adjusting oxygen, CO_2 transport parameters, blood volumes, urine creatinine clearance, protein/creatinine ratios and other parameters. Can a radial basis neural network be applied to accurately predict the body surface from gender, age, weight and height?

Example

The body surfaces of 90 persons were calculated using direct photometric measurements. These previously measured outcome data will be used as the so called learning sample, and the computer will be commanded to teach itself making predictions about the body surface from the predictor variables gender, age, weight and height. The first 20 patients are underneath. The entire data file is in "radialbasisnn".

1,00	13,00	30,50	138,50	10,072,90
0,00	5,00	15,00	101,00	6189,00
0,00	0,00	2,50	51,50	1906,20
1,00	11,00	30,00	141,00	10,290,60
1,00	15,00	40,50	154,00	13,221,60
0,00	11,00	27,00	136,00	9654,50
0,00	5,00	15,00	106,00	6768,20
1,00	5,00	15,00	103,00	6194,10
1,00	3,00	13,50	96,00	5830,20
0,00	13,00	36,00	150,00	11,759,00
0,00	3,00	12,00	92,00	5299,40
1,00	0,00	2,50	51,00	2094,50
0,00	7,00	19,00	121,00	7490,80
1,00	13,00	28,00	130,50	9521,70
1,00	0,00	3,00	54,00	2446,20
0,00	0,00	3,00	51,00	1632,50
0,00	7,00	21,00	123,00	7958,80
1,00	11,00	31,00	139,00	10,580,80
1,00	7,00	24,50	122,50	8756,10
1,00	11,00	26,00	133,00	9573,00

Var 1 gender
Var 2 age
Var 3 weight (kg)
Var 4 height (m)
Var 5 body surface measured (cm^2)

The Computer Teaches Itself to Make Predictions

The SPSS module Neural Networks is used for training and outcome prediction. It uses XML (exTended Markup Language) files to store the neural network. Start by opening the data file.

Command

click Transform....click Random Number Generators....click Set Starting Point....click Fixed Value (2000000)....click OK....click Analyze.... Neural Networks....Radial Basis Function....Dependent Variables: enter Body surface measured....Factors: enter gender, age, weight, and height....Partitions: Training 7....Test 3....Holdout 0....click Output: mark Description....Diagram....Model summary....Predicted by observed chart....Case processing summary ....click Save: mark Save predicted value of category for each dependent variable....automatically generate unique names....click Export....mark Export synaptic weights estimates to XML file....click Browse....File Name: enter "exportradialbasisnn" and save in the appropriate folder of your computer....click OK.

The output warns that in the testing sample some cases have been excluded from analysis, because of values not occurring in the training sample. Minimizing the output sheets shows the data file with predicted values. They are pretty much the same as the measured body surface values. We will use linear regression to estimate the association between the two.

Command

Analyze....Regresssion....Linear....Dependent: bodysurface ....Independent: RBF_PredictedValue....OK.

The output sheets show that the r-value is 0.931, p < 0.0001. The saved XML file will now be used to compute the body surface in six individual patients.

gender	age	weight	height
1,00	9,00	29,00	138,00
1,00	1,00	8,00	76,00
,00	15,00	42,00	165,00
1,00	15,00	40,00	151,00
1,00	1,00	9,00	80,00
1,00	7,00	22,00	123,00

gender
age (years)
weight (kg)
height (m)

Enter the above data in a new SPSS data file.

Command
Utilities. . . .click Scoring Wizard. . . .click Browse. . . .click Select. . . .Folder: enter
the exportradialbasisnn.xml file. . . .click Select. . . .in Scoring Wizard click Next. . . .
click Use value substitution. . . .click Next. . . .click Finish.

The underneath data file now gives the body surfaces computed by the neural
network with the help of the XML file.

gender	age	weight	height	predicted body surface
1,00	9,00	29,00	138,00	9219,71
1,00	1,00	8,00	76,00	5307,81
,00	15,00	42,00	165,00	13,520,13
1,00	15,00	40,00	151,00	13,300,79
1,00	1,00	9,00	80,00	5170,13
1,00	7,00	22,00	123,00	8460,05

gender
age (years)
weight (kg)
height (m)
predicted body surface (cm^2)

Conclusion

Radial basis neural networks can be readily trained to provide accurate body surface
values of individual patients.

Note

More background, theoretical and mathematical information of neural networks is
available in Machine learning in medicine part one, Chaps. 12 and 13, entitled
"Artificial intelligence, multilayer perceptron" and "Artificial intelligence, radial
basis functions", pp. 145–156 and 157–166, Springer Heidelberg Germany 2013,
and in the Chap. 55 of the current book.

Chapter 69
Automatic Modeling of Drug Efficacy Prediction (250 Patients)

General Purpose

SPSS modeler is a work bench for automatic data mining (Chap. 66) and modeling (see also the Chap. 70). So far it is virtually unused in medicine, and mainly applied by econo−/sociometrics. Automatic modeling of continuous outcomes computes the ensembled result of a number of best fit models for a particular data set, and provides better sensitivity than the separate models do. This chapter is to demonstrate its performance with drug efficacy prediction. Ensembled correlation coefficients are computed for the purpose.

Background

IBM SPSS Modeler is a data mining and text analytics software application from IBM. It is used to build predictive models and conduct other analytic tasks. It has a visual interface which allows users to leverage statistical and data mining algorithms without programming. It has already been used in this edition in the Chap. 66. IBM SPSS Modeler is a data mining and text analytics software application from IBM. It is used to build predictive models and conduct other analytic tasks. It has a visual interface which allows users to leverage statistical and data mining algorithms without programming. One of its main aims from the outset was to get rid of unnecessary complexity in data transformations, and to make complex predictive models very easy to use. The first version incorporated decision trees, and neural

This chapter was previously published in "Machine learning in medicine-cookbook 2" as Chap.18, 2014.

Electronic Supplementary Material The online version of this chapter (https://doi.org/10.1007/978-3-030-33970-8_69) contains supplementary material, which is available to authorized users.

© Springer Nature Switzerland AG 2020
T. J. Cleophas, A. H. Zwinderman, *Machine Learning in Medicine – A Complete Overview*, https://doi.org/10.1007/978-3-030-33970-8_69

networks through backpropagation, which could both be trained without underlying knowledge of how those techniques worked. Backpropagation is the central mechanism by which neural networks learn. It is the messenger telling the network whether or not the net made a mistake when it made a prediction. To propagate is to transmit something (light, sound, motion or information) in a particular direction or through a particular medium. IBM SPSS Modeler was originally named Clementine by its creators, Integral Solutions Limited. This name continued for a while after SPSS's acquisition of the product. SPSS later changed the name to SPSS Clementine, and then later to PASW Modeler. Following IBM's 2009 acquisition of SPSS, the product was renamed IBM SPSS Modeler, its current name.

Specific Scientific Question

The expression of a cluster of genes can be used as a functional unit to predict the efficacy of cytostatic treatment. Can ensembled modeling with three best fit statistical models provide better precision than the separate analysis with single statistical models does.

Example

A 250 patients' data file includes 28 variables consistent of patients' gene expression levels and their drug efficacy scores. Only the first 12 patients are shown underneath. The entire data file is in extras.springer.com, and is entitled "ensembledmodelcontinuous". All of the variables were standardized by scoring them on 11 points linear scales. The following genes were highly expressed: the genes 1–4, 16–19, and 24–27.

Example 533

G1	G2	G3	G4	G16	G17	G18	G19	G24	G25	G26	G27	O
8,00	8,00	9,00	5,00	7,00	10,00	5,00	6,00	9,00	9,00	6,00	6,00	7,00
9,00	9,00	10,00	9,00	8,00	8,00	7,00	8,00	8,00	9,00	8,00	8,00	7,00
9,00	8,00	8,00	8,00	8,00	9,00	7,00	8,00	9,00	8,00	9,00	9,00	8,00
8,00	9,00	8,00	9,00	6,00	7,00	6,00	4,00	6,00	6,00	5,00	5,00	7,00
10,00	10,00	8,00	10,00 9,00	10,00	10,00	8,00	8,00	9,00	9,00	9,00	8,00	
7,00	8,00	8,00	8,00	8,00	7,00	6,00	5,00	7,00	8,00	8,00	7,00	6,00
5,00	5,00	5,00	5,00	5,00	6,00	4,00	5,00	5,00	6,00	6,00	5,00	5,00
9,00	9,00	9,00	9,00	8,00	8,00	8,00	8,00	9,00	8,00	3,00	8,00	8,00
9,00	8,00	9,00	8,00	9,00	8,00	7,00	7,00	7,00	7,00	5,00	8,00	7,00
10,00	10,00	10,00	10,00 10,00	10,00	10,00	10,00	10,00	8,00	8,00	10,00	10,00	
2,00	2,00	8,00	5,00	7,00	8,00	8,00	8,00	9,00	3,00	9,00	8,00	7,00
7,00	8,00	8,00	7,00	8,00	6,00	6,00	7,00	8,00	8,00	8,00	7,00	7,00

G1	G2	G3	G4	G16	G17	G18	G19	G24	G25	G26	G27	O
8,00	8,00	9,00	5,00	7,00	10,00	5,00	6,00	9,00	9,00	6,00	6,00	7,00
9,00	9,00	10,00	9,00	8,00	8,00	7,00	8,00	8,00	9,00	8,00	8,00	7,00
9,00	8,00	8,00	8,00	8,00	9,00	7,00	8,00	9,00	8,00	9,00	9,00	8,00
8,00	9,00	8,00	9,00	6,00	7,00	6,00	4,00	6,00	6,00	5,00	5,00	7,00
10,00	10,00	8,00	10,00	9,00	10,00	10,00	8,00	9,00	9,00	9,00	9,00	8,00
7,00	8,00	8,00	8,00	8,00	7,00	6,00	5,00	7,00	8,00	8,00	7,00	6,00
5,00	5,00	5,00	5,00	5,00	6,00	4,00	5,00	5,00	6,00	6,00	5,00	5,00
9,00	9,00	9,00	9,00	8,00	8,00	8,00	8,00	9,00	8,00	3,00	8,00	8,00
9,00	8,00	9,00	8,00	9,00	8,00	7,00	7,00	7,00	7,00	5,00	8,00	7,00
10,00	10,00	10,00	10,00	10,00	10,00	10,00	10,00	10,00	8,00	8,00	10,00	10,00
2,00	2,00	8,00	5,00	7,00	8,00	8,00	8,00	9,00	3,00	9,00	8,00	7,00
7,00	8,00	8,00	7,00	8,00	6,00	6,00	7,00	8,00	8,00	8,00	7,00	7,00

G = gene (gene expression levels), O = outcome (score)

Step 1 Open SPSS Modeler (14.2)

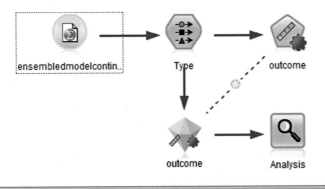

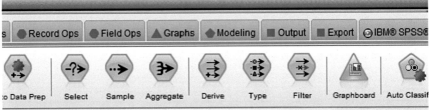

Step 2 The Statistics File Node

The canvas is, initially, blank, and above a screen view is of the final "completed ensemble" model, otherwise called stream of nodes, which we are going to build. First, in the palettes at the bottom of the screen full of nodes, look and find the **Statistics File node**, and drag it to the canvas. Double-click on it....Import file: browse and enter the file "ensembledmodelcontinuous" ....click OK. The graph below shows that the data file is open for analysis.

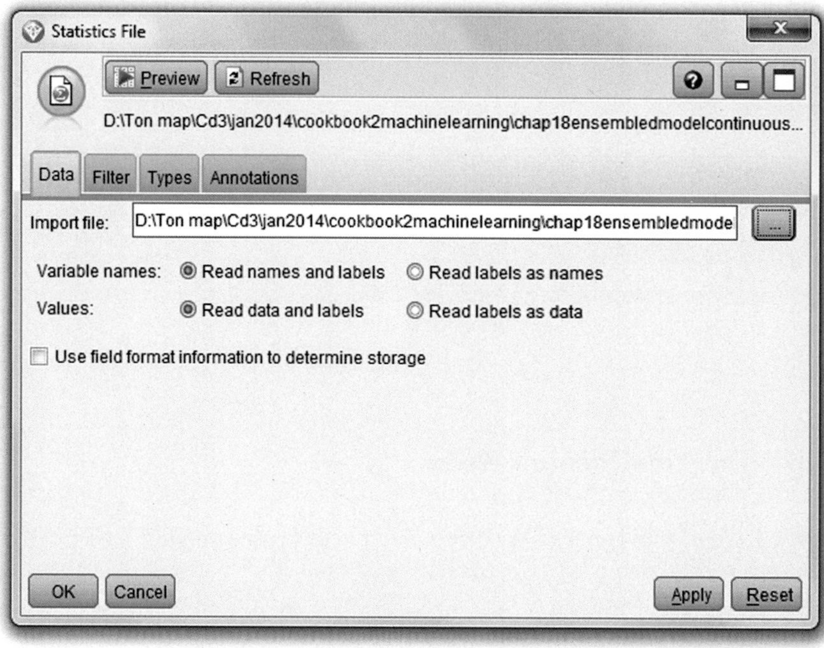

Step 3 The Type Node

In the palette at the bottom of screen find Type node and drag to the canvas....right-click on the Statistics File node....a Connect symbol comes up....click on the Type node....an arrow is displayed....double-click on the Type Node....after a second or two the underneath graph with information from the Type node is observed. Type nodes are used to access the properties of the variables (often called fields here) like type, role, unit etc. in the data file. As shown below, the variables are appropriately set: 14 predictor variables, 1 outcome (= target) variable, all of them continuous.

Field	Measurement	Values	Missing	Check	Role
geneone	Continuous	[0.0,10.0]		None	Input
genetwo	Continuous	[0.0,10.0]		None	Input
genethree	Continuous	[0.0,10.0]		None	Input
genefour	Continuous	[3.0,10.0]		None	Input
genesixteen	Continuous	[0.0,10.0]		None	Input
genesevente...	Continuous	[0.0,10.0]		None	Input
geneeighteen	Continuous	[0.0,10.0]		None	Input
genenineteen	Continuous	[0.0,10.0]		None	Input
genetwentyf	Continuous	[0.0,10.0]		None	Input

○ View current fields   ○ View unused field settings

Step 4 The Auto Numeric Node

Now, click the Auto Numeric node and drag to canvas and connect with the Type node using the above connect-procedure. Click the Auto Numeric node, and the underneath graph comes up. . . .now click Model. . . .select Correlation as metric to rank quality of the various analysis methods used. . . . the additional manoeuvres are as indicated below. . . .in Numbers of models to use: type the number 3.

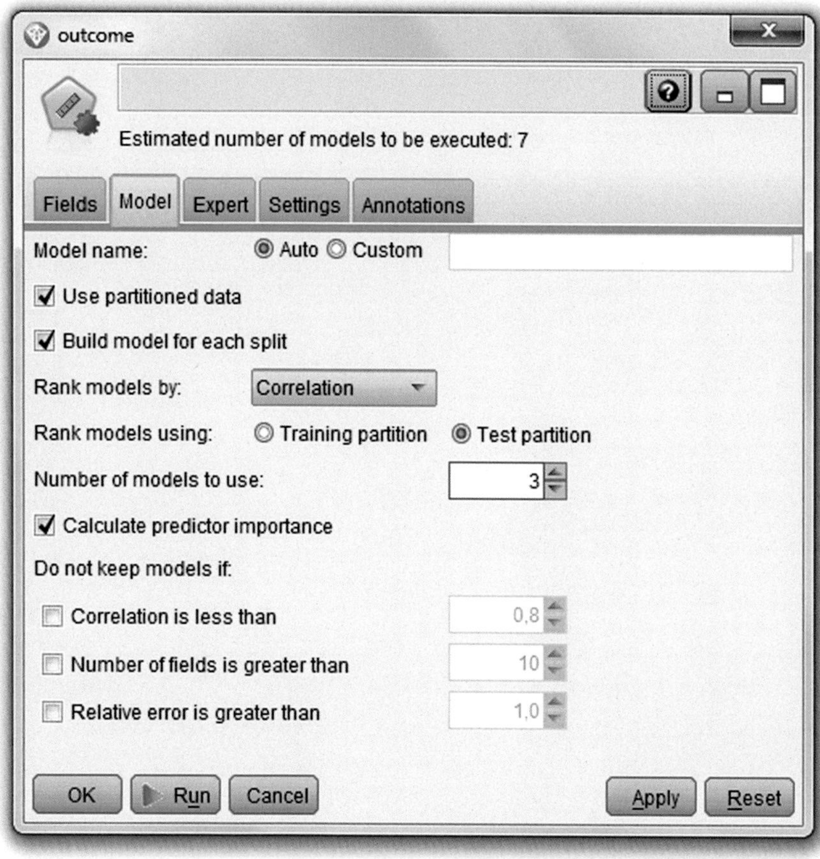

Step 5 The Expert Node

Then click the Expert tab. It is shown below. Out of 7 statistical models the three best fit ones are used by SPSS modeler for the ensembled model.

The 7 statistical models include:

1. Linear regression (Regression)
2. Generalized linear model (Generalized. . . .)
3. K nearest neighbor clustering (KNN Algorithm)
4. Support vector machine (SVM)
5. Classification and regression tree (C&R Tree)
6. Chi square automatic interaction detection (CHAID Tree)
7. Neural network (Neural Net)

More background information of the above methods are available at

1. SPSS for Starters Part One, Chap.5, Linear regression, pp. 15–18, Springer Heidelberg Germany 2010
2. The Chaps. 20 and 21 of current book.
3. Chap.1 of current work.

4. Machine Learning in Medicine Part Two, Chap.15, Support vector machines, pp. 155–161, Springer Heidelberg Germany, 2013.
5. Chap. 53 of current book.
6. Machine Learning in Medicine Part Three, Chap.14, Decision trees, pp. 137–150, Springer Heidelberg Germany 2013.
7. Machine Learning in Medicine Part One, Chap.12, Artificial intelligence, multi-layer perceptron modeling, pp. 145–154, Springer Heidelberg Germany 2013.

All of the seven above references are from the same authors as the current work.

Step 6 The Settings Tab

In the above graph click the Settings tab….click the Run button….now a gold nugget is placed on the canvas….click the gold nugget….the model created is shown below.

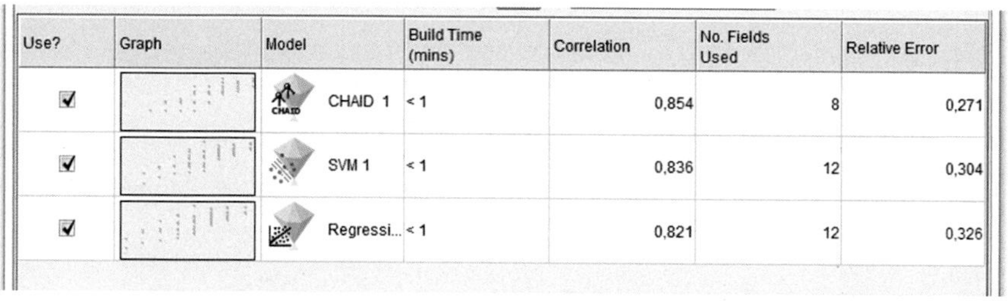

Use?	Graph	Model	Build Time (mins)	Correlation	No. Fields Used	Relative Error
✔		CHAID 1	< 1	0,854	8	0,271
✔		SVM 1	< 1	0,836	12	0,304
✔		Regressi...	< 1	0,821	12	0,326

The correlation coefficients of the three best models are over 0.8, and, thus, pretty good. We will now perform the ensembled procedure.

Step 7 the Analysis Node

Find in the palettes below the screen the Analysis node and drag it to the canvas. With the above connect procedure connect it with the gold nugget….click the Analysis node.

Comparing $XR-outcome with outcome

Minimum Error	-2,878
Maximum Error	3,863
Mean Error	-0,014
Mean Absolute Error	0,77
Standard Deviation	1,016
Linear Correlation	0,859
Occurrences	250

The above table is shown and gives the statistics of the ensembled model created. The ensembled outcome is the average score of the scores from the three best fit statistical models. Adjustment for multiple testing and for variance stabilization with Fisher transformation is automatically carried out. The ensembled outcome (named the $XR-outcome) is compared with the outcomes of the three best fit statistical models, namely, CHAID (chi square automatic interaction detector), SVM (support vector machine), and Regression (linear regression). The ensembled correlation coefficient is larger (0.859) than the correlation coefficients from the three best fit models (0.854, 0.836, 0.821), and so ensembled procedures make sense, because they can provide increased precision in the analysis. The ensembled model can now be stored as an SPSS Modeler Stream file for future use in the appropriate folder of your computer. For the readers' convenience it is in extras.springer.com, and it is entitled "ensembledmodelcontinuous".

Conclusion

In the example given in this chapter, the ensembled correlation coefficient is larger (0.859) than the correlation coefficients from the three best fit models (0.854, 0.836, 0.821), and, so, ensembled procedures do make sense, because they can provide increased precision in the analysis.

Note

SPSS Modeler is a software program entirely distinct from SPSS statistical software, though it uses most if not all of the calculus methods of it. It is a standard software package particularly used by market analysts, but, as shown, can, perfectly, well be applied for exploratory purposes in medical research. It is also applied in the Chaps. 66 and 70.

Chapter 70
Automatic Modeling for Clinical Event Prediction (200 Patients)

General Purpose

SPSS modeler is a work bench for automatic data mining (Chap. 66) and modeling (see also the Chap. 69). So far it is virtually unused in medicine, and mainly applied by econo−/sociometrists. Automatic modeling of binary outcomes computes the ensembled result of a number of best fit models for a particular data set, and provides better sensitivity than the separate models do. This chapter is to demonstrate its performance with clinical event prediction. Ensembled accuracies are computed for the purpose.

Background

IBM SPSS Modeler is a data mining and text analytics software application from IBM. It is used to build predictive models and conduct other analytic tasks. It has a visual interface which allows users to leverage statistical and data mining algorithms without programming. It has already been used in this edition in the Chaps. 66 and 69. IBM SPSS Modeler is a data mining and text analytics software application from IBM. It is used to build predictive models and conduct other analytic tasks. It has a visual interface which allows users to leverage statistical and data mining algorithms without programming. One of its main aims from the outset was to get rid of unnecessary complexity in data transformations, and to make complex predictive models very easy to use. The first version incorporated decision trees, and neural

---

This chapter was previously published in "Machine learning in medicine-cookbook 2" as Chap.19, 2014.

Electronic Supplementary Material The online version of this chapter (https://doi.org/10.1007/978-3-030-33970-8_70) contains supplementary material, which is available to authorized users.

networks through backpropagation, which could both be trained without underlying knowledge of how those techniques worked. Backpropagation is the central mechanism by which neural networks learn. It is the messenger telling the network whether or not the net made a mistake when it made a prediction. To propagate is to transmit something (light, sound, motion or information) in a particular direction or through a particular medium. IBM SPSS Modeler was originally named Clementine by its creators, Integral Solutions Limited. This name continued for a while after SPSS's acquisition of the product. SPSS later changed the name to SPSS Clementine, and then later to PASW Modeler. Following IBM's 2009 acquisition of SPSS, the product was renamed IBM SPSS Modeler, its current name.

Specific Scientific Question

Multiple laboratory values can predict events like health, death, morbidities etc. Can ensembled modeling with four best fit statistical models provide better precision than the separate analysis with single statistical models does.

Example

A 200 patients' data file includes 11 variables consistent of patients' laboratory values and their subsequent outcome (death or alive). Only the first 12 patients are shown underneath. The entire data file is in extras.springer.com, and is entitled "ensembledmodelbinary".

Death	ggt	asat	alat	bili	ureum	creat	c-clear	esr	crp	leucos
,00	20,00	23,00	34,00	2,00	3,40	89,00	−111,00	2,00	2,00	5,00
,00	14,00	21,00	33,00	3,00	2,00	67,00	−112,00	7,00	3,00	6,00
,00	30,00	35,00	32,00	4,00	5,60	58,00	−116,00	8,00	4,00	4,00
,00	35,00	34,00	40,00	4,00	6,00	76,00	−110,00	6,00	5,00	7,00
,00	23,00	33,00	22,00	4,00	6,10	95,00	−120,00	9,00	6,00	6,00
,00	26,00	31,00	24,00	3,00	5,40	78,00	−132,00	8,00	4,00	8,00
,00	15,00	29,00	26,00	2,00	5,30	47,00	−120,00	12,00	5,00	5,00
,00	13,00	26,00	24,00	1,00	6,30	65,00	−132,00	13,00	6,00	6,00
,00	26,00	27,00	27,00	4,00	6,00	97,00	−112,00	14,00	6,00	7,00
,00	34,00	25,00	13,00	3,00	4,00	67,00	−125,00	15,00	7,00	6,00
,00	32,00	26,00	24,00	3,00	3,60	58,00	−110,00	13,00	8,00	6,00
,00	21,00	13,00	15,00	3,00	3,60	69,00	−102,00	12,00	2,00	4,00

death = death yes no (0 = no)
ggt = gamma glutamyl transferase (u/l)

asat = aspartate aminotransferase (u/l)
alat = alanine aminotransferase (u/l)
bili = bilirubine (micromol/l)
ureum = ureum (mmol/l)
creat = creatinine (mmicromol/l)
c-clear = creatinine clearance (ml/min)
esr = erythrocyte sedimentation rate (mm)
crp = c-reactive protein (mg/l)
leucos = leucocyte count $(.10^9 /l)$

Step 1 Open SPSS Modeler (14.2)

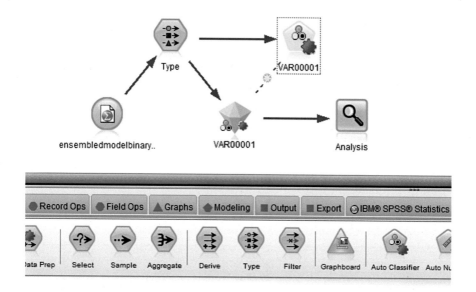

Step 2 The Statistics File Node

The canvas is, initially, blank, and above is given a screen view of the completed ensembled model, otherwise called stream of nodes, which we are going to build. First, in the palettes at the bottom of the screen full of nodes, look and find the **Statistics File node**, and drag it to the canvas, pressing the mouse left side. Double-click on this node....Import file: browse and enter the file "chap19ensembledmodelbinary" ....click OK. The graph below shows, that the data file is open for analysis.

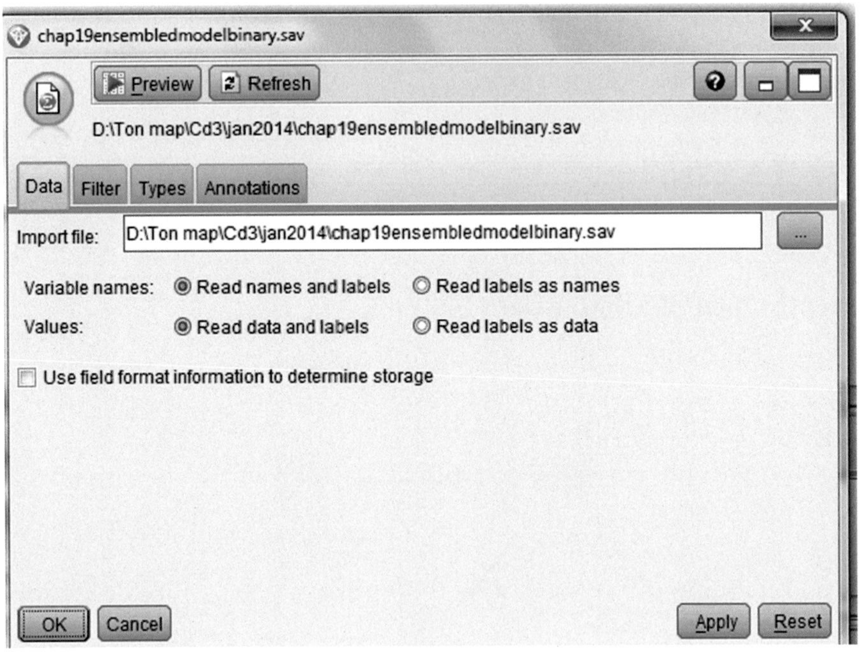

Step 3 The Type Node

In the palette at the bottom of screen find Type node and drag to the canvas. . . .right-click on the Statistics File node. . . .a Connect symbol comes up. . . .click on the Type node. . . .an arrow is displayed. . . .double-click on the Type Node. . . .after a second or two the underneath graph with information from the Type node is observed. Type nodes are used to access the properties of the variables (often called fields here) like type, role, unit etc. in the data file. As shown below, 10 predictor variables (all of them continuous) are appropriately set. However, VAR 00001 (death) is the outcome (= target) variable, and is binary. Click in the row of variable VAR00001 on the measurement column and replace "Continuous" with "Flag". Click Apply and OK. The underneath figure is removed and the canvas is displayed again.

Step 4 The Auto Classifier Node

Now, click the Auto Classifier node and drag to the canvas, and connect with the Type node using the above connect-procedure. Click the Auto Classifier node, and the underneath graph comes up. . . .now click Model. . . .select Lift as Rank model of the various analysis models used. . . . the additional manoeuvres are as indicated below. . . .in Numbers of models to use: type the number 4.

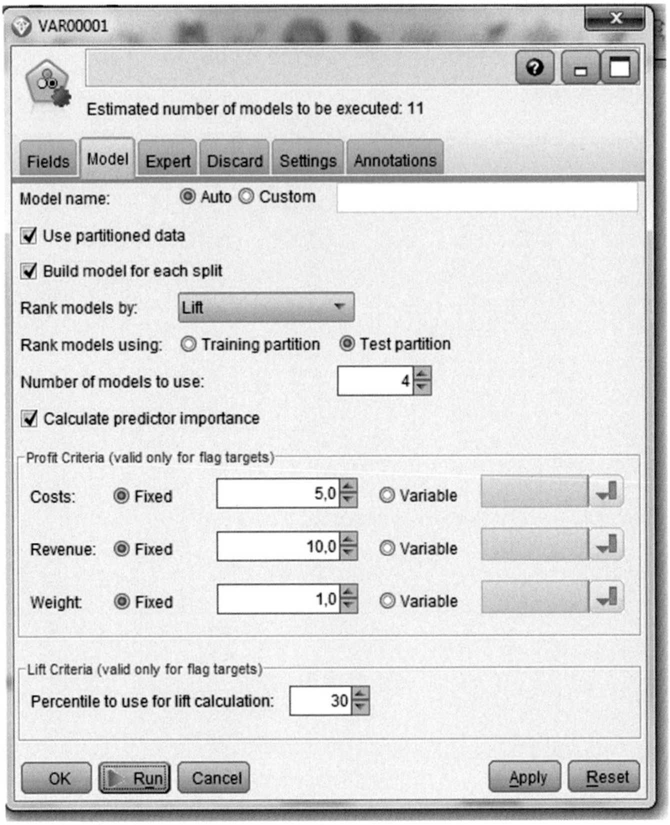

Step 5 The Expert Tab

Then click the Expert tab. It is shown below. Out of 11 statistical models the four best fit ones are selected by SPSS modeler for constructing an ensembled model.

The 11 statistical analysis methods for a flag target (= binary outcome) include:

1. C5.0 decision tree (C5.0).
2. Logistic regression (Logist r. . .).
3. Decision list (Decision. . . .)
4. Bayesian network (Bayesian. . . .)
5. Discriminant analysis (Discriminant).
6. K nearest neighbors algorithm (KNN Alg. . .).
7. Support vector machine (SVM).
8. Classification and regression tree (C&R Tree).
9. Quest decision tree (Quest Tr. . . .)
10. Chi square automatic interaction detection (CHAID Tree).
11. Neural network (Neural Net).

More background information of the above methods are available at .

1. Chapter 15 of current work, Automatic data mining for the best treatment of a Disease.
2. SPSS for Starters Part One, Chap.11, Logistic regression, pp. 39–42, Springer Heidelberg Germany 2010.
3. Decision list models identify high and low performing segments in a data file,
4. Machine Learning in Medicine Part Two, Chap.16, Bayesian networks, pp. 163–170, Springer Heidelberg Germany, 2013.
5. Machine Learning in Medicine Part One, Chap.17, Discriminant analysis for supervised data, pp. 215–224, Springer Heidelberg Germany 2013.
6. Chapter 4 of current work, Nearest neighbors for classifying new medicines.
7. Machine Learning in Medicine Part Two, Chap.15, Support vector machines, pp. 155–161, Springer Heidelberg Germany, 2013.
8. Chapter 53 of current work.
9. QUEST (Quick Unbiased Efficient Statistical Trees) are improved decision trees for binary outcomes.
10. Machine Learning in Medicine Part Three, Chap.14, Decision trees, pp. 137–150, Springer Heidelberg Germany 2013.
11. Machine Learning in Medicine Part One, Chap.12, Artificial intelligence, multilayer perceptron modeling,pp. 145–154, Springer Heidelberg Germany 2013.

All of the above references are from the same authors as the current work.

Step 6 The Settings Tab

In the above graph click the Settings tab....click the Run button....now a gold nugget is placed on the canvas....click the gold nugget....the model created is shown below.

Use?	Graph	Model	Build Time (mins)	Max Profit	Max Profit Occurs in (%)	Lift{Top 30%}	Overall Accuracy (%)	No. Fields Used	Area Under Curve
✔		Ba... < 1		405	34	2,645	76,423	10	0,995
✔		KN... < 1		447	39	2,645	80,081	10	0,998
✔		Lo... < 1		425	37	2,645	76,829	10	0,994
✔		Ne... < 1		440	36	2,645	78,862	10	0,998

The overall accuracies (%) of the four best fit models are over 0.8, and are, thus, pretty good. We will now perform the ensembled procedure.

Step 7 The Analysis Node

Find in the palettes at the bottom of the screen the Analysis node and drag it to the canvas. With above connect procedure connect it with the gold nugget....click the Analysis node.

Correct	241	97,97%
Wrong	5	2,03%
Total	246	

The above table is shown and gives the statistics of the ensembled model created. The ensembled outcome is the average accuracy of the accuracies from the four best fit statistical models. In order to prevent overstated certainty due to overfitting, bootstrap aggregating ("bagging") is used. The ensembled outcome (named the $XR-outcome) is compared with the outcomes of the four best fit statistical models, namely, Bayesian network, k Nearest Neighbor clustering, Logistic regression, and Neural network. The ensembled accuracy (97.97%) is much larger than the accuracies of the four best fit models (76.423, 80,081, 76,829, and 78,862%), and, so, ensembled procedures make sense, because they provide increased precision in the analysis. The computed ensembled model can now be stored in your computer in the form of an SPSS Modeler Stream file for future use. For the readers' convenience it is in extras.springer.com, and entitled "ensembledmodelbinary".

Conclusion

In the example given in this chapter, the ensembled accuracy is larger (97,97%) than the accuracies from the four best fit models (76,423, 80,081, 76,829, and 78,862%), and so ensembled procedures make sense, because they can provide increased precision in the analysis.

Note

SPSS modeler is a software program entirely distinct from SPSS statistical software, though it uses most if not all of the calculus methods of it. It is a standard software package particularly used by market analysts, but, as shown, can perfectly well be applied for exploratory purposes in medical research. It is also applied in the Chaps. 66 and 69.

Chapter 71
Automatic Newton Modeling in Clinical Pharmacology (15 Alfentanil Dosages, 15 Quinidine Time-Concentration Relationships)

General Purpose

Traditional regression analysis selects a mathematical function, and, then, uses the data to find the best fit parameters. For example, the parameters a and b for a linear regression function with the equation $y = a + bx$ have to be calculated according to

$$b = \text{regression coefficient} = \frac{\sum (x - \bar{x})(y - \bar{y})}{\sum (x - \bar{x})^2}$$

$$a = \text{intercept} = \bar{y} - b\bar{x}$$

With a quadratic function, $y = a + b_1 x + b_2 x^2$ (and other functions) the calculations are similar, but more complex. Newton's method works differently. Instead of selecting a mathematical function and using the data for finding the best fit parameter-values, it uses arbitrary parameter-values for a, b_1, b_2, and, then, iteratively measures the distance between the data and the modeled curve until the shortest distance is obtained. Calculations are much more easy than those of traditional regression analysis, making the method, particularly, interesting for comparing multiple functions to one data set. Newton's method is mainly used for computer solutions of engineering problems, but is little used in clinical research. This chapter is to assess whether it is also suitable for the latter purpose.

This chapter was previously published in "Machine learning in medicine-cookbook 2" as Chap. 20, 2014.

Electronic Supplementary Material The online version of this chapter (https://doi.org/10.1007/978-3-030-33970-8_71) contains supplementary material, which is available to authorized users.

Background

Isaac Newton died in London UK in 1727. As a physicist Isaac Newton invented his laws of motion, and of gravitation. But he was more. Particularly he was a mathematician who invented differentiations, which are the basis of Newton's methods reviewed in this chapter.

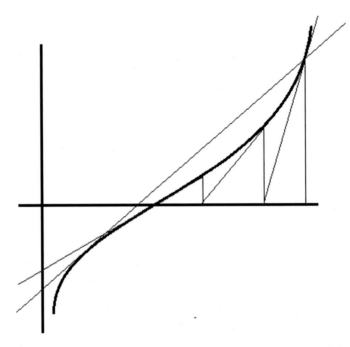

Newton's method is explained in the above figure. Four tangential lines to a non-linear curve are drawn. The left tangential line crosses the non-linear curve. Here a new tangential is drawn. This one crosses the x-axis, and at this point a new tangential is drawn. This is repeated and soon a tangential is established that crosses the x-axis at $y = 0$ (the root of the function). Only four iterations were required to find the root (zero-point) of this non-linear function. Mathematically, each iteration can be described as:

$$x_{n+1} = x_n - f\ x_n / f'\ x_n, \text{ where } f'\ x_n \text{ is the first derivative of } f\ x$$

Just like traditional regression analysis Newton's method determines the best fit values of the parameters a, b_1, b_2 for the data given. Both methods used the so-called least squares for the purpose. If the y values of each data point are called the y_{values} and the y values of the function's curve are called y_{curve}, then the goal is to minimize the so-called *residual sum of squares* function:

$$SS = sum (y_{data} - y_{curve})^2.$$

Traditional linear regressions use the smallest sums of squares method as criterion for best fit of the data to the function's curve. The method is called the least squares method. This method is only valid with Gaussian distributions of uncertainty, but in biology this is a common assumption. In order to establish a best fit more accurately and rapidly than traditional regression analysis does, Newton's method is helpful. It is explained in above figure. Four tangential lines to a non-linear curve are drawn. The left tangential line crosses the non-linear curve. Here a new tangential is drawn. This one crosses the x-axis, and at this point a new tangential is drawn. This is repeated and soon a tangential is established that crosses the x-axis at y = 0 (the root of the function). Only four iterations were required to find the root (zero-point) of this non-linear function. Mathematically, each iteration can be described as already shown above:

$$x_{n+1} = x_n - f\, x_n / f'\, x_n, \text{where } f'\, x_n \text{ is the first derivative of f x.}$$

An appropriate software program including the most common and interesting functions is now required, and for each of these functions the best fit parameters a, b_1, b_2 etc. are calculated. The magnitude of the residual sum of squares SS is used as criterion for level of fit. Finally, of all best fit functions the one with the smallest overall SS is identified as the ultimately best function for the given data. This method should be more powerful than traditional regression methods, because, instead of a single function, hundreds of them are checked simultaneously.

Specific Scientific Question

Can Newton's methods provide appropriate mathematical functions for dose-effectiveness and time-concentration studies?

Examples

Dose-Effectiveness Study

Alfentanil dose x-axis mg/m^2	effectiveness y-axis [1- pain scale]
0,10	0,1701
0,20	0,2009
0,30	0,2709
0,40	0,2648
0,50	0,3013
0,60	0,4278
0,70	0,3466
0,80	0,2663
0,90	0,3201
1,00	0,4140
1,10	0,3677
1,20	0,3476
1,30	0,3656
1,40	0,3879
1,50	0,3649

The above table gives the data of a dose-effectiveness study. Newton's algorithm is performed. We will the online Nonlinear Regression Calculator of Xuru's website (This website is made available by Xuru, the world largest business network based in Auckland CA, USA. We simply copy or paste the data of the above table into the spreadsheet given be the website, then click "allow comma as decimal separator" and click "calculate". Alternatively the SPSS file available at extras.springer.com entitled "newtonmethod" can be opened if SPSS is installed in your computer and the copy and paste commands are similarly given.

Since Newton's method can be applied to (almost) any function, most computer programs fit a given dataset to over 100 functions including Gaussians, sigmoids, ratios, sinusoids etc. For the data given 18 significantly ($P < 0.05$) fitting non-linear functions were found, the first 6 of them are shown underneath.

	Non-linear function	residual sum of squares	P value
1.	$y = 0.42 \, x / (x + 0.17)$	0.023	0.003
2.	$y = -1 / (38.4 \, x + 1)^{0.12} + 1$ 0.024	0.003	
3.	$y = 0.08 \ln x + 0.36$	0.025	0.004
4.	$y = 0.40 \, e^{-0.11/x}$ 0.025	0.004	
5.	$y = 0.36 \, x^{\, 0.26}$	0.027	0.004
6.	$y = -0.024 / x + 0.37$	0.029	0.005

The first one gives the best fit. Its measure of certainty, given as residual sum of squares, is 0.023. It is the function of a hyperbola:

$$y = 0.42\,x/(x + 0.17).$$

This is convenient, because, dose-effectiveness curves are, often, successfully assessed with hyperbolas mimicking the Michaelis-Menten equation. The parameters of the equation can be readily interpreted as effectiveness$_{maximum}$ = 0.42, and dissociation constant = 0.17. It is usually very laborious to obtain these parameters from traditional regression modeling of the quantal effect histograms and cumulative histograms requiring data samples of at least 100 or so to be meaningful. The underneath figure shows an Excel graph of the fitted non-linear function for the data, using Newton's method (the best fit curve is here a hyperbola). A cubic spline goes smoothly through every point, and does this by ensuring that the first and second derivatives of the segments match those that are adjacent.

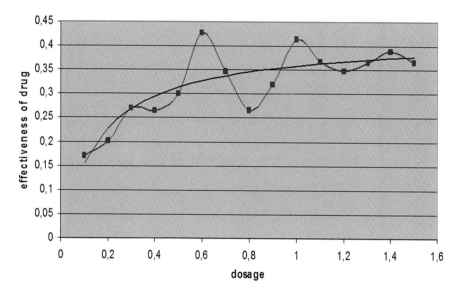

The Newton's equation better fits the data than traditional modeling with linear, logistic, quadratic, and polynomial modeling does as shown underneath.

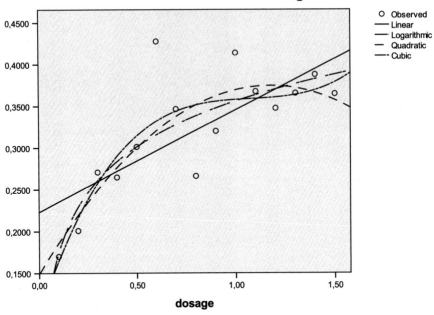

Time Concentration Study

Time	quinidine concentration
x-axis hours	µg/ml
0,10	0,41
0,20	0,38
0,30	0,36
0,40	0,34
0,50	0,36
0,60	0,23
0,70	0,28
0,80	0,26
0,90	0,17
1,00	0,30
1,10	0,30
1,20	0,26
1,30	0,27
1,40	0,20
1,50	0,17

The above table gives the data of a time-concentration study. Again a non-linear regression using Newton's algorithm is performed. We use the online Nonlinear Regression Calculator of Xuru's website. We copy or paste the data of the above table into the spreadsheet, then click "allow comma as decimal separator" and click "calculate". Alternatively the SPSS file available at extras.springer.com entitled "newtonmethod" can be opened if SPSS is installed in your computer and the copy and paste commands are similarly given. For the data given 10 statistically significantly ($P < 0.05$) fitting non-linear functions were found and shown. For further assessment of the data an exponential function, which is among the first 5 shown by the software, is chosen, because relevant pharmacokinetic parameters can be conveniently calculated from it:

$$y = 0.41 \ e^{-0.48 \ x}.$$

This function's measure of uncertainty (residual sums of squares) value is 0.027, with a p-value of 0.003). The following pharmacokinetic parameters are derived:

$$0.41 = C_0 = (\text{administration dosage drug})/(\text{distribution volume})$$

$$-0.48 = \text{elimination constant}.$$

Below an Excel graph of the exponential function fitted to the data is given. Also, a cubic spline curve going smoothly through every point and to be considered as a perfect fit curve is again given. It can be observed from the figure that the exponential function curve matches the cubic spline curve well.

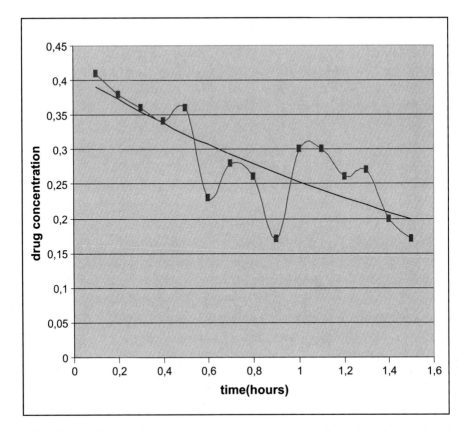

The Newton's equation fits the data approximately equally well as do traditional best fit models with linear, logistic, quadratic, and polynomial modeling shown underneath. However, traditional models do not allow for the computation of pharmacokinetic parameters.

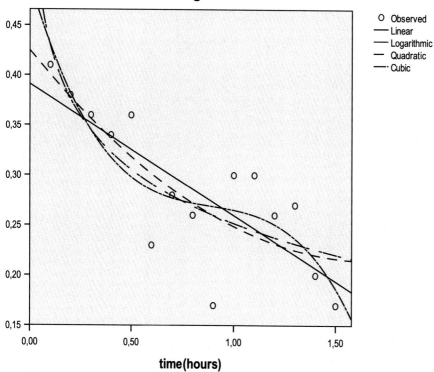

Conclusion

Newton's methods provide appropriate mathematical functions for dose-effectiveness and time-concentration studies.

Note

More background theoretical and mathematical information of Newton's methods are in Machine learning in medicine part three, Chap.16, Newton's methods, pp. 161–172, Springer Heidelberg Germany, 2013, from the same authors.

Chapter 72
Spectral Plots for High Sensitivity Assessent of Periodicity (6 Years' Monthly C Reactive Protein Levels)

General Purpose

In clinical research times series often show many peaks and irregular spaces.

Spectral plots is based on traditional Fourier analyses, and may be more sensitive than traditional autocorrelation analysis in this situation.

Background

A spectral plot is a graph which allows to examine the cyclic structure, in the frequency domain, of a time series. A time series represents a progression of some parameter in time. In technical terms, a spectral plot is a smoothed Fourier transform of the auto-covariance function of the time series.

Spectral plots were introduced in 2007 by the 46 year old Banerjee, professor in economics from Harvard. He gave the following more broad description.

A basic question in biology and other fields is, to identify the characteristic properties that on one hand are shared by structures from a particular realm, like gene regulation, protein–protein interaction or neural networks or foodwebs, and that on the other hand distinguish them from other structures.

He applied a general method, based on the spectrum of the normalized Laplacian graph, that yields representations, the spectral plots, that allowed him to find and visualize such properties systematically. Visualizations as shown underneath for a wide range of biological networks are convenient and can compare them with those

This chapter was previously published in "Machine learning in medicine-cookbook 3" as Chap. 9, 2014.

Electronic Supplementary Material The online version of this chapter (https://doi.org/10.1007/978-3-030-33970-8_72) contains supplementary material, which is available to authorized users.

T. J. Cleophas, A. H. Zwinderman, *Machine Learning in Medicine – A Complete Overview*, https://doi.org/10.1007/978-3-030-33970-8_72

for networks derived from theoretical schemes. The differences he found were quite striking and suggest that the search for universal properties of biological networks should be complemented by an understanding of more specific features of biological organization principles at different scales.

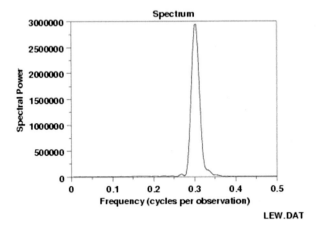

LEW.DAT

Specific Scientific Question

To assess whether, in monthly C reactive Protein (CRP) levels with inconclusive scattergrams and autocorrelation analysis, spectral plot methodology is able to demonstrate periodicity even so.

Example

A data file of 6 years' mean monthly CRP levels from a target population was assessed for seasonality. The first 2 years' values are given underneath. The entire data file is in "spectralanalysis" as available on the internet at extras.springer.com.

First day of month   CRP level (mg/l)
1993/07/01   1.29
1993/08/01   1.43
1993/09/01   1.54
1993/10/01   1.68
1993/11/01   1.54

Example   563

1993/12/01	2.78
1994/01/01	1.27
1994/02/01	1.26
1994/03/01	1.26
1994/04/01	1.54
1994/05/01	1.13
1994/06/01	1.60
1994/07/01	1.47
1994/08/01	1.78
1994/09/01	2.69
1994/10/01	1.91
1994/11/01	1.74
1994/12/01	3.11

Start by opening the data file in SPSS.

Command

Click Graphs....click Legacy Dialogs....click Scatter/Dot.... Click Simple Scatter.....click Define....y-axis: enter "mean crp mg/l"....x-axis: enter date.... click OK.

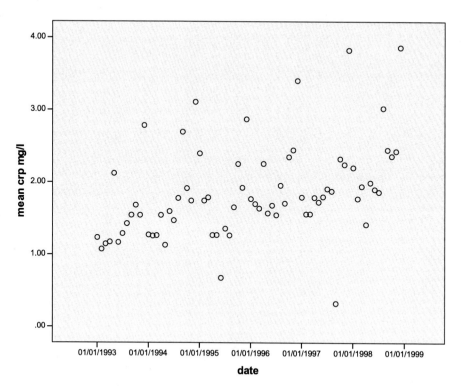

In the output the above figure is displayed. Many peaks and irregularities are observed, and the presence of periodicity is not unequivocal.

Subsequently, autocorrelation coefficients are computed.

Command
click   Analyze. . . .click   Forecast. . . .click   Autocorrelations. . . .Variables: enter "mean crp mg/l". . . .click OK.

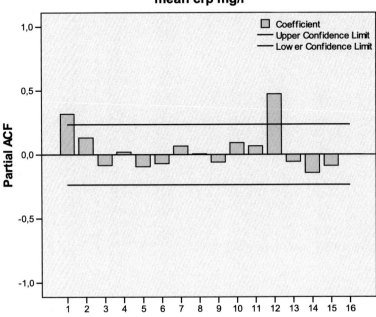

In the output the above autocorrelation coefficients (partial ACFs) by month are given. It suggests the presence of periodicity. However, this conclusion is based on a single value, i.e., the 12th month value, and, for concluding unequivocal periodicity not only autocorrelation coefficients significantly larger than 0 but also significantly smaller than 0 should have been observed.

Spectral plots may be helpful for support.

Example 565

Command

Analyze....Forecasting....Spectral Analysis....select CRP and enter into Variable (s)....select Spectral density in Plot....click Paste....change in syntax text: TSET PRINT-DEFAULT into TSET PRINT-DETAILED.... click Run....click All.

In the output sheets underneath the *periodogram* is observed (upper part) with mean CRP values on the y-axis and frequencies on the x-axis. Of the peaks CRP-values observed the first one has a frequency of slightly less than 0.1. We assumed that CRP had an annual periodicity. Twelve months are in a year, months is the unit applied. As period is the inverted value of frequency a period of 12 months would equal a frequency of $1/12 = 0.0833$. An annual periodicity would produce a peak CRP-value with a frequency of $1/12 = 0.0833$. Indeed, the table underneath shows that at a frequency of 0.0833 the highest CRP value is observed. However, many more peaks are observed, and how to interpret them. For that purpose we use *spectral density analysis* (lower figure underneath).

Periodogram of CRP by Frequency

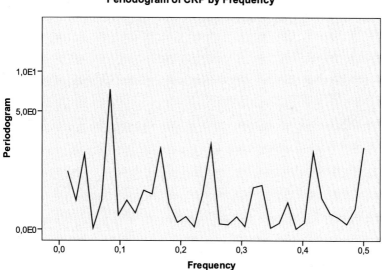

Univariate Statistics

Series Name:mean crp mg/l

	Frequency	Period	Sine Transform	Cosine Transform	Periodogram	Spectral Density Estimate
1	,00000		,000	1,852	,000	8,767
2	,01389		-,197	,020	1,416	12,285
3	,02778		-,123	,012	,552	9,223
4	,04167		-,231	,078	2,144	10,429
5	,05556		,019	,010	,016	23,564
6	,06944		-,040	-,117	,552	22,985
7	,08333		-,365	,267	7,355	19,519
8	,09722		-,057	-,060	,243	20,068
9	,11111		-,101	-,072	,556	20,505
10	,12500		-,004	-,089	,286	5,815
11	,13889		,065	-,135	,811	10,653
12	,15278		-,024	,139	,715	10,559
13	,16667		-,257	,039	2,425	10,187
14	,18056		-,090	-,075	,495	8,850
15	,19444		-,054	-,016	,115	7,313
16	,20833		,010	,077	,218	3,508
17	,22222		-,021	,027	,041	8,345
18	,23611		-,137	,031	,711	8,341
19	,25000		-,272	-,007	2,675	8,037
20	,26389		,050	-,005	,090	8,398
21	,27778		-,037	,026	,075	6,880
22	,29167		-,077	,010	,218	2,932
23	,30556		,019	-,031	,047	4,871
24	,31944		,018	-,156	,892	4,779
25	,33333		-,140	-,084	,959	4,523
26	,34722		-,003	-,026	,024	5,532
27	,36111		,029	-,045	,102	3,569
28	,37500		,048	-,109	,512	1,693
29	,38889		,007	,014	,009	6,608
30	,40278		-,017	,053	,110	7,769
31	,41667		-,194	-,157	2,246	7,280
32	,43056		-,098	-,086	,611	7,694
33	,44444		-,023	-,085	,279	7,592
34	,45833		-,039	,063	,199	3,440
35	,47222		,044	,019	,084	7,609
36	,48611		-,101	-,014	,375	7,867
37	,50000		,000	-,263	2,494	7,631

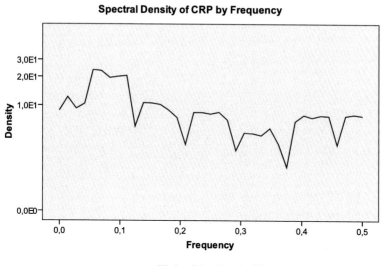

Spectral Density of CRP by Frequency

Window: Tukey-Hamming (5)

The spectral density curve is a filtered, otherwise called smoothed, version of the usual periodogram with irregularities beyond a given threshold (noise) filtered out. The above spectral density curve shows 5 distinct peaks with a rather regular pattern. The lowest frequency simply displays the yearly peak at a frequency of 0.0833. The other peaks at higher frequencies are the result of the Fourier model consistent of sine and cosine functions, and do not indicate additional periodicities. Even so much so that they demonstrate the absence of further periodicities.

Conclusion

Seasonal patterns are assumed in many fields of medicine. Usually, the mean differences between the data of different seasons or months are used. E.g., the number of hospital admissions in the month of January may be roughly twice that of July. However, biological processes are full of variations and the possibility of chance findings can not be fully ruled out. Autocorrelations can be adequately used for the purpose. It is a technique that cuts time curves into pieces. These pieces are, subsequently, compared with the original data-curve using linear regression analysis. Autocorrelation coefficients significantly larger and smaller than 0 must be observed in order to conclude periodicity. If not, spectral analysis is often helpful.

It displays a peak outcome at the frequency of the expected periodicity (months, years, weeks etc). The current chapter shows that spectral analysis can be adequately used with very irregular patterns and inconclusive autocorrelation analysis, and is able to demonstrate unequivocal periodicities where visual methods like scatter-grams and traditional methods like autocorrelations are inconclusive.

A limitation of spectral analysis is the variance problem. The periodogram's variance does not decrease with increased sample sizes. However, smoothing using the spectral density function, is sample size dependent, and therefore, reduces the variance problem.

Note

More background, theoretical and mathematical information of spectral analysis and autocorrelations is given in Machine learning in medicine part three, Chap. 15, Spectral plots, pp. 151–160, Springer Heidelberg Germany 2013, and in Machine learning in medicine part one, Chap. 10, Seasonality assessments, pp. 113–126, Springer Heidelberg Germany, 2013, both from the same authors.

Chapter 73
Runs Test for Identifying Best Regression Models (21 Estimates of Quantity and Quality of Patient Care)

General Purpose

R-square values are often used to test the appropriateness of diagnostic models.

However, in practice, pretty large r-square values (squared correlation coefficients) may be observed even if data do not fit the model very well. This chapter assesses whether the runs test is a better alternative to the traditional r-square test for addressing the differences between the data and the best fit regression models.

Background

After the statisticians Wald from Hungary 1950 and Wolfowitz from Poland 1981 the runs test has been named. It is a non-parametric statistical test that checks a randomness hypothesis for a two-valued data sequence. More precisely, it can be used to test the hypothesis that the elements of the sequence are mutually independent. A run of a sequence is a maximal non-empty segment of the sequence consisting of adjacent equal elements. For example, the 22-element-long sequence

$$+ + + + - - - + + + - - + + + + + + - - - -$$

consists of 6 runs, 3 of which consist of "+" and the others of "−". The run test is based on the null hypothesis that each element in the sequence is independently drawn from the same distribution. Under the null hypothesis, the number of runs in a

This chapter was previously published in "Machine learning in medicine-cookbook 3" as Chap. 10, 2014.

Electronic Supplementary Material The online version of this chapter (https://doi.org/10.1007/978-3-030-33970-8_73) contains supplementary material, which is available to authorized users.

© Springer Nature Switzerland AG 2020
T. J. Cleophas, A. H. Zwinderman, *Machine Learning in Medicine – A Complete Overview*, https://doi.org/10.1007/978-3-030-33970-8_73

sequence of N elements is a random variable whose conditional distribution given the observation of N_+ positive values and N_- negative values $(N = N_+ + N_-)$ is normal.

Primary Scientific Question

A real data example was given comparing quantity of care with quality of care scores.

Example

Doctors were assessed for the relationship between their quantity and quality of care. The quantity of care was estimated with the numbers of daily interventions like endoscopies and small operations per doctor, the quality of care with quality of care scores. The data file is given below, and is also available in "runstest" on the internet at extras.springer.com.

Quantity of care	Quality of care
19,00	2,00
20,00	3,00
23,00	4,00
24,00	5,00
26,00	6,00
27,00	7,00
28,00	8,00
29,00	9,00
29,00	10,00
29,00	11,00
28,00	12,00
27,00	13,00
27,00	14,00
26,00	15,00
25,00	16,00
24,00	17,00
23,00	18,00
22,00	19,00
22,00	20,00
21,00	21,00
21,00	22,00

Quantity of care = numbers of daily interventions per doctor; Quality of care = quality of care scores

Example 571

The relationship seemed not to be linear, and curvilinear regression in SPSS was used to find the best fit curve to describe the data and eventually use them as prediction model. First, we will make a graph of the data.

Command

Analyze....Graphs....Chart builder....click: Scatter/Dot....Click quality of care and drag to the Y-Axis....Click Intervention per doctor and drag to the X-Axis.... OK.

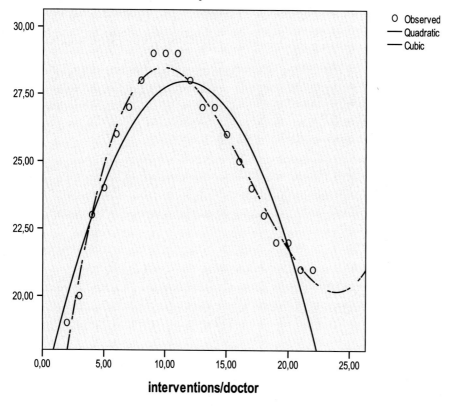

qual care score

The above figure shows the scattergram of the data. A non-linear relationship is indeed suggested, and the curvilinear regression option in SPSS was helpful to find the best fit model.

Command

Analyze....Regression....Curve Estimation....mark: Quadratic, Cubic....mark: Display ANOVA Table....OK.

The quadratic (best fit second order, parabolic, relationship) and cubic (best fit third order, hyperbolic, relationship) were the best options, with very good r-squares and p-values <0.0001 as shown in the table given by the software.

Model Summary and Parameter Estimates

Dependent Variable:qual care score

Equation	Model Summary					Parameter Estimates			
	R Square	F	df1	df2	Sig.	Constant	b1	b2	b3
Quadratic	,866	58,321	2	18	,000	16,259	2,017	-,087	
Cubic	,977	236,005	3	17	,000	10,679	4,195	-,301	,006

The independent variable is interventions/doctor.

The runs test requires the residues from respectively the best fit quadratic and the cubic models of the data (instead of - and + distances from the modeled curves (the residues) to be read from the above figure, the values 0 and 1 have to be added as separate variables used in SPSS).

Quantity of care	Quality of care	Residues quadratic model	Residues cubic model
19,00	2,00	0,00	1,00
20,00	3,00	0,00	0,00
23,00	4,00	1,00	1,00
24,00	5,00	0,00	0,00
26,00	6,00	1,00	0,00
27,00	7,00	1,00	0,00
28,00	8,00	1,00	0,00
29,00	9,00	1,00	1,00
29,00	10,00	1,00	1,00
29,00	11,00	1,00	1,00
28,00	12,00	1,00	1,00
27,00	13,00	0,00	0,00
27,00	14,00	0,00	1,00
26,00	15,00	0,00	1,00
25,00	16,00	0,00	0,00
24,00	17,00	0,00	0,00
23,00	18,00	0,00	0,00
22,00	19,00	0,00	0,00
22,00	20,00	1,00	1,00
21,00	21,00	1,00	0,00
21,00	22,00	1,00	1,00

Command

Analyze....Nonparametric tests....Runs Test....move the runsquadratic model residues variable to Test Variable List....click Options....click Descriptives.... click Continue....click Cut Point....mark Median....click OK.

Example   573

The output table shows that in the runs test the quadratic model differs from the actual data with $p = 0.02$. It means that the quadratic model is systematically different from the data.

Runs Test

	runsquadratic model
Test Value[a]	1,00
Cases < Test Value	10
Cases >= Test Value	11
Total Cases	21
Number of Runs	6
Z	-2,234
Asymp. Sig. (2-tailed)	,026
Exact Sig. (2-tailed)	,022
Point Probability	,009

a. Median

When the similar procedure is followed for the best fit cubic model, the result is very insignificant with a p-value of 1.00. The cubic model was, thus, a much better predicting model for the data than the quadratic model.

Runs Test 2

	runscubicmo del
Test Value[a]	,4762
Cases < Test Value	11
Cases >= Test Value	10
Total Cases	21
Number of Runs	11
Z	,000
Asymp. Sig. (2-tailed)	1,000
Exact Sig. (2-tailed)	1,000
Point Probability	,165

a. Mean

Conclusion

The runs test is appropriate both for testing whether fitted theoretical curves are systematically different or not from a given data set. The fit of regression models is traditionally assessed with r-square tests. However, the runs test is more appropriate for the purpose, because large r-square value do not exclude poor systematic data fit, and because the runs test assesses the entire pattern in the data, rather than mean distances between data and model.

Note

More background, theoretical and mathematical information of the runs test is given in Machine learning in medicine part three, Chap. 13, Runs test, pp. 127–135, Springer Heidelberg Germany 2013, from the same authors.

Chapter 74
Evolutionary Operations for Process Improvement (8 Operation Room Air Condition Settings)

General Purpose

Evolutionary operations (evops) try and find improved processes by exploring the effect of small changes in an experimental setting. It stems from evolutionary algorithms (see Machine learning in medicine part three, Chap. 2, Evolutionary operations, pp. 11–18, Springer Heidelberg Germany, 2013, from the same authors), which uses rules based on biological evolution mechanisms where each next generation is slightly different and generally somewhat improved as compared to its ancestors. It was developed in the 1950s by George E. P. Box. Evop methodology introduces experimental designs and improvements, while an ongoing full-scale manufacturing process continues to produce satisfactory results. It is, currently, widely used not only in genetic research, but also in chemical and technical processes. So much so that the internet nowadays offers free evop calculators suitable not only for the optimization of the above processes, but also for the optimization of your pet's food, your car costs, and many other daily life standard issues. This chapter is, to assess how evops can be helpful to optimize the air quality of operation rooms.

This chapter was previously published in "Machine learning in medicine-cookbook 3" as Chap. 11, 2014.

Electronic Supplementary Material The online version of this chapter (https://doi.org/10.1007/978-3-030-33970-8_74) contains supplementary material, which is available to authorized users.

Background

Evolutionary algorithms are, thus, optimization algorithms that are based on mechanisms inspired by biological evolution such as mutation, recombination and selection. These algorithms are normally used in high-dimensional spaces with thousands of variables and they do well, because the algorithms do not use assumptions on the shape of the criterion-function that is to be optimized. There is however no guarantee, that an evolutionary algorithm finds the optimum, and therefore they are especially useful, when an approximate solution is acceptable. There are many machine learning techniques that use similar evolutionary operations. Among these are genetic programming to search for the best computer program, neuroevolution to search for the best neural networks, and (3) genetic algorithms to search for the best subset of variables. The R Statistical Software Package *Subselect* is convenient, but in this chapter we will, simply, use multiple linear regressions in SPSS statistical software with numbers of infectious diseases as outcome and three factors to identify the significant predictors.

Specific Scientific Question

The air quality of operation rooms is important for infection prevention. Particularly, the factors (1) humidity (30–60%), (2) filter capacity (70–90%), and (3) air volume change (20–30% per hour) are supposed to be important determinants. Can an evolutionary operation be used for process improvement.

Example

Eight operation room air condition settings were investigated, and the results are underneath.

Example   577

Operation Setting	humidity (30% = 1, 60% = 4)	filter capacity (70% = 1, 90% = 3)	air volume change (20% = 1, 30% = 3)	infections number of
1	1	1	1	99
2	2	1	1	90
3	1	2	1	75
4	2	2	1	73
5	1	1	2	99
6	2	1	2	99
7	1	2	2	61
8	2	2	2	52

We will use multiple linear regression in SPSS with the number of infections as outcome and the three factors as predictors to identify the significant predictors.

First, the data file available as "evops" in extras.springer.com is opened in SPSS.

Command

Analyze....Regression....Linear....Dependent: enter "Var00004".... Independent(s): enter "Var00001–00003)"....click OK.

The underneath table in the output shows that all of the determinants are statistically significant at $p < 0.10$. A higher humidity, filtering level, and air volume change better prevents infections.

Coefficients^a

Model		Unstandardized Coefficients B	Std. Error	Standardized Coefficients Beta	t	Sig.
1	(Constant)	103,250	18,243		5,660	,005
	hunidity1	-12,250	3,649	-,408	-3,357	,028
	filter capacity1	-21,250	3,649	-,707	-5,824	,004
	airvolume change1	15,750	3,649	,524	4,317	,012

a. Dependent Variable: infections 1

In the next 8 operation settings higher determinant levels were assessed.

Operation Setting	humidity (30% = 1, 60% = 4)	filter capacity (70% = 1, 90% = 3)	air volume change (20% = 1, 30% = 3)	infections number of
1	3	2	2	51
2	4	2	2	45
3	3	3	2	33
4	4	3	2	26
5	3	2	3	73
6	4	2	3	60
7	3	3	3	54
8	4	3	3	31

We will use again multiple linear regression in SPSS with the number of infections as outcome and the three factors as predictors to identify the significant predictors.

Command:

Analyze. . . .Regression. . . .Linear. . . .Dependent: enter "Var00008". . . . Independent(s): enter "Var00005–00007)". . . .click OK.

Coefficients^a

Model		Unstandardized Coefficients		Standardized Coefficients	t	Sig.
		B	Std. Error	Beta		
1	(Constant)	145,500	15,512		9,380	,001
	humidity2	-5,000	5,863	-,145	-,853	,442
	filter capacity2	-31,500	5,863	-,910	-5,373	,006
	airvolume change2	-6,500	5,863	-,188	-1,109	,330

a. Dependent Variable: infections2

The underneath table in the output shows that only Var 00006 (the filter capacity) is still statistically significant. Filter capacity 3 performs better than 2, while humidity levels and air volume changes were not significantly different. We could go one step further to find out how higher levels would perform, but for now we will conclude that humidity level 2–4, filter capacity level 3, and air flow change level 2–4 are efficacious level combinations. Higher levels of humidity and air flow change is not meaningful. An additional benefit of a higher level of filter capacity cannot be excluded, but requires additional testing.

Conclusion

Evolutionary operations can be used to improve the process of air quality maintenance in operation rooms. This methodology can similarly be applied for finding the best settings for numerous clinical, and laboratory settings. We have to add that interaction between the predictors was not taken into account in the current example. For a meaningful assessment of 2- and 3-factor interactions larger samples would be required, however. Moreover, we have clinical arguments that no important interactions are to be expected.

Note

More background, theoretical and mathematical information of evops is given in Machine learning in medicine part three, Chap. 2, Evolutionary operations, pp. 11–18, Springer Heidelberg Germany, 2013, from the same authors.

Chapter 75
Bayesian Networks for Cause Effect Modeling (600 Patients)

General Purpose

Bayesian networks are probabilistic graphical models using nodes and arrows, respectively representing variables, and probabilistic dependencies between two variables. Computations in a Bayesian network are performed using weighted likelihood methodology and marginalization, meaning that irrelevant variables are integrated or summed out. Additional theoretical information is given in Machine Learning in medicine part two, Chap. 16, Bayesian networks, pp. 163–170, Springer Heidelberg Germany, 2013, from the same authors). This chapter is to assess if Bayesian networks is able to determine direct and indirect predictors of binary outcomes like morbidity/mortality outcomes.

Background

The term Bayesian network was coined by Judea Pearl in 1985 to emphasize

- the often subjective nature of the input information,
- the reliance on Bayes' conditioning as the basis for updating information,
- the distinction between causal and evidential modes of reasoning.

In the late 1980s Pearl's work entitled "Probabilistic Reasoning in Intelligent Systems and Neapolitan's Probabilistic Reasoning in Expert Systems" summarized their properties and established them as a field of study. A Bayesian network (BN) is

---

This chapter was previously published in "Machine learning in medicine-cookbook 3" as Chap. 12, 2014.

Electronic Supplementary Material The online version of this chapter (https://doi.org/10.1007/978-3-030-33970-8_75) contains supplementary material, which is available to authorized users.

T. J. Cleophas, A. H. Zwinderman, *Machine Learning in Medicine – A Complete Overview*, https://doi.org/10.1007/978-3-030-33970-8_75

a tool to describe and analyze multivariate distributions. The tool is member of the family of probabilistic graphical models. Despite its association, Bayesian networks do not necessarily use Bayesian statistical methods for data-analysis, the name refers rather to the way conditional and marginal probability distributions are related to one another. Bayesian networks are sometimes used in conjunction with Bayesian statistical methods, especially when prior knowledge is analyzed together with data, but this is not unique for BNs. Graphical models in general, and Bayesian networks too, have been proposed especially to deal with complex data (−analysis), and with an eye towards causal interpretations. This is achieved by combining graph theory, probability theory, statistics, and computer science. Bayesian networks have been used in many different fields, for instance, in the Microsoft Windows system and the NASA mission control. In biomedicine the main applications seems to be in expert systems, in bioinformatics applications in genetics, and in identifying gene-regulatory networks.

Primary Scientific Question

Longevity is multifactorial, and logistic regression is adequate to assess the chance of longevity in patients with various predictor scores like physical, psychological, and family scores. However, some factors may have both direct and indirect effects. Can a best fit Bayesian network demonstrate not only direct but also indirect effects of factors on the outcome?

Example

In 600 patients, 70 years of age, a score sampling of factors predicting longevity was performed. The outcome was death after 10 years of follow-up. The first 12 patients are underneath, the entire data file is in "longevity", and is available at extras. springer.com. We will first perform a logistic regression of these data using SPSS statistical software. Start by opening SPSS. Enter the above data file.

Variables

1	2	3	4	5	6
death	econ	psychol	physic	family	educ
0	70	117	76	77	120
0	70	68	76	56	114
0	70	74	71	57	109
0	90	114	82	79	125
0	90	117	100	68	123
0	70	74	100	57	121
1	70	77	103	62	145

0	70	62	71	56	100
0	90	86	88	65	114
0	90	77	88	61	111
0	110	56	65	59	130
0	70	68	50	60	118

death (0 = no)
econ = economy score
psychol = psychological score
physic = physical score
family = familial risk score of longevity
educ = educational score

Binary Logistic Regression in SPSS

Command

Analyze....Regression....Binary Logistic....Dependent: enter "death"....Covariates: enter "econ, psychol, physical, family, educ"....OK.

The underneath output table shows the results. With p < 0.10 as cut-off for statistical significance, all of the covariates, except economical score, were significant predictors of longevity (death), although both negative and positive b-values were observed.

Variables in the Equation

		B	S.E.	Wald	df	Sig.	Exp(B)
Step 1ª	ecom	,003	,006	,306	1	,580	1,003
	psychol	-,056	,009	43,047	1	,000	,946
	physical	-,019	,007	8,589	1	,003	,981
	family	,045	,017	7,297	1	,007	1,046
	educ	,017	,009	3,593	1	,058	1,018
	Constant	-,563	,922	,373	1	,541	,569

a. Variable(s) entered on step 1: ecom, psychol, physical, family, educ.

For these data we hypothesized that all of these scores would independently affect longevity. However, indirect effects were not taken into account, like the effect of psychological on physical scores, and the effect of family on educational scores etc. In order to assess both direct and indirect effects, a Bayesian network DAG (directed acyclic graph) was fitted to the data. The Konstanz information miner (Knime) was used for the analysis. In order to enter the SPSS data file in Knime, an excel version of the data file is required. For that purpose open the file in SPSS and follow the commands.

Command in SPSS

click File....click Save as....in "Save as" type: enter Comma Delimited (∗.csv)....
click.

Save.

For convenience the excel file has been added to extras.springer.com, and is, just
like the SPSS file, entitled "longevity".

Konstanz Information Miner (Knime)

In Google enter the term "knime". Click Download and follow instructions. After
completing the pretty easy download procedure, open the knime workbench by
clicking the knime welcome screen. The center of the screen displays the workflow
editor like the canvas in SPSS modeler. It is empty, and can be used to build a stream
of nodes, called workflow in knime. The node repository is in the left lower angle of
the screen, and the nodes can be dragged to the workflow editor simply by left-
clicking. The nodes are computer tools for data analysis like visualization and
statistical processes. Node description is in the right upper angle of the screen.
Before the nodes can be used, they have to be connected with the file reader and
with one another by arrows drawn again simply by left clicking the small triangles
attached to the nodes. Right clicking on the file reader enables to configure from your
computer a requested data file.....click Browse.....and download from the appropriate folder a csv type Excel file. You are almost set for analysis now, but in order to
perform a Bayesian analysis Weka software 3.6 for windows (statistical software
from the University of Waikato (New Zealand) is required. Simply type the term
Weka software, and find the site. The software can be freely downloaded from the
internet, following a few simple instructions, and it can, subsequently, be readily
opened in Knime. Once it has been opened, it is stored in your Knime node
repository, and you will be able to routinely use it.

Knime Workflow

A knime workflow for the analysis of the above data example is built, and the final
result is shown in the underneath figure, by dragging and connecting as explained
above.

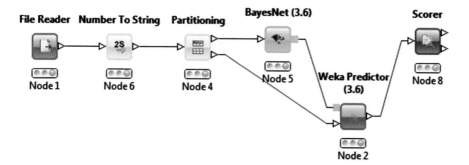

In the node repository click and type File Reader and drag to workflow editor in the node repository click again File reader....click the ESCbutton of your computer....in the node repository click again and type Number to String....the node is displayed....drag it to the workflow editor....perform the same kind of actions for all of the nodes as shown in the above figure....connect, by left clicking, all of the nodes with arrows as indicated above....click File Reader....click Browse....and type the requested data file ("longevity.csv")....click OK....the data file is given....right click all of the nodes and then right click Configurate and execute all of the nodes by right clicking the nodes and then the texts "Configurate" and "Execute"....the red lights will successively turn orange and then green....right click the Weka Predictor node....right click the Weka Node View....right click Graph.

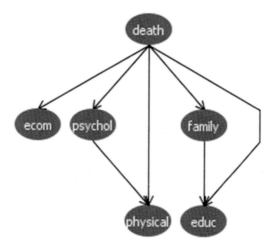

The above graph, a socalled directed acyclic graph (DAG) shows the Bayesian network obtained from the analysis. This best fitting DAG was, obviously, more complex than expected from the logistic model. Longevity was directly determined by all of the 5 predictors, but additional indirect effects were between physical and psychological scores, and between educational and family scores. In order to assess the validity of the Bayesian model, a confusion matrix and accuracy statistics were computed.

Right click the Scorer node....right click Confusion matrix.

Confusion Matrix

Table "spec_name" - Rows: 2	Spec - Columns: 2	Properties	Flow Variables

Row ID	0	1
0	295	70
1	91	44

The observed and predicted values are summarized. Subsequently, right click Accuracy statistics.

Accuracy Statistics

Table "default" - Rows: 3	Spec - Columns: 11	Properties	Flow Variables							
Row ID	TruePo...	FalsePo...	TrueNe...	FalseN...	D Recall	D Precision	D Sensitivity	D Specifity
0	295	91	44	70	0.808	0.764	0.808	0.326
1	44	70	295	91	0.326	0.386	0.326	0.808
Overall	?	?	?	?	?	?	?	?

The sensitivity of the Bayesian model to predict longevity was pretty good, 80.8%. However, the specificity was pretty bad. "No deaths" were rightly predicted in 80.8% of the patients, "deaths", however, were rightly predicted in only 32.6% of the patients.

Conclusion

Bayesian networks are probabilistic graphical models for assessing cause effect relationships. This chapter is to assess if Bayesian networks is able to determine direct and indirect predictors of binary outcomes like morbidity/mortality outcomes. As an example a longevity study is used. Longevity is multifactorial, and logistic regression is adequate to assess the chance of longevity in patients with various predictor scores like physical, psychological, and family scores. However, factors may have both direct and indirect effects. A best fit Bayesian network demonstrated not only direct but also indirect effects of the factors on the outcome.

Note

More background, theoretical and mathematical information of Bayesian networks is in Machine learning in medicine part two, Chap. 16, Bayesian networks, pp. 163–170, Springer Heidelberg Germany, 2013, from the same authors.

Chapter 76
Support Vector Machines for Imperfect Nonlinear Data (200 Patients with Sepsis)

General Purpose

Support vector machines is a simplified cluster program that does not apply all observations but rather the difficult observations lying close to the separation lines. The basic aim of support vector machines is to construct the best fit separation line (or with three dimensional data separation plane), separating cases and controls as good as possible. Discriminant analysis (Chap. 22), classification trees or decision trees (Chap. 8), and neural networks (Chap. 55), are alternative methods for the purpose, but support vector machines are generally more stable and sensitive, although heuristic studies to indicate when they perform better are missing. Support vector machines are also often used in automatic modeling that computes the ensembled results of several best fit models see the Chaps. 69 and 70).

This chapter uses the Konstanz information miner (Knime), a free data mining software package developed at the University of Konstanz, and also used in the Chaps. 7 and 8.

This chapter was previously published in "Machine learning in medicine-cookbook 3" as Chap. 13, 2014.

Electronic Supplementary Material The online version of this chapter (https://doi.org/10.1007/978-3-030-33970-8_76) contains supplementary material, which is available to authorized users.

Background

Basic aim of SVMs is to construct a hyperplane formed by the set of patient characteristics that separates the cases and controls as good as possible. For two dimensional data this hyperplane is the best fit separation line, for three dimensional data the best fit separation plane. For multidimensional data hyperplanes equally exist, although they are difficult to imagine. The aim of SVMs is similar to that of neural networks (and other techniques), but SVMs are usually better capable of finding the best fit hyperplane and are also more easily extended to patterns that are not linearly separable. This latter is done by transforming the data into "a new space" by Kernel functions, as non-parametric way to estimate random variables.

Consider the bivariate scatterplot of two patient-characteristics in the underneath Fig. A, where cases are denoted by crosses and controls by dots. A linear hyperplane is defined as $a*X_1 + b*X_2$, and "a" and "b" are weights associated with the two patient-characteristics. The object is to find "a", "b" and "c" such that $a*X_1 + b*X_2 \leq c$ for all controls and $a*X_1 + b*X_2 > c$ for cases. There are often many different solutions for "a", "b" and "c" and the left figure (Fig. A) shows three different hyperplanes that separate cases and controls equally well. The object of any classification technique is to find the optimal hyperplane, but the various techniques differ in which observations are used to define what is optimal. Regression models and neural networks apply all of the observations, but SVMs use only the "difficult" observations that are lying close to the optimal hyperplane (denoted as the "decision boundary"); these observations are called the support vectors. The rationale of this choice may be argued by the fact that the decision boundary will not change very much if the "easy" observations are removed from the dataset whereas the decision boundary will change dramatically if one or more of the difficult observations are removed. Therefore, the difficult observations or support vectors are the critical observations in the dataset. SVMs choose the hyperplane that maximizes the distance "d" from it to the difficult observations on either side (right side Fig. (B)). The starting points of the support vectors denoted as v_1, v_2, and v_3 are in the figure. All three vector arrows meet in the origin. One line through the starting points of v_2 and v_3 is drawn, and one parallel line through the starting point of v_1. The best fit hyperplane line is midway between the two parallel lines, distance d in Fig. B. The distance from the hyperplane line to the origin is an important estimator in SVM statistics, and is expressed just like t-values in t-tests in a standardized way: if d = w (weight), and the distance from the hyperplane line to the origin = b, then the distance from the hyperplane line to the origin equals b/w (expressed in "w-units"). In order to extent this fairly simple procedure to more complex situations like multidimensional data and non linear data, a more general notation is prefered. It is given underneath.

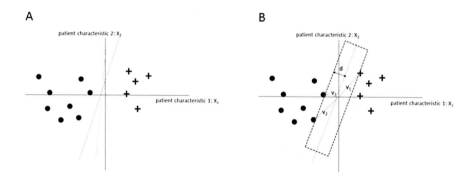

A

B

Hyperplanes H are defined as $w'x_i + b \leq -1$ for controls and $w'x_i + b \geq 1$ for cases, where x_i is the vector of all patient-characteristics of patient i, w is a vector with weights and b is called a bias term and is comparable to an intercept of regression models. The optimal set of weights is determined so that the distance "d" is maximized. It turns out that this is equivalent to minimizing the Euclidean norm $\|w\|^2$ subject to the condition that there are no observations in the margin: $w'x_i + b \leq -1$ for controls and $w'x_i + b \geq 1$ for cases, or $y_i(w'x_i) \geq 1$ when $y_i = 1$ for cases and $y_i = -1$ for controls. This is a quadratic programming problem that can be solved by, for instance, the Lagrangian multiplier method.

This algorithm has been extended for situations where no hyperplane exists that can split the cases and controls. The so-called soft margin method chooses a hyperplane that separates the cases and controls as good as possible, but still maximizing the distance "d" to the nearest cleanly split observations. The method introduces slack-variables ξ_i that represent the degree of misclassification: $y_i(w'x_i) \geq 1-\xi_i$. Instead of minimizing $\|w\|^2$ now $0.5\|w\|^2 + C*\Sigma_i\xi_i$ is minimized where the constant C is a penalty-parameter that regulates the amount of misclassification that is accepted.

In some cases where no linear separation exists, a non-linear function might exist that is capable of linear separation. Take for instance the situation of the following sequence of cases and controls ranked on a single patient-characteristic:

$$+ + + + \bullet\bullet\bullet\bullet\bullet + + + +$$

Apparently, some cases have low values of the characteristic and other cases have high values, whereas controls have values in the middle of the distribution. There exists no linear hyperplane that separates cases and controls, but a simple quadratic function will easily do the job (underneath figure).

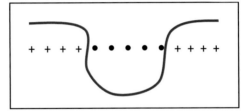

This situation is not unlikely; take for instance a patient-characteristic such as body temperature: both when it is increased and when it is decreased, the risk of having a (infectious) disease might be large.

Transformations are, usually, considered through Kernel functions $K(x_i, x_j)$ of the inner products of the patient-characteristics of two observations x_i and x_j. The usual Kernel functions that are considered, are the polynomial Kernel function $(x_i'x_j + 1)^p$, the radial basis function $\exp.(-\|x_i - x_j\|^2/2\sigma^2)$ and the sigmoid function $\tanh(\kappa\, x_i'x_j - \delta)$. The different transformations are characterized by parameters p, σ, and (κ, δ).

The effectiveness of a SVM for any application depends (next to that of the data) on the possibility to specify appropriate Kernel-functions, Kernel parameters, and soft margin C. Commonly, one starts with a Gaussian Kernel and then a grid search is performed for the parameters C and σ. Overfitting is a realistic danger for SVMs and it is crucial to do a form of double (and repeated) cross validation to select the optimal Kernels, parameters and C values and estimate the classification ability of the SVM.

Several software packages exist to develop a support vector machine. The free R system has an implementation in the package e1071. SPSS offers SVM models in the SPSS modeler package, SAS offers SVMs in their enterprise Miner package. It is also available in the standalone machine-learning program Weka (http://weka. wikispaces.com/Primer), as well as the Konstanz information miner (Knime) applied in this text. All of them offer SVM models for binary and multiclass classification as well as support vector regression analysis and SVM models for novelty detection.

Primary Scientific Question

Is support vector machines adequate to classify cases and controls in a cohort of admitted because of sepsis?

Example

Two hundred patients were admitted because of sepsis. The laboratory values and the outcome death or alive were registered. We wish to use support vector machines to predict from the laboratory values the outcome, death or alive, including information on the error rate. The data of the first 12 patients are underneath. The entire data file is in extras.springer.com. Konstanz information miner (Knime) does not use SPSS files, and, so, the file has to be transformed into a csv excel file (click Save As....in "Save as" type: replace SPSS Statistics(∗sav) with SPSS Statistics (∗csv). For convenience the csv file is in extras.springer.com and is entitled "svm".

Death 1= yes	Ggt	asat	alat	bili	ureum	creat	c-clear	esr	crp	leucos
var1	var2	var3	var4	var5	var6	var7	var8	var9	Var10	var11
0	20	23	34	2	3,4	89	-111	2	2	5
0	14	21	33	3	2	67	-112	7	3	6
0	30	35	32	4	5,6	58	-116	8	4	4
0	35	34	40	4	6	76	-110	6	5	7
0	23	33	22	4	6,1	95	-120	9	6	6
0	26	31	24	3	5,4	78	-132	8	4	8
0	15	29	26	2	5,3	47	-120	12	5	5
0	13	26	24	1	6,3	65	-132	13	6	6
0	26	27	27	4	6	97	-112	14	6	7
0	34	25	13	3	4	67	-125	15	7	6
0	32	26	24	3	3,6	58	-110	13	8	6
0	21	13	15	3	3,6	69	-102	12	2	4

Var 1	death 1 = yes
Var 2	gammagt (Var = variable) (U/l)
Var 3	asat (U/l)
Var 4	alat (U/l)
Var 5	bili (mumol/l)
Var 6	ureum (mmol/l)
Var 7	creatinine (mumol/l)
Var 8	creatinine clearance (ml/min)
Var 9	esr (erythrocyte sedimentation rate) (mm)
Var 10	c-reactive protein (mg/l)
Var 11	leucos (x10^9 /l)

Knime Data Miner

In Google enter the term "knime". Click Download and follow instructions. After completing the pretty easy download procedure, open the knime workbench by clicking the knime welcome screen. The center of the screen displays the workflow editor like the canvas in SPSS modeler. It is empty, and can be used to build a stream of nodes, called workflow in knime. The node repository is in the left lower angle of the screen, and the nodes can be dragged to the workflow editor simply by left-clicking. The nodes are computer tools for data analysis like visualization and statistical processes. Node description is in the right upper angle of the screen. Before the nodes can be used they have to be connected with the file reader and with one another by arrows drawn again simply by left clicking the small triangles attached to the nodes. Right clicking on the file reader enables to configure from your computer a requested data file.

Knime Workflow

A knime workflow for the analysis of the above data example will be built, and the final result is shown in the underneath figure.

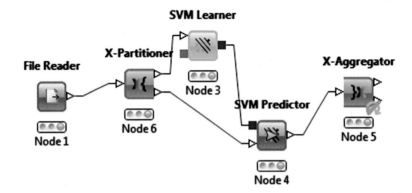

File Reader Node

In the node repository find the node File Reader. Drag the node to the workflow editor by left clicking....click Browse....and download from extras.springer.com the csv type Excel file entitled "svm". You are set for analysis now. By left clicking the node the file is displayed. The File Reader has chosen Var 0006 (ureum) as S variable (dependent). However, we wish to replace it with Var 0001 (death yes = 1)....click the column header of Var 0006....mark "Don't include column in output"....click OK....in the column header of Var 0001 leave unmarked "Don't include column in output"click OK.

The outcome variable is now rightly the Var 0001 and is indicated with S, the Var 0006 has obtained the term "SKIP"between brackets.

The Nodes X-Partitioner, SVM Learner, SVM Predictor, X-Aggregator

Find the above nodes in the node repository and drag them to the workflow editor and connect them with one another according to the above figure. Configurate and execute all them by right clicking the nodes and the texts "Configurate" and "Execute". The red lights under the nodes get, subsequently, yellow and, then, green. The miner has accomplished its task.

Error Rates

Right click the X-Aggregator node once more, and then right click Error rates. The underneath table is shown. The svm model is used to make predictions about death or not from the other variables of your file. Nine random samples of 25 patients are shown. The error rates are pretty small, and vary from 0–12.5%. We should add that other measures of uncertainty like sensitivity or specificity are not provided by knime.

Error rates - 0:5 - X-Aggregator

File

Table "default" - Rows: 10 | Spec - Columns: 3 | Properties | Flow Variables

Row ID	D Error in %	Size of ...	Error C...
fold 0	4	25	1
fold 1	4	25	1
fold 2	4.167	24	1
fold 3	12	25	3
fold 4	4.167	24	1
fold 5	8	25	2
fold 6	12	25	3
fold 7	0	24	0
fold 8	8	25	2
fold 9	12.5	24	3

Prediction Table

Right click the x-aggregator node once more, and then right click Prediction Table.. The underneath table is shown. The svm model is used to make predictions about death or not from the other variables of your file.

The left column gives the outcome values (death yes $= 1$), the right one gives the predicted values. It can be observed that the two results very well match one another.

	Prediction table - 0:5 - X-Aggregator										

File

Table "default" - Rows: 246 | Spec - Columns: 11 | Properties | Flow Variables

Row ID	S i=čVAR...	i VAR00...	i VAR00...	i VAR00...	i VAR00...	i VAR00...	i VAR00...	i VAR00...	i VAR00...	i VAR00...	S Predicti...
Row 4	0	23	33	22	4	95	-120	9	6	6	0
Row 6	0	15	29	26	2	47	-120	12	5	5	0
Row 9	0	34	25	13	3	67	-125	15	7	6	0
Row 14	0	19	16	9	4	80	-113	8	4	7	0
Row 18	0	24	24	27	4	84	-120	15	6	6	0
Row 36	0	19	236	15	2	78	-113	7	6	6	0
Row 42	0	27	17	27	4	98	-101	14	4	3	0
Row 47	0	15	17	15	2	89	-112	13	9	6	0
Row 62	0	16	14	19	4	67	-102	14	7	2	0
Row 64	0	14	14	27	2	76	-109	18	5	5	0
Row 66	0	16	27	29	3	77	-102	14	4	6	0
Row 67	0	24	25	24	2	69	-110	16	5	7	0
Row 68	0	21	29	25	4	78	-112	15	7	4	0
Row 73	0	21	15	13	2	92	-120	17	7	4	0
Row 114	1	900	759	856	287	532	-8	109	103	23	1
Row 144	1	376	459	389	135	267	-29	97	33	20	1
Row 151	1	169	154	267	75	244	-50	42	21	15	1
Row 155	1	175	250	276	95	231	-41	36	28	15	1
Row 170	1	276	230	156	79	235	-54	34	23	15	1
Row 181	1	75	84	145	39	137	-66	28	18	14	1

Conclusion

The basic aim of support vector machines is to construct the best fit separation line (or with three dimensional data separation plane), separating cases and controls as good as possible. This chapter uses the Konstanz information miner, a free data mining software package developed at the University of Konstanz, and also used in the Chaps. 1 and 2. The example shows that support vector machines is adequate to predict the presence of a disease or not in a cohort of patients at risk of a disease.

Note

More background, theoretical and mathematical information of support vector machines is given in Machine in medicine part two, Chap. 14, Support vector machines, pp. 155–162, Springer Heidelberg Germany, from the same authors.

Chapter 77
Multiple Response Sets for Visualizing Clinical Data Trends (811 Patient Visits)

General Purpose

Multiple response methodology answers multiple qualitative questions about a single group of patients, and uses for the purpose summary tables. The method visualizes trends and similarities in the data, but no statistical test is given.

Background

The term "multiple-response"refers to the situation, when people are allowed to tick more than one answer option for a question. Multiple response analysis is a frequency analysis, when there can be more than one response per participant to a survey question. For example, survey instructions such as: "Tick all responses that apply." A multiple response set is a special construct within a data file. You can define and save multiple response sets in IBM® SPSS® Statistics data files, but you cannot import or export multiple response sets from/to other file formats.

Multiple Response Analysis allows you to create frequency and crosstabulation tables for user-defined "multiple response sets". When a survey question can be answered multiple valid times, such as questions which note "Check all that apply", multiple variables are necessary to capture all the responses. This collection of variables is called a multiple response set. The variables of a multiple response set are coded as dichotomies or categories. In a multiple dichotomy set, a separate variable is created for each of the valid responses to the question. Each variable has

This chapter was previously published in "Machine learning in medicine-cookbook 3" as Chap. 14, 2014.

Electronic Supplementary Material The online version of this chapter (https://doi.org/10.1007/978-3-030-33970-8_77) contains supplementary material, which is available to authorized users.

© Springer Nature Switzerland AG 2020

T. J. Cleophas, A. H. Zwinderman, *Machine Learning in Medicine – A Complete Overview*, https://doi.org/10.1007/978-3-030-33970-8_77

two possible values, which indicate whether or not the response was selected by the survey taker. In a multiple category set, a separate variable is created for each response given by the survey taker, up to the maximum number of responses given by any survey taker. Multiple category sets are most often used when the maximum number of responses given by any survey taker is significantly less than the number of possible responses.

The analysis of complex survey data involving multiple response sets has been investigated since the early seventies. An unsolved problem till today is the presence of multiple dependencies between the different variables in these datasets. In 1981 the statisticians Rao and Scott from the university of Auckland developed a corrected/adjusted version of a typical Pearson chi-square. It is used for example to account for the violations of equal probability across Likert scale responses in survey data. It is a very complicated concept, and it is not available in SPSS statistical software. Other software programs like R, SAS, and Matlab can be used as an alternative.

Specific Scientific Question

Can multiple response sets better than traditional frequency tables demonstrate results that could be selected for formal trend tests.

Example

An 811 person health questionnaire addressed the reasons for visiting general practitioners (gps) in 1 month. Nine qualitative questions addressed various aspects of health as primary reasons for visits. SPSS statistical software was used to analyze the data.

Example599

ill	alcohol	weight	tired	cold	family	mental	physical	social	no
0	0	1	1	0	0	0	0	1	0
1	1	1	1	1	1	1	1	1	0
0	0	0	0	0	0	0	0	0	1
1	0	0	1	0	0	0	0	0	0
1	0	0	0	1	1	1	1	0	0
0	0	0	0	0	1	1	1	0	0
0	0	0	0	0	0	0	0	0	1
1	1	0	1	1	1	1	1	1	0
0	0	0	0	0	0	1	0	0	0
1	1	0	1	0	1	1	1	1	0
0	0	0	0	0	0	0	0	0	1
0	0	0	0	0	1	1	1	0	0
1	1	0	1	1	1	0	1	1	0
1	0	0	0	1	0	1	0	0	0
1	0	0	1	0	0	0	1	1	0

ill = ill feeling
alcohol = alcohol abuse
weight = weight problems
tired + tiredness
cold = common cold
family = family problem
mental = mental problem
physical = physical problem
social = social problem
no = no answer

The first 15 patient data are given. The entire data file is entitled "multipleresponse", and can be downloaded from extras.springer.com. SPSS statistical software is used for analysis. We will start by the descriptive statistics.

Command
Descriptive Statistics....Frequencies....Variables: enter the variables between illfeeling" to "no answer"....click Statistics....click Sum....click Continue.... click OK.

The output is in the underneath 10 tables. It is pretty hard to observe trends across the Tables. Also redundant information as given is not helpful for overall conclusion about the relationships between the different questions.

illfeeling

		Frequency	Percent	Valid Percent	Cumulative Percent
Valid	No	420	43,3	51,8	51,8
	Yes	391	40,3	48,2	100,0
	Total	811	83,6	100,0	
Missing	System	159	16,4		
Total		970	100,0		

alcohol

		Frequency	Percent	Valid Percent	Cumulative Percent
Valid	No	569	58,7	70,2	70,2
	Yes	242	24,9	29,8	100,0
	Total	811	83,6	100,0	
Missing	System	159	16,4		
Total		970	100,0		

weight problem

		Frequency	Percent	Valid Percent	Cumulative Percent
Valid	No	597	61,5	73,6	73,6
	Yes	214	22,1	26,4	100,0
	Total	811	83,6	100,0	
Missing	System	159	16,4		
Total		970	100,0		

tiredness

		Frequency	Percent	Valid Percent	Cumulative Percent
Valid	No	511	52,7	63,0	63,0
	Yes	300	30,9	37,0	100,0
	Total	811	83,6	100,0	
Missing	System	159	16,4		
Total		970	100,0		

Example 601

cold

		Frequency	Percent	Valid Percent	Cumulative Percent
Valid	No	422	43,5	52,0	52,0
	Yes	389	40,1	48,0	100,0
	Total	811	83,6	100,0	
Missing	System	159	16,4		
Total		970	100,0		

family problem

		Frequency	Percent	Valid Percent	Cumulative Percent
Valid	No	416	42,9	51,3	51,3
	Yes	395	40,7	48,7	100,0
	Total	811	83,6	100,0	
Missing	System	159	16,4		
Total		970	100,0		

mental problem

		Frequency	Percent	Valid Percent	Cumulative Percent
Valid	No	410	42,3	50,6	50,6
	Yes	401	41,3	49,4	100,0
	Total	811	83,6	100,0	
Missing	System	159	16,4		
Total		970	100,0		

physical problem

		Frequency	Percent	Valid Percent	Cumulative Percent
Valid	No	402	41,4	49,6	49,6
	Yes	409	42,2	50,4	100,0
	Total	811	83,6	100,0	
Missing	System	159	16,4		
Total		970	100,0		

social problem

		Frequency	Percent	Valid Percent	Cumulative Percent
Valid	No	518	53,4	63,9	63,9
	Yes	293	30,2	36,1	100,0
	Total	811	83,6	100,0	
Missing	System	159	16,4		
Total		970	100,0		

no answer

		Frequency	Percent	Valid Percent	Cumulative Percent
Valid	,00	722	74,4	89,0	89,0
	1,00	89	9,2	11,0	100,0
	Total	811	83,6	100,0	
Missing	System	159	16,4		
Total		970	100,0		

In order to find out more about trends in de data a multiple response analysis will be performed next.

Command

Analyze....Multiple Response....Define Variable Sets....move "ill feeling, alcohol, tiredness, cold, family problem, mental problem, physical problem, social problem" from Set Definition to Variables in Set....Counted Values enter 1.... Name enter "health"....Label enter "health"....Multiple Response Set: click Add....click Close....click Analyze....Multiple Response....click Frequencies ....move $health from Multiple Response Sets to Table(s)....click OK.

The underneath Case Summary table show that of all visitants 25.6% did not answer any question, here called the missing cases.

Case Summary

	Cases					
	Valid		Missing		Total	
	N	Percent	N	Percent	N	Percent
$health[a]	722	74,4%	248	25,6%	970	100,0%

a. Dichotomy group tabulated at value 1.

Example 603

$health Frequencies

		Responses		Percent of Cases
		N	Percent	
health[a]	illfeeling	391	12,9%	54,2%
	alcohol	242	8,0%	33,5%
	weight problem	214	7,1%	29,6%
	tiredness	300	9,9%	41,6%
	cold	389	12,8%	53,9%
	family problem	395	13,0%	54,7%
	mental problem	401	13,2%	55,5%
	physical problem	409	13,5%	56,6%
	social problem	293	9,7%	40,6%
Total		3034	100,0%	420,2%

a. Dichotomy group tabulated at value 1.

The letter N gives the numbers of yes-answers per question, "Percent of Cases" gives the yes-answers per question in those who answered at least once (missing data not taken into account), and Percent gives the percentages of these yes-answers per question.

The above output shows the number of patients who answered yes to at least one question. Of all visitants 25.6% did not answer any question, here called the missing cases. In the second table the letter N gives the numbers of yes-answers per question, "Percent of Cases" gives the yes-answers per question in those who answered at least once (missing data not taken into account), and "Percent" gives the percentages of these yes-answers per question. The gp consultation burden of mental and physical problems was about twice the size of that of alcohol and weight problems. Tiredness and social problems were in-between. In order to assess these data against all visitants, the missing cases have to be analyzed first.

Command
Transform....Compute Variable....Target Variable: type "none"....Numeric Expression: enter "1-max(illfeeling , ..., social problem)" ....click Type and Label....LabelL enter "no answer"....click Continue....click OK....Analyze ....Multiple Response ....Define Variable sets....click Define Multiple Response Sets....click $health....move "no answer" to Variables in Set....click Change.... click Close.

The data file now contains the novel "no answer" variable and a novel multiple response variable including the missing cases but the latter is not shown. It is now also possible to produce crosstabs with the different questions as rows and other variables like personal characteristics as columns. In this way the interaction with the personal characteristics can be assessed.

Command

Analyze....Multiple Response....Multiple Response Crosstabs....Rows: enter $health....Columns: enter ed. (= level of education)....click Define Range.... Minimum: enter 1....Maximum: enter 5....Continue....Click Options....Cell Percentages: click Columns.... click Continue....click OK.

$health*ed Crosstabulation

			Level of education					Total
			no highschool	highschool	college	university	completed university	
health[a]	illfeeling	Count	45	101	87	115	43	391
		% within ed	27,6%	43,3%	50,9%	60,2%	81,1%	
	alcohol	Count	18	55	52	83	34	242
		% within ed	11,0%	23,6%	30,4%	43,5%	64,2%	
	weight problem	Count	13	51	43	82	25	214
		% within ed	8,0%	21,9%	25,1%	42,9%	47,2%	
	tiredness	Count	10	55	71	122	42	300
		% within ed	6,1%	23,6%	41,5%	63,9%	79,2%	
	cold	Count	71	116	85	96	21	389
		% within ed	43,6%	49,8%	49,7%	50,3%	39,6%	
	family problem	Count	75	118	84	93	25	395
		% within ed	46,0%	50,6%	49,1%	48,7%	47,2%	
	mental problem	Count	78	112	91	94	26	401
		% within ed	47,9%	48,1%	53,2%	49,2%	49,1%	
	physical problem	Count	78	123	87	95	26	409
		% within ed	47,9%	52,8%	50,9%	49,7%	49,1%	
	social problem	Count	11	67	68	111	36	293
		% within ed	6,7%	28,8%	39,8%	58,1%	67,9%	
	no answer	Count	39	29	13	6	2	89
		% within ed	23,9%	12,4%	7,6%	3,1%	3,8%	
Total		Count	163	233	171	191	53	811

Percentages and totals are based on respondents.

a. Dichotomy group tabulated at value 1.

The output table gives the results. Various trends are observed. E.g., there is a decreasing trend of patients not answering any question with increased levels of education. Also there is an increasing trend of ill feeling, alcohol problems, weight problems, tiredness and social problems with increased levels of education. If we wish to test whether the increasing trend of tiredness with increased level of education is statistically significant, a formal trend test can be performed.

Command

Analyze....Descriptive Statistics....Crosstabs....Rows: enter tiredness....

Columns: enter level of education....click Statistics....mark Chi-square.... click Continue....click OK.

Underneath a formal trend test is given. It tests whether an increasing trend of tiredness is associated with increased levels of education.

Chi-Square Tests

	Value	df	Asymp. Sig. (2-sided)
Pearson Chi-Square	185,824[a]	4	,000
Likelihood Ratio	202,764	4	,000
Linear-by-Linear Association	184,979	1	,000
N of Valid Cases	811		

a. 0 cells (,0%) have expected count less than 5. The minimum expected count is 19,61.

In the output chi-square tests are given. The linear-by-linear association data show a chi-square value of 184.979 and 1 degree of freedom. This means that a statistically very significant linear trend with $p < 0.0001$ is in these data.

Also interactions and trends of any other health problems with all of the other variables including gender, age, marriage, income, period of constant address or employment can be similarly analyzed.

Conclusion

The answers to a set of multiple questions about a single underlying disease / condition can be assessed as multiple dimensions of a complex variable. Multiple response methodology is adequate for the purpose. The most important advantage of the multiple response methodology versus traditional frequency table analysis is that it is possible to observe relevant trends and similarities directly from data tables. A disadvantage is that only summaries but no statistical tests are given, but observed trends can, of course, be, additionally, tested statistically with formal trend tests.

Note

More background, theoretical and mathematical information of multiple response sets are in Machine Learning in medicine part three, Chap. 11, pp. 105–115, Multiple response sets, Springer Heidelberg Germany, 2013, from the same authors.

Chapter 78
Protein and DNA Sequence Mining

General Purpose

This chapter is to demonstrate, that sequence similarity searching of aminoacids and DNA is a method, that can be applied by almost anybody for finding similarities between his/her sequences and the sequences known to be associated with different clinical effects.

Background

Sequence similarity searching is a method that can be applied by almost anybody for finding similarities between his/her query sequences of amino acids and DNA and the sequences known to be associated with different clinical effects. The latter have been included in database systems like the BLAST (Basic Local Alignment Search Tool) database system from the US National Center of Biotechnology Information (NCBI), and the MOTIF data base system, a joint website from different European and American institutions, and they are available through the internet for the benefit of individual researchers trying and finding a match for novel sequences from their own research. In the figure underneath an example is given of a string applied for example in bioinformatics to describe DNA strands composed of nitrogenous bases.

This chapter was previously published in "Machine learning in medicine-cookbook 3" as Chap.15, 2014.

T. J. Cleophas, A. H. Zwinderman, *Machine Learning in Medicine – A Complete Overview*, https://doi.org/10.1007/978-3-030-33970-8_78

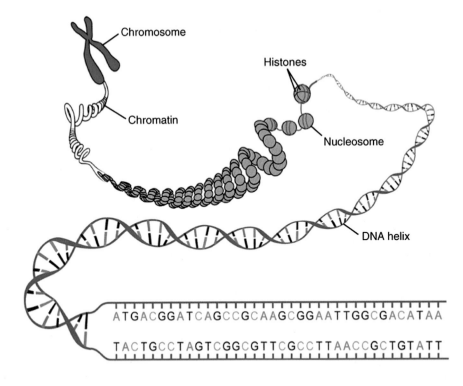

ATGACGGATCAGCCGCAAGCGGAATTGGCGACATAA

TACTGCCTAGTCGGCGTTCGCCTTAACCGCTGTATT

Specific Scientific Question

Abbreviations for amino acids

Amino acid	Three-letter abbreviation	One-letter symbol
Alanine	Ala	A
Arginine	Arg	R
Asparagine	Asn	N
Aspartic acid	Asp	D
Asparagine or aspartic acid	Asx	B
Cysteine	Cys	C
Glutamine	Gln	Q
Glutamic acid	Glu	E
Glutamine or glutamic acid	Glx	Z
Glycine	Gly	G
Histidine	His	H
Isoleucine	Ile	I
Leucine	Leu	L
Lysine	Lys	K
Methionine	Met	M
Phenylalanine	Phe	F
Proline	Pro	P
Serine	Ser	S
Threonine	Thr	T
Tryptophan	Trp	W
Tyrosine	Tyr	Y
Valine	Val	V

In this chapter amino acid sequences are analyzed, but nucleic acids sequences can similarly be assessed. The above table gives the one letter abbreviations of amino acids. The specific scientific question is: can sequence similarity search be applied for finding similarities between the sequences found in your own research and the sequences known to be associated with different clinical effects.

Data Base Systems on the Internet

The BLAST (http://blast.ncbi.nlm.nih.gov/Blast.cgi) program reports several terms:

1. Max score = best bit score between query sequence and database sequence (the bit score = the standardized score, i.e. the score that is independent of any unit).
2. Total score = best bit score if some amino acid pairs in the data have been used more often than just once.
3. Query coverage = percentage of amino acids used in the analysis.
4. E-value = expected number of large similarity alignment scores.

If the E-value is very small for the score observed, then a chance finding can be rejected. The sequences are then really related. An E-value = p-value adjusted for multiple testing = the chance that the association found is a chance finding. It indicates that the match between a novel and already known sequence is closer than could happen by chance, and that the novel and known sequence are thus homologous (philogenetically from the same ancestor, whatever that means).

Example 1

We isolated the following amino acid sequence: serine, isoleucine, lysine, leucine, tryptophan, proline, proline. The one letter abbreviation code for this sequence is SIKLWPP. The BLAST Search site is explored, while giving the following commands.

Open BLAST Search site at appropriate address (Reference 1).
　Choose Protein BLAST
　Click Enter Sequences and enter the amino acid sequence SIKLWPP
　Click BLAST
The output tables use the term blast hit which means here a database sequence selected by the provider's software to be largely similar to the unknown sequence, and the term query, which means here an unknown sequence that the investigator has entered for sequence testing against known sequences from the database. The output tables report.

1. No putative conserved domains have been detected.
2. In the Distribution of 100 Blast Hits on the Query sequence all of the Blast Hits have a very low alignment score (<40).
3. In spite of the low scores their precise alignment values are given next, e.g. the best one has

　a max score of 21.8,
　total score of 21.8,
　query coverage of 100%, and

Example 2   611

adjusted p-value of 1956 (not significant).

As a contrast search the MOTIF Search site is explored. We command.

Open MOTIF Search site at appropriate address (MOTIF Search. http://www.genome.jp/tools/motif).

Choose: Searching Protein Sequence Motifs

Click: Enter your query sequence and enter the amino acid sequence SIKLWPP.

Select motif libraries: click various databases given

Then click Search.

The output table reports: 1 motif found in PROSITE database (found motif PKC_PHOSPHO_SITE; description: protein kinase C phosphorylation site). Obviously, it is worthwhile to search other databases if one does not provide any hits.

Example 2

We wish to examine a 12 amino acid sequence that we isolated at our laboratory, use again BLAST. We command.

Open BLAST Search site at appropriate address (Reference 1).

Choose Protein BLAST

Click Enter Sequences and enter the amino acid sequence ILVFMCWLVFQC

Click BLAST

The output tables report

1. No putative conserved domains have been detected.
2. In the Distribution of 100 Blast Hits on the Query sequence all of the Blast Hits have a very low alignment score (<40).
3. In spite of the low scores their precise alignment values are given next. Three of them have a significant alignment score at $p < 0.05$ with

max scores of 31.2,

total scores 31.2,

query cover of around 60%, and

E-values (adjusted p-values) of 4.1, 4.1, and 4.5.

Parts of the novel sequence have been aligned to known sequences of proteins from a streptococcus and a nocardia bacteria and from caenorhabditis, a small soil-dwelling nematode. These findings may not seem clinically very relevant, and may be due to type I errors, with low levels of statistical significance, or material contamination.

Example 3

A somewhat larger amino acid sequence (25 letters) is examined using BLAST. We command.

   Open BLAST Search site at appropriate address (Reference 1).
   Choose Protein BLAST
   Click Enter Sequences and enter the amino acid sequence
SIKLWPPSQTTRLLLVERMANNLST
   Click BLAST
   The output tables report the following.

1. Putative domains have been detected. Specific hits regard the WPP superfamily. The WPP domain is a 90 amino acid protein that serves as a transporter protein for other protein in the plant cell from the cell plasma to the nucleus.
2. In the Distribution of 100 Blast Hits on the Query sequence all of the Blast Hits have a very high alignment score (80–200 for the first 5 hits, over 50 for the remainder, all of them statistically very significant).
3. Precise alignment values are given next. The first 5 hits have the highest scores: with

   max scores of 83.8,
   total scores of 83.8,
   Cover queries of 100%,
   p-values of 4 e^{-17}, which is much smaller than 0.05 (5%).

   All of them relate to the WPP superfamily sequence.
   The next 95 hits produced Max scores and Total scores from 68.9 to 62.1, query coverages from 100 to 96%. and adjusted p-values from 5 e^{-12} to 1 e^{-9}, which is again much smaller than 0.05 (5%).

   4. We can subsequently browse through the 95 hits to see if anything of interest for our purposes can be found. All of the alignments as found regarded plant proteins like those of grasses, maize, nightshade and other plants, no alignments with human or veterinary proteins were established.

Example 4

A 27 amino acid sequence from a laboratory culture of pseudomonas is examined using BLAST. We command.

   Open BLAST Search site at appropriate address (Reference 1).
   Choose Protein BLAST
   Click Enter Sequences and enter the amino acid sequence
MTDLNIPHTHAHLVDAFQALGIRAQAL
   Click BLAST
   The output tables report

1. No putative domains have been detected.
2. The 100 blast hit table shows, however, a very high alignment score for gentamicin acetyl transferase enzyme, recently recognized as being responsible for resistance of pseudomonas to gentamicin. The ailments values were

max score
total score of 85.5,
query coverage of 100%,
adjusted p-value of 1 e^{-17}, and so statistically very significant.

3. In the Distribution of the 99 remaining Blast Hits only 5 other significant alignment were detected with

max score and total scores from 38.5 to 32.9,
query coverages 55 to 92%,
adjusted p-values between 0.08 and 4.5 (all of them 5%).

The significant alignments regarded bacterial proteins including the gram negative bacterias, rhizobium, xanthomonas, and morganella, and a mite protein. This may not clinically be very relevant, but our novel sequence was derived from a pseudomonas culture, and we know now that this particular culture contains pathogens very resistant to gentamicin.

Conclusion

Sequence similarity searching is a method that can be applied by almost anybody for finding similarities between his/her query sequences and the sequences known to be associated with different clinical effects.

With sequence similarity searching the use of p-values to distinguish between high and low similarity is relevant. Unlike the BLAST interactive website, the MOTIFinteractive website does not give them, which hampers inferences from the alignments to be made.

Note

More background, theoretical and mathematical information of protein and DNA sequence mining is given in Machine learning in medicine part two, Chap. 17, pp. 171–185, Protein and DNA sequence mining, Springer Heidelberg Germany 2013, from the same authors.

Chapter 79
Iteration Methods for Crossvalidations (150 Patients with Pneumonia)

General Purpose

In the Chap. 8 of this book validation of a decision tree model is performed splitting a data file into a training and a testing sample. This method performed pretty well with a sensitivity of 90–100% and an overall accuracy of 94%. However, measures of error of predictive models like the above one are based on residual methods, assuming a priori defined data distributions, particularly normal distributions. Machine learning data file may not meet such assumptions, and distribution free methods of validation, like crossvalidations may be more safe.

Background

Crossvalidation, sometimes called rotation estimation, or out of sample testing, is any of various model validation techniques for assessing how the results of a statistical analysis will generalize to an independent data set. It is mainly used in settings where the goal is prediction, and one wants to estimate how accurately a predictive model will perform in practice. In a prediction problem, a model is usually given a dataset of known data on which training is run (training dataset), and a dataset of unknown data (or first seen data) against which the model is tested (called the validation dataset or testing set). The goal of crossvalidation is to test the model's

This chapter was previously published in "Machine learning in medicine-cookbook 3" as Chap. 16, 2014.

Electronic Supplementary Material The online version of this chapter (https://doi.org/10.1007/978-3-030-33970-8_79) contains supplementary material, which is available to authorized users.

ability to predict new data that was not used in estimating it, in order to flag problems like overfitting or selection bias and to give an insight on how the model will generalize to an independent dataset (i.e., an unknown dataset, for example from a real problem.

Crossvalidation involves partitioning a sample into complementary subsets, performing the analysis on one subset (called the training set), and validating the analysis on the other subset (called the validation set or testing set). In order to reduce variability, multiple rounds of crossvalidation are performed using different partitions, and the validation results are averaged over the rounds to give an estimate of the model's predictive performance. Crossvalidation thus averaged measures of fitness in prediction to derive a more accurate estimate of model prediction performance. The underneath figure, taken from the public domain (Wikipedia Cross-Validations), should explain how things work.

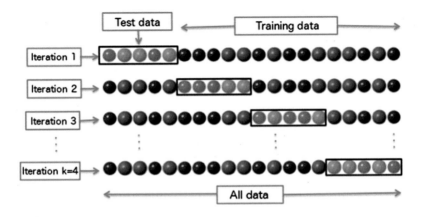

Primary Scientific Question

How does crossvalidation of the data from Chap. 3 perform as compared to the residual method used in the scorer node of the Konstanz information miner (Knime)?

Example

The data file from Chap. 8 is used once more. Four inflammatory markers (CRP (C-reactive protein), ESR (erythrocyte sedimentation rate), leucocyte count (leucos), and fibrinogen) were measured In 150 patients. Based on x-ray chest clinical severity was classified as A (mild infection), B (medium severity), C (severe infection). A major scientific question was to assess what markers were the best predictors of the severity of infection.

CRP	leucos	fibrinogen	ESR	x-ray severity
120,00	5,00	11,00	60,00	A
100,00	5,00	11,00	56,00	A
94,00	4,00	11,00	60,00	A
92,00	5,00	11,00	58,00	A
100,00	5,00	11,00	52,00	A
108,00	6,00	17,00	48,00	A
92,00	5,00	14,00	48,00	A
100,00	5,00	11,00	54,00	A
88,00	5,00	11,00	54,00	A
98,00	5,00	8,00	60,00	A
108,00	5,00	11,00	68,00	A
96,00	5,00	11,00	62,00	A
96,00	5,00	8,00	46,00	A
86,00	4,00	8,00	60,00	A
116,00	4,00	11,00	50,00	A
114,00	5,00	17,00	52,00	A

CRP = C-reactive protein (mg/l)
leucos = leucyte count ($*10^9$ /l)
fibrinogen = fibrinogen level (mg/l
ESR = erythrocyte sedimentation rate (mm)
x-ray severity = x-chest severity pneumonia score (A − C = mild to severe)

The first 16 patients are in the above table, the entire data file is in "decisiontree" and can be obtained from "extras.springer.com"on the internet.

Downloading the Knime Data Miner

In Google enter the term "knime". Click Download and follow instructions. After completing the pretty easy download procedure, open the knime workbench by clicking the knime welcome screen. The center of the screen displays the workflow editor like the canvas in SPSS modeler. It is empty, and can be used to build a stream of nodes, called workflow in knime. The node repository is in the left lower angle of the screen, and the nodes can be dragged to the workflow editor simply by left-clicking. Start by dragging the file reader node to the workflow. The nodes are computer tools for data analysis like visualization and statistical processes. Node description is in the right upper angle of the screen. Before the nodes can be used, they have to be connected with the file reader node and with one another by arrows drawn again simply by left clicking the small triangles attached to the nodes. Right clicking on the file reader node enables to configure from your computer a requested data file....click Browse....and download from the appropriate folder a csv type Excel file. You are set for analysis now.

Note: the above data file cannot be read by the file reader node as it is an SPSS file, and must first be saved as an csv type Excel file. For that purpose command in SPSS: click File....click Save as....in "Save as type: enter Comma Delimited (∗. csv)....click Save. For your convenience it is available in extras.springer.com, and is also entitled "decisiontree".

Knime Workflow

A knime workflow for the analysis of the above data example is built, and the final result is shown in the underneath figure.

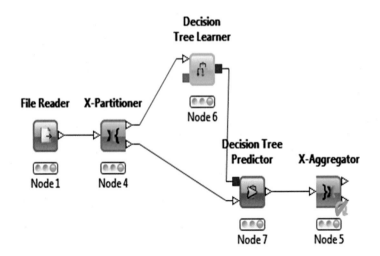

In the node repository click X-Partitioner, Decision Tree Learner, Decision Tree Predictor and X-Aggregator and drag them to the workflow editor. If you have difficulty finding the nodes (the repository contains hundreds of nodes), you may type their names in the small window at the top of the node repository box, and its icon and name will immediately appear. Connect, by left clicking, all of the nodes with arrows as indicated above....Configurate and execute all of the nodes by right clicking the nodes and then the texts "Configurate" and "Execute"....the red lights will successively turn orange and then green....right click the Decision Tree Predictor again....right click the text "View: Decision Tree View". The decision tree comes up, and it is, obviously, identical to the one of Chap. 8.

Crossvalidation

If you, subsequently, right click the Decision Tree Predictor, and then click Classsified Data, a table turns up of 15 randomly selected subjects from your test sample. The predicted values are identical to the measured ones. And, so, for this selection the Decision Tree Predictor node performed well.

Row ID	İ ï»¿CRP	İ leucos	İ fibrinogen	İ ESR	S xrayse...	S Predicti...
Row5	108	6	17	48	A	A
Row20	108	6	11	60	A	A
Row28	104	4	11	58	A	A
Row39	102	5	11	56	A	A
Row94	112	14	44	76	B	B
Row103	126	19	59	68	C	C
Row111	128	18	62	70	C	C
Row112	136	18	68	72	C	C
Row113	114	17	65	60	C	C
Row120	138	19	74	99	C	C
Row126	124	16	59	84	C	C
Row137	128	18	59	44	C	C
Row138	120	16	59	98	C	C
Row144	134	19	80	100	C	C
Row145	134	17	74	64	C	C

Next, right click the x-aggregator node, and then click Prediction table. The results of 10 iterative random samples of 15 subjects from your test sample are simultaneously displayed. Obviously, virtually all of the predictions were in agreement with the measured values. Subsequently, right click the node again, and then click Error rates.

⚠ Error rates - 0:5 - X-Aggregator			
File			
Table "default" - Rows: 10	Spec - Columns: 3	Properties	Flow Variables
Row ID	**D Error in %**	**❙ Size of ...**	**❙ Error C...**
fold 0	6.667	15	1
fold 1	6.667	15	1
fold 2	6.667	15	1
fold 3	20	15	3
fold 4	0	15	0
fold 5	0	15	0
fold 6	6.667	15	1
fold 7	6.667	15	1
fold 8	0	15	0
fold 9	0	15	0

The above table comes up. It shows the error rates of the above 10 iterative random samples. The result is pretty good. Virtually, all of them have 0 or 1 erroneous value.

The crossvalidation can also be performed with a novel validation set. For that purpose you need a novel file reader node, and the novel validation set has to be configured and executed. Furthermore, you need to copy and paste the above Aggregator node, and you need to connect the output port of the above Decision Tree Predictor node to the input port of Aggregator node.

Conclusion

In Chap. 8 of this volume validation of a decision tree model was performed splitting a data file into a training and testing sample. This method performed pretty well with an overall accuracy of 94%. However, the measure of error is based on the normal distribution assumption, and data may not meet this assumption. Crossvalidation is a distribution free method, and may here be a more safe, and less biased approach to validation.

It performed very well, with errors mostly 0 and 1 out of 15 cases. We should add that Knime does not provide sensitivity and specificity measures here.

Note

More background, theoretical and mathematical information of validations and crossvalidations is given in:

Statistics applied to clinical studies 5th edition, Springer Heidelberg Germany.

Chapter 46, Validating qualitative diagnostic tests, pp. 509–517, 2012,
Chapter 47 Uncertainty of qualitative diagnostic tests, pp. 519–525, 2012,
Chapter 50 Validating quantitative diagnostic tests, pp. 545–552, 2012,
Chapter 51 Summary of validation procedures for diagnostic tests, pp. 555–568, 2012.

Machine learning in medicine part one, Springer Heidelberg Germany.

Chapter 1 Introduction to machine learning, p 5, 2012,
Chapter 3 Optimal scaling: discretization, p 28, 2012,
Chapter 4 Optimal scaling, regularization including ridge, lasso, and elastic net regression, p 41, 2012.

All of the above publications are from the same authors as the current work.

Chapter 80
Improving Parallel-Groups with Different Sample Sizes and Variances (5 Parallel-Group Studies)

General Purpose

Unpaired t-tests are traditionally used for testing the significance of difference between parallel-groups according to

$$t - value = (mean_1 - mean_2)/\surd(SD_1/N_1 + SD_2/N_2)$$

where mean, SD, N are respectively the mean, the standard deviation and the sample size of the parallel groups.

Many calculators on the internet (e.g., the P value calculator-GraphPad) can tell you whether the t-value is significantly smaller than 0.05, and, thus, whether there is a statistically significant difference between the parallel groups.

E.g., open Google and type p-value calculator for t-test....click Enter....click P value calculator -GraphPad....select P from t....t: enter computed t-value....DF: compute $N_1 + N_2 - 2$ and enter the result....click Compute P.

This procedure assumes that the two parallel groups have equal variances. However in practice this is virtually never entirely true. This chapter is to assess tests accounting the effect of different variances on the estimated p-values.

Background

In statistics, Welch's t-test, or unequal variances t-test, is a two-sample location test which is used to test the hypothesis that two populations have equal means. It is named for its creator, Bernard Lewis Welch (1947), and is an adaptation of Student's

This chapter was previously published in "Machine learning in medicine-cookbook 3" as Chap.17, 2014.

t-test, and is more reliable when the two samples have unequal variances and/or unequal sample sizes. These tests are often referred to as "unpaired" or "independent samples" t-tests, as they are typically applied when the statistical units underlying the two samples being compared are non-overlapping. Given that Welch's t-test has been less popular than Student's t-test, and may be less familiar to readers, a more informative name is "Welch's unequal variances t-test"or "unequal variances t-test" for brevity.

Primary Scientific Question

Two methods for adjustment of different variances and different sample sizes are available, the pooled t-test which assumes that the differences in variances are just residual, and that the two variances are equal, and the Welch's test which assumes that they are due to a real effect, like a difference in treatment effect with comcomitant difference in spread of the data. How are the results of the two adjustment procedures.

Examples

In the underneath table the t- test statistics and p-values of 5 parallel-group studies with differences in the means, standard deviations (SDs) and sample sizes (Ns) are given. In the examples 2, 3, 4, and 5 respectively the Ns, SDs, means, and SDs have been changed as compared to example 1.

means	SDs	Ns	unadjusted		adjusted(pooled)		Welch's adjust	
			t value	p value	t value	p value	t value	p value
1. 50/40	5/3	100/200	1.715/0.087		1.811/0.071		1.715/0.088	
2.		10/20	1.715/0.092		1.814/0.080		1.715/0.100	
3.	10/3		0.958/0.339		1.214/0.226		0.958/0.340	
4. 60/40			3.430/0.007		3.662/0.000		3.430/0.001	
5.	6/2		1.581/0.115		1.963/0.051		1.581/0.117	

Open Google and type GraphPad Software QuickCalcs t test calculator. . . .mark: Enter mean, SEM, N. . . .mark: Unpaired test. . . .label: type Group 1. . . .mean: type

50. . . .SEM: type 5. . . .N: type 100. . . .label: type Group 2. . . . mean: type 40. . . . SEM: type 3. . . .N: type 200. . . .click Calculate now.

In the output an adjusted t-value of 1.811 is given and a p-value of 0.071, slightly better than the unadjusted p-value of 0.087. Next a Welch's t-test will be performed using the same procedure as above, but with Welch's Unpaired t-test marked instead of just Unpaired t-test. The output sheet shows that the p-value is now worse than the unadjusted p-value instead of better.

In the examples 2–5 slightly different means, SDs, and Ns were used but, otherwise, the data were the same. After computations it can be observed that in all of the examples the adjusted test using pooled variances produced the best p-values. This sometimes lead to a statistically significant effect while the other two test are non-significant, for example with data 5 (p-value = 0.05). The Welch's adjustment produced the worst p-value, while the unadjusted produced the best statistics.

Conclusion

Two methods for adjustment of different variances and different sample sizes are available, the pooled t-test which assumes that the differences in variances are just residual, and the Welch's test which assumes that they are real differences. From 5 examples it can be observed that the t-tests using pooled variances consistently produced the best p-values sometimes leading to a statistically significant result in otherwise statistically insignificant data. In contrast, the Welch's adjustment consistently produced the worst result. The pooled t-test is probably the best option if we have clinical arguments for residual differences in variances, while the Welch's test would be a scientifically better option, if it can be argued that differences in variance were due to real clinical effects. Moreover, the Welch's test would be more in agreement with the general feature of advanced statistical analyses: tests taking special effects in the data into account are associated with larger p-values (more uncertainties).

Note

More background, theoretical and mathematical information of improved t-tests are in Statistics applied to clinical studies, Chap. 2, The analysis of efficacy data, pp. 15–40, Springer Heidelberg Germany 5th edition, 2012, from the same authors.

Chapter 81
Association Rules Between Exposure and Outcome (50 and 60 Patients)

General Purpose

Traditional analysis of exposure outcome relationships is only sensitive with strong relationships. This chapter is to assess whether association rules, based on conditional probabilities, may be more sensitive in case of weak relationships.

Background

Association rule mining, at a basic level, involves the use of machine learning models to analyze data for patterns, or co-occurrence, in a database. Association rules are created by searching data for frequent if-then patterns and using the criteria support and confidence to identify the most important relationships. Examples of important rules and their algebraic functions are underneath (frq = frequency, Supp = Support).

This chapter was previously published in "Machine learning in medicine-cookbook 3" as Chap. 18, 2014.

Electronic Supplementary Material The online version of this chapter (https://doi.org/10.1007/978-3-030-33970-8_81) contains supplementary material, which is available to authorized users.

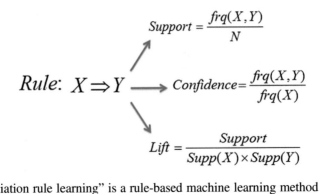

"Association rule learning" is a rule-based machine learning method for discovering interesting relations between variables in large databases. It is intended to identify strong rules discovered in databases using some measures of interestingness. Based on the concept of strong rules, Agrawal, computer scientist at Microsoft in 1993, introduced association rules for discovering regularities between products in large-scale transaction data recorded by point-of-sale (POS) systems in supermarkets. For example, the rule found in the sales data of a supermarket would indicate that if a customer buys onions and potatoes together, they are likely to also buy hamburger meat. Such information can be used as the basis for decisions about marketing activities such as, e.g., promotional pricing or product placements. In addition to the above example from market basket analysis association rules are employed today in many application areas including Web usage mining, intrusion detection, continuous production, and bioinformatics. In contrast with sequence mining, association rule learning typically does not consider the order of items either within a transaction or across transactions.

Primary Scientific Question

Is association rule analysis better sensitive than regression analysis and paired chi-square tests are for demonstrating significant exposure effects.

Example

The proportions observed in a sample are equal to chances or probabilities. If you observe a 40% proportion of healthy patients, then the chance or probability (P) of being healthy in this group is 40%. With two variables, e.g., healthy and happy, the symbol ∩ is often used to indicate "and" (both are present). Underneath a hypothesized example of 5 patients, with 3 of them having overweight and 2 of them coronary artery disease (CAD), is given.

Example 629

Patient	overweight (predictor)	coronary artery disease
	X	Y
1	1	0
2	0	1
3	0	0
4	1	1
5	1	0

Support rule
Support $= P\ X \cap Y = 1/5 = 0.2$

Confidence rule
Confidence $= P\ X \cap Y/P\ Y = [1/5] / [2/5] = 0.5$

Lift rule (or lift-up rule)
Lift $= P\ X \cap Y/[P\ X \times P\ Y] = [1/5]/[2/5 \times 2/5] = 1.25$

Conviction rule
Conviction $= [1 - P\ Y]/[1 - P\ X \cap Y/P\ Y] = [1 - 2/5]/[1 - 0.5] = 1.20$

I. The support gives the proportion of patients with both overweight and CAD in the entire population. A support of 0.0 would mean that overweight and CAD are mutually elusive, a support of x.y would mean that the two factors are independent of one another.

II. The confidence gives the fraction of patients with both CAD and overweight in those with CAD. This fraction is obviously larger than that in the entire population, because it rose from 0.2 to 0.5.

III. The lift compares the observed proportion of patients with both overweight and CAD with the expected proportion if CAD and overweight would have occurred independently of one another. Obviously, the observed value is larger than expected, 1.25 versus 1.00, suggesting that overweight does contribute to the risk of CAD.

IV. Finally, the conviction compares the patients with no-CAD in the entire population with those with both no-CAD and the presence of overweight. The ratio is larger than 1.00, namely 1.20. Obviously, the benefit of no-CAD is better for the entire population than it is for the subgroup with overweight.

In order to assess whether the computed values, like 0.2 and 1.25, are significantly different from 0.0 and 1.0 confidence intervals have to be calculated. We will use the McCallum-Layton calculator for proportions, freely available from the Internet (Confidence interval calculator for proportions. www.mccallum-layton.co.uk/).

The calculations will somewhat overestimate the true confidence intervals, because the true confidence intervals are here mostly composed of two or more proportions, and this is not taken into account. Therefore, doubling the p-values may be more adequate (Bonferroni adjustment), but with very small p-values we need not worry.

Example One

A data set of 50 patients with coronary artery disease or not (1 = yes) and overweight as predictor (1 = yes) is given underneath.

Patient	Overweight	Coronary artery disease
1	1,00	0,00
2	0,00	1,00
3	0,00	0,00
4	1,00	1,00
5	0,00	0,00
6	1,00	0,00
7	0,00	1,00
8	0,00	0,00
9	1,00	1,00
10	0,00	0,00
11	1,00	0,00
12	0,00	1,00
13	0,00	0,00
14	1,00	1,00
15	0,00	0,00

The first 15 patients are given. The entire data file are the Variables A and B of the data file entitled "associationrule", and are in extras.springer.com.

20/50 of the patients have overweight (predictor), 20/50 have CAD. A paired binary test (McNemar's test) shows no significant difference between the two columns (p = 1.0). Binary logistic regression with the predictor as independent variable is equally insignificant (b = 0.69, p = 0.241).

Applying association rules we find a support of 0.2 and confidence of 0.5. The lift is 1.25 and the conviction is 1.20. The McCallum calculator gives the confidence intervals, respectively 10–34, 36–64, 110–145, and 107–137%. All of these 95% confidence intervals indicate a very significant difference from respectively 0% (support and confidence) and 100% (lift and conviction) with p-values <0.001 (Bonferroni adjusted p < 0.002) Indeed, the predictor overweight had a very significant positive effect on the risk of CAD.

Example Two

A data set of 60 patients with coronary artery disease or not (1 = yes) with overweight and "being manager" as predictors (1 = yes).

Patient	Overweight	Manager	Coronary artery disease
1	1,00	1,00	0,00
2	0,00	0,00	1,00
3	1,00	1,00	0,00
4	0,00	1,00	1,00
5	0,00	0,00	0,00
6	1,00	1,00	1,00
7	1,00	1,00	0,00
8	0,00	0,00	1,00
9	1,00	1,00	0,00
10	0,00	1,00	1,00
11	0,00	0,00	0,00
12	1,00	1,00	1,00
13	1,00	1,00	0,00
14	0,00	0,00	1,00
15	1,00	1,00	0,00

The first 15 patients are given. The entire data file are the variables C, D, and E of the data file entitled "associationrule", and is in extras.springer.com.

Instead of a single x –variable now 2 of them are included. 30/60 of the patients have overweight, 40/60 are manager, and 30/60 have CAD. A paired binary test (Cochran's test) shows no significant difference between the three columns (p = 0.082). Binary logistic regression with the two predictors as independent variables is equally insignificant (b-values are − 21.9 and 21.2, p-values are 0.99 and 0.99).

Applying association rules we find a support of 0.1666 and confidence of 0.333. The lift is 2.0 and the conviction is 1.25. The McCallum calculator gives the confidence intervals. Expressed as percentages they are respectively, 8–29, 22–47, and 159–270 and 108–136%. All of these 95% confidence intervals indicate a very significant difference from respectively 0% (support and confidence) and 100% (lift and conviction) with p-values <0.001 (Bonferroni adjusted p < 0.002 or < 0.003). Indeed, the predictors overweight and being manager had a statistically very significant effect on the risk of CAD.

Conclusion

Association rule analysis is more sensitive than regression analysis and paired chi-square tests, and is able to demonstrate significant predictor effects, when the other methods are not. It can also include multiple variables and very large datasets and is a welcome methodology for clinical predictor research.

Note

More background, theoretical and mathematical information of association rules are in Machine learning in medicine part two, Chap. 11, pp. 105–113, Springer Heidelberg Germany, 2013, from the same authors.

Chapter 82
Confidence Intervals for Proportions and Differences in Proportions (100 and 75 Patients)

General Purpose

Proportions, fractions, percentages, risks, hazards are all synonymous terms to indicate what part of a population had events like death, illness, complications etc. Instead of p-values, confidence intervals are often calculated. If you obtained many samples from the same population, 95% of them would have their mean results between the 95% confidence intervals. And, likewise, samples from the same population with their proportions outside the 95% confidence intervals means that they are significantly different from the population with a probability of 5% ($p < 0.05$). This chapter is to assess how confidence intervals can be computed.

Background

Jerzy Neyman, a mathematician from Poland who died in Oakland CA 1981, introduced the term "confidence intervals" in a 1937, a time when statisticians published papers in journals like "Philosophical Transactions". In statistics, a confidence interval (CI) is a type of interval estimate, computed from the statistics of the observed data, that might contain the true value of an unknown population parameter. The interval has an associated confidence level that, loosely speaking, quantifies the level of confidence that the parameter lies in the interval. More strictly speaking, the confidence level represents the frequency (i.e. the proportion) of possible confidence intervals that contain the true value of the unknown population parameter. In other words, if confidence intervals are constructed using a given confidence level from an infinite number of independent sample statistics, the proportion of

---

This chapter was previously published in "Machine learning in medicine-cookbook 3" as Chap.19, 2014.

those intervals that contain the true value of the parameter will be equal to the confidence level. Confidence intervals consist of a range of potential values of the unknown population parameter. However, the interval computed from a particular sample does not necessarily include the true value of the parameter. Based on the (usually taken) assumption that observed data are random samples from a true population, the confidence interval obtained from the data is also random. The confidence level is designated prior to examining the data. Most commonly, the 95% confidence level is used. However, other confidence levels can be used, for example, 90% and 99%. Factors affecting the width of the confidence interval include the size of the sample, the confidence level, and the variability in the sample. A larger sample will tend to produce a better estimate of the population parameter, when all other factors are equal. A higher confidence level will tend to produce a broader confidence interval.

Primary Scientific Question

P-values give the type I error, otherwise called the chance of finding a difference where there is none. Confidence intervals tell you the same, but, in addition, they give the range in which the true outcome value lies, and the direction and strength of it. Are confidence intervals more relevant for exploratory studies than p-values, because of the additional information provided.

Example

If in two parallel groups of respectively 100 and 75 patients the numbers of patients with an event are 75 and 50, according to a z-test or chi-square test (see Statistics Applied to Clinical Studies 5th edition, Chap. 3, The analysis of safety data, pp. 41–60, 2012, Springer Heidelberg Germany, from the same authors), then the p-value of difference will be 0.23. This means that we have 23% chance of a type one error, and that this chance is far too large to be statistically significant ($p > 0.05$).

In the two above groups the proportions are respectively $75/100 = 0.750$ and $50/75 = 0.667$. The standard errors of these proportions can be calculated from the equation

$$\text{standard errors} = \pm\sqrt{(p(1-p)/\sqrt{n})}$$

where p = proportion and n = sample size.

Example   635

$$95\% \text{confidence intervals} = \pm 1.96\sqrt{(p(1-p)/\sqrt{n})}$$

If you have little affinity with computations, then plenty calculators on the internet are helpful.

Confidence Intervals of Proportions

We will use the free "Matrix Software". Open Google and type Standard Error (SE) of Sample Proportion Calculator-Binomial Standard Deviation....click Enter....click Matrix Software....in Calculate SE Sample Proportion of Standard deviation type 0.75 for Proportion of successes (p)....type 100 for Number of Observations (n)....click Calculate....

The binomial SE of the Sample proportion	$= \pm 0.04330127....$
The 95% confidence interval of this proportion	$= \pm 1.96 \times 0.04330127$
	$= \pm 0.08487$
	$=$ between 0.66513 and 0.83487

Similarly the 95% confidence interval of the data from group 2 can be calculated.

Confidence Intervals of Differences in Proportions

In order to calculate the confidence interval of the differences between the above two proportions, we will use the free Vassarstats. Open Google en type http://vassarstats. net/prop2_ind.html....click enter....select The Confidence Interval for the Difference Between Two Independent Proportions....Larger Proportion: k_a (number of observations with event) =: type 75....n_a (total number of observations) =: type 100....click Calculate.

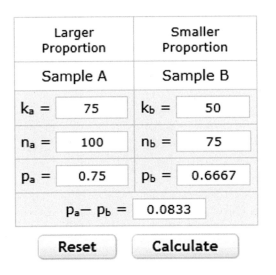

Larger Proportion		Smaller Proportion	
Sample A		Sample B	
k_a =	75	k_b =	50
n_a =	100	n_b =	75
p_a =	0.75	p_b =	0.6667
	$p_a - p_b$ =	0.0833	

Reset   Calculate

95% confidence interval: no continuity correction			
Lower limit =	-0.0505	Upper limit =	0.2183

95% confidence interval: including continuity correction			
Lower limit =	-0.0584	Upper limit =	0.2263

The output is given above. p_a an p_b are the proportions, $p_a - p_b$ the difference. The 95% confidence interval is between -0.0505 and 0.2183.

Proportions are yes/no data, e.g., a proportion of 75 subjects out of 100 had an event. The normal distribution is used for the calculation of the p-values and confidence intervals. In order to test yes/no data with a normal distribution, a continuity correction can be used to improve the quality of the analysis. In the example given the 75/100 in your sample indicates that the real event rate in your entire population of, e.g., 1000 may be between 745 and 755/1000. Because 745/1000 is, of course, smaller than 750/1000, it would make sense to use the proportion 745/1000 for the calculation of the confidence interval instead of 750/1000. This procedure is called the continuity correction, and as shown above it produces somewhat wider confidence intervals, and, thus, more uncertainty in your data. Unfortunately, higher quality is often associated with larger levels of uncertainty.

Conclusion

Proportions are used to indicate what part of a population had events. Instead of p-values to tell you whether your observed proportion is statistically significantly different from a proportion of 0.0, 95% confidence intervals are often calculated. If you obtained many samples from the same population, 95% of them would have their result between the 95% confidence intervals. And, likewise, samples from the same population having their proportions outside the 95% confidence intervals means that they are significantly different from the population with a probability of 5% ($p < 0.05$). P-values give the type I error, otherwise called the chance of finding a difference where there is none, or the chance of erroneously rejecting the null-hypothesis. Confidence intervals tell you the same, but, in addition, they give you the range in which the true outcome value lies, and the direction and strength of it. Particularly, for data mining of exploratory studies the issue of null-hypothesis testing with p-values is generally less important than information on the range in which the true outcome value lies, and the direction and strength of it.

Note

More background, theoretical and mathematical information of proportions and their confidence intervals is given in Statistics applied to clinical studies 5th edition, Chap. 3, The analysis of safety data, pp. 41–60, 2012, Springer Heidelberg Germany, from the same authors.

Chapter 83
Ratio Statistics for Efficacy Analysis of New Drugs (50 Patients)

General Purpose

Treatment efficacies are often assessed as differences from baseline. However, better treatment efficacies may be observed in patients with high baseline-values than in those with low ones. This was, e.g., the case in the Progress study, a parallel-group study of pravastatin versus placebo (see Statistics applied to clinical studies 5th edition, Chap. 17, Logistic and Cox regression, Markov models, and Laplace transformations, pp. 199–218, Springer Heidelberg Germany, 2012, from the same authors) . This chapter assesses the performance of ratio statistics for that purpose.

Background

Ratio statistics is applied in social research for many decades, and, so far, little in health research. Social Research is a method used by social scientists and researchers to learn about people and societies so that they can design products/services that cater to various needs of the people. Ratio data is defined as quantitative data, having the same properties as interval data, with an equal and definitive ratio between each dataset and absolute "zero" being a treated as a point of origin. In other words, there can be no negative numerical value in ratio data. A problem with ratios is that they usually suffer from overdispersion and that they therefore should be differently assessed from normal distribution assessments. Three estimators are often assessed with ratio statistics.

This chapter was previously published in "Machine learning in medicine-cookbook 2" as Chap. 20, 2014.

Electronic Supplementary Material The online version of this chapter (https://doi.org/10.1007/978-3-030-33970-8_83) contains supplementary material, which is available to authorized users.

T. J. Cleophas, A. H. Zwinderman, *Machine Learning in Medicine – A Complete Overview*, https://doi.org/10.1007/978-3-030-33970-8_83

1. First medians (values in the middle) are applied.
2. Second, the index of dispersion, otherwise called dispersion index, coefficient of dispersion, relative variance, or variance-to-mean ratio (VMR), like the coefficient of variation is often used. It is a normalized measure of the dispersion of a probability distribution, and it is a measure used to quantify whether a set of observed occurrences are clustered or dispersed compared to a standard statistical model. It is defined as the ratio of the variance to the mean.
3. A third estimator often applied is the concentration coefficient. It assumes that you are assessing the distribution of a variable (say social transfers) when the units of analysis are ranked by another variable (say gross income). For example, if C > G, the variable measured by G increases inequality.

Primary Scientific Question

The differences of treatment efficacy and baseline may be the best fit test statistic, if the treatment efficacies are independent of baseline. However, if not, then ratios of the two may fit the data better.

Example

A 50-patient 5-group parallel-group study was performed with 5 different cholesterol-lowering compounds. The first 12 patients of the data file is underneath. The entire data file is entitled "ratiostatistics" and is in extra.springer.com.

Variable

1	2	3	4
Baseline cholesterol (mmol/l)	Treatment cholesterol (mmol/l)	Treatment group no.	Baseline minus treatment cholesterol level (mmol/l)
6.10	5.20	1.00	.90
7.00	7.90	1.00	-.90
8.20	3.90	1.00	4.30
7.60	4.70	1.00	2.90
6.50	5.30	1.00	1.20
8.40	5.40	1.00	3.00
6.90	4.20	1.00	2.70
6.70	6.10	1.00	.60
7.40	3.80	1.00	3.60
5.80	6.30	1.00	-.50
6.20	4.30	2.00	1.90
7.10	6.80	2.00	.30

Example   641

Start by opening the above data file in SPSS statistical software.

Command:

Graphs. . . .Legacy Dialogs. . . . .Error Bar. . . .mark Summaries of groups of cases. . . . click Define. . . .Variable: enter "baseline minus treatment". . . .Category Axis: enter Treatment group. . . .Confidence interval for mean: Level enter 95%. . . .click OK.

The underneath graph shows that all of the treatments were excellent and significantly lowered cholesterol levels as shown by the 95% confidence intervals. T-tests are not needed here.

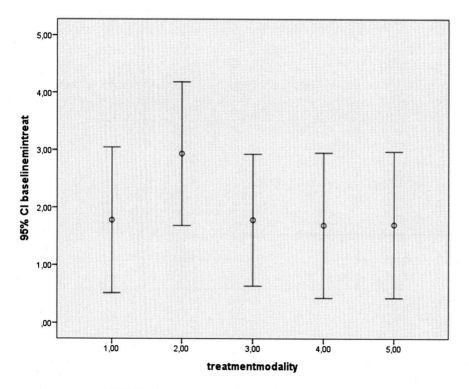

A one-way ANOVA (treatment modality as predictor and "baseline minus treatment" as outcome) will be performed to assess whether any of the treatments significantly outperformed the others.

Command

Analyze. . . .Compare means. . . .One-Way ANOVA. . . .Dependent List: enter "baseline minus treatment". . . .Factor: enter Treatment group. . . .click OK.

ANOVA

baselinemintreat

	Sum of Squares	df	Mean Square	F	Sig.
Between Groups	10,603	4	2,651	,886	,480
Within Groups	134,681	45	2,993		
Total	145,284	49			

According the above table the differences between the different treatment were statistically insignificant. And, so, according to the above analysis all treatments were excellent and no significance difference between any of the groups were observed. Next, we will try and find out whether ratio statistics can make additional observations.

Command

Analyze....Descriptive Statistics....Ratio....Numerator: enter "treatment".... Denominator: enter "baseline"....Group Variable: enter "treatmentmodality (treatment group)"....click Statistics....mark Median....mark COD (coefficient of dispersion)....Concentration Index: Low Proportion: type 0.8....High Proportion: type 1.2....click Add....Percent of Median: enter 20....click Add....click Continue....click OK.

The underneath table is shown.

Ratio Statistics for treatment / baseline

			Coefficient of Concentration	
Group	Median	Coefficient of Dispersion	Percent between 0.8 and 1.2 inclusive	Within 20% of Median inclusive
1.00	.729	.265	50.0%	50.0%
2.00	.597	.264	22.2%	44.4%
3.00	.663	.269	36.4%	54.5%
4.00	.741	.263	50.0%	50.0%
5.00	.733	.267	50.0%	50.0%
Overall	.657	.282	42.0%	38.0%

A problem with ratios is, that they usually suffer from overdispersion, and, therefore, the spread in the data must be assessed differently from that of normal distributions. First medians are applied, which is not the mean value but the values in the middle of all values. Assessment of spread is then estimated with.

(1) the coefficient of dispersion,
(2) the percentual coefficient of concentration (all ratios within 20% of the median are included),
(3) the interval coefficient of concentration (all ratios between the ratio 0.8*median and 1.2*median are included (* = symbol of multiplication).

The coefficients (2) and (3) are not the same, if the distribution of the ratios are very skewed.

The above table shows the following.

Treatment 1 (Group 1) performs best with 60% reduction of cholesterol after treatment, treatment 4 performs worst with only 74% reduction of cholesterol after treatment. The coefficient (1) is a general measure of variability of the ratios and the coefficient (3) shows the same but is more easy to interpret: around 50% Of the individual ratios are within 20% distance from the median ratio. The coefficient (2) gives the % of individual ratios between the interval of 0.8 and 1.2 * median ratio. Particularly, groups 2 and 3 have small coefficients indicating little concentration of the individual ratios here. Group 2 may produce the best median ratio, but is also least concentrated, and is thus more uncertain than, e.g., groups 1, 4, 5.

It would make sense to conclude from these observations that treatment group 1 with more certainty is a better treatment choice than treatment group 2.

Conclusion

Treatment efficacies are often assessed as differences from baseline. However, better treatment efficacies may be observed in patients with high baseline-values than in those with low ones. The differences of treatment efficacy and baseline may be the best fit test statistic, if the treatment efficacies are independent of baseline. However, if not, then ratios of the two may fit the data better, and allow for relevant additional conclusions.

Note

More background, theoretical and mathematical information of treatment efficacies that are not independent of baseline is given in Statistics applied to clinical studies 5th edition, Chap.17, Logistic and Cox regression, Markov models, and Laplace transformations, pp. 199–218, Springer Heidelberg Germany, 2012, from the same authors.

Chapter 84
Fifth Order Polynomes of Circadian Rhythms (1 Patient with Hypertension)

General Purpose

This chapter is to assess, whether polynomial analysis can visualize circadian patterns of blood pressure in individual patients with hypertension, and, thus, be helpful for making a precise diagnosis of the type of hypertension, like borderline, diastolic, systolic, white coat, no dipper hypertension).

Background

Ambulatory blood pressure measurements and other circadian phenomena are traditionally analyzed using mean values of arbitrarily separated daytime hours. The poor reproducibility of these mean values undermines the validity of this diagnostic tool. In 1998 our group demonstrated that polynomial regression lines of the 4th to 7th order generally provided adequate reliability to describe the best fit circadian sinusoidal patterns of ambulatory blood pressure measurements (Van de Luit et al., Eur J Intern Med 1998; 9: 99–103 and 251–256).

We should add that the terms multinomial and polynomial are synonymous. However, in statistics terminology is notoriously confusing, and multinomial analyses are often, though not always, used to indicate logistic regression models with multiple outcome categories. In contrast, polynomial regression analyses are often used to name the extensions of simple linear regression models with multiple order instead of first order relationships between the x and y values (Chap.16, Curvilinear regression, pp. 187–198, in: Statistics applied to clinical studies 5th edition, Springer Heidelberg Germany 2012, from the same authors as the current work). Underneath,

Electronic Supplementary Material The online version of this chapter (https://doi.org/10.1007/978-3-030-33970-8_84) contains supplementary material, which is available to authorized users.

T. J. Cleophas, A. H. Zwinderman, *Machine Learning in Medicine – A Complete Overview*, https://doi.org/10.1007/978-3-030-33970-8_84

polynomial regression equations of the first to fiftth order are given with y as dependent and x as independent variables.

$y = a + bx$ first order (linear) relationship
$y = a + bx + cx^2$ second order (parabolic) relationship
$y = a + bx + cx^2 + dx^3$ third order (hyperbolic) relationship
$y = a + bx + cx^2 + dx^3 + ex^4$ fourth order (sinusoidal) relationship
$y = a + bx + cx^2 + dx^3 + ex^4 + fx^5$ fifth order relationship

This chapter is to assess whether this method can readily visualize circadian patterns of blood pressure in individual patients with hypertension, and, thus, be helpful for making a precise diagnosis of the type of hypertension, like borderline, diastolic, systolic, white coat, no dipper hypertension).

Primary Scientific Question

Can 5th order polynomes visualize the ambulatory blood pressure pattern of individual patients?

Example

In an untreated patient with mild hypertension ambulatory blood pressure measurement was performed using a light weight portable equipment (Space Lab Medical Inc., Redmond WA) every 30 min for 24 h. The first 10 measurements are underneath, the entire data file is entitled "polynomials" and is in extras.springer.com.

Blood pressure mm Hg	Time (30 min intervals)
205,00	1,00
185,00	2,00
191,00	3,00
158,0 0	4,00
198,00	5,00
135,00	6,00
221,00	7,00
170,00	8,00
197,00	9,00
172,00	10,00
188,00	11,00
173,00	12,00

Example   647

SPSS statistical software will be used for polynomial modeling of these data. Open the data file in SPSS.

Command:

Analyze....General   Linear   Model....Univariate....Dependent: enter   y (mm Hg).... Covariate(s): enter x (min)....click: Options....mark: Parameter Estimates....click Continue....click Paste....in "/Design = x."replace x with a 5th order polynomial equation tail (∗ is sign of multiplication)

$$x \: x ∗ x \: x ∗ x ∗ x \: x ∗ x ∗ x ∗ x \: x ∗ x ∗ x ∗ x ∗ x$$

....then click the green triangle in the upper graph row of your screen.

The underneath table is in the output sheets, and gives you the partial regression coefficients (B values) of the 5th order polynomial with blood pressure as outcome and with time as independent variable ($-7135E-6$ indicates 0.000007135, which is a pretty small B value. However, in the equation it will have to be multiplied with x^5, and a large very large term will result even so.

Parameter Estimates

Dependent Variable:y

Parameter	B	Std. Error	t	Sig.	95% Confidence Interval	
					Lower Bound	Upper Bound
Intercept	206,653	17,511	11,801	,000	171,426	241,881
x	-9,112	6,336	-1,438	,157	-21,858	3,634
x∗x	,966	,710	1,359	,181	-,463	2,395
x∗x∗x	-,047	,033	-1,437	,157	-,114	,019
x∗x∗x∗x	,001	,001	1,471	,148	,000	,002
x∗x∗x∗x∗x	-7,135E-6	4,948E-6	-1,442	,156	-1,709E-5	2,819E-6

Parameter Estimates

Dependent Variable:yy

Parameter	B	Std. Error	t	Sig.	95% Confidence Interval	
					Lower Bound	Upper Bound
Intercept	170,284	11,120	15,314	,000	147,915	192,654
x	-7,034	4,023	-1,748	,087	-15,127	1,060
x∗x	,624	,451	1,384	,173	-,283	1,532
x∗x∗x	-,027	,021	-1,293	,202	-,069	,015
x∗x∗x∗x	,001	,000	1,274	,209	,000	,001
x∗x∗x∗x∗x	-3,951E-6	3,142E-6	-1,257	,215	-1,027E-5	2,370E-6

The entire equations can be written from the above B values:

$$y = 206.653 - 9112x + 0.966x^2 - 0.47x^3 + 0.001x^4 + 0.000007135x^5$$

This equation is entered in the polynomial grapher of David Wees available on the internet at "davidwees.com/polygrapher/", and the underneath graph is drawn. This graph is speculative as none of the x terms is statistically significant. Yet, the actual data have a definite patterns with higher values at daytime and lower ones at night. Sometimes even better fit curve are obtained by taking higher order polynomes like 5th order polynomes as previously tested by us (see the above section General Purpose). We should add that in spite of the insignificant p-values in the above tables the two polynomes are not meaningless. The first one suggests some white coat effect, the second one suggests normotension and a normal dipping pattern. With machine learning meaningful visualizations can sometimes be produced of your data, even if statistics are pretty meaningless.

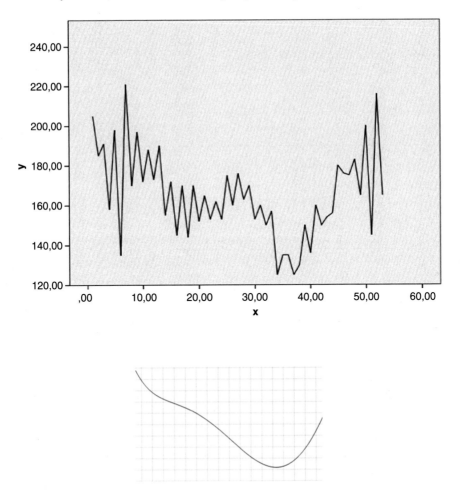

Example   649

24 h ABPM recording (30 min measures) of untreated subject with hypertension and 5th order polynome (suggesting some white coat effect).

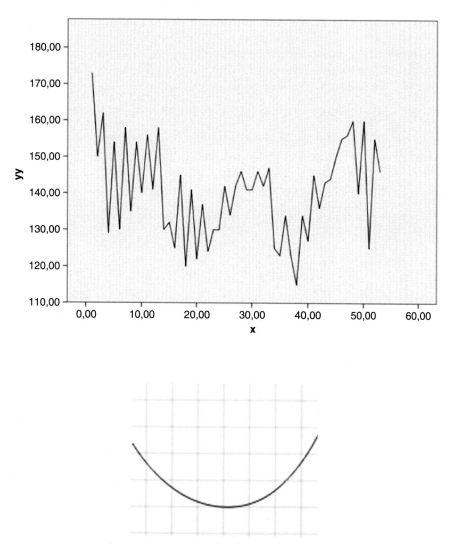

24 h ABPM recording (30 min measures) of the above subject treated and 5th order polynome (suggesting normotension and a normal dipping pattern).

Conclusion

Polynomes of ambulatory blood pressure measurements can be applied for visualizing not only hypertension types but also treatment effects, see underneath graphs of circadian patterns in individual patients (upper row) and groups of patients on different treatments (Figure from Cleophas et al., Chap.16, Curvilinear regression, pp. 187–198, in: Statistics applied to clinical studies 5th edition, Springer Heidelberg Germany 2012, with permission from the editor).

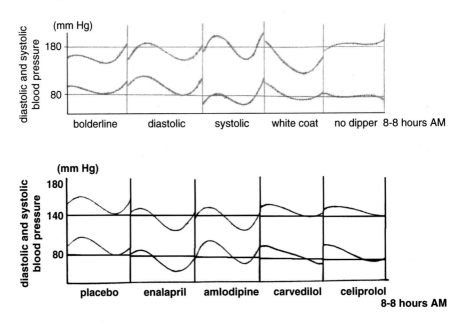

Note

More background, theoretical and mathematical information of polynomes is given in Chap.16, Curvilinear regression, pp. 187–198, in: Statistics applied to clinical studies 5th edition, Springer Heidelberg Germany 2012, from the same authors.

Chapter 85
Gamma Distribution for Estimating the Predictors of Medical Outcome Scores (110 Patients)

General Purpose

The gamma frequency distribution is suitable for statistical testing of nonnegative data with a continuous outcome variable and fits such data often better than does the normal frequency distribution.

Background

The gamma frequency distribution is adequate for statistical testing of nonnegative data with a continuous outcome variable and fits such data often better than does the normal frequency distribution, particularly when magnitudes of benefits or risks is the outcome, like costs. It is often used in marketing research.

By readers not fond of Maths the next few lines can be skipped.

The gamma frequency distribution ranges, like the Poisson distribution for rate assessments, from 0-∞. It is bell-shaped, like the normal distribution, but not as symmetric, looking a little like the chi-square distribution. Its algebraic approximation resembles and is given underneath.

$$y = e^{-1/2} x^2 \text{ (standardized normal distribution)}$$

$$y = (\lambda x)^r / \gamma * e^{-\lambda x} \text{ (gamma distribution)}$$

where

Electronic Supplementary Material The online version of this chapter (https://doi.org/10.1007/978-3-030-33970-8_85) contains supplementary material, which is available to authorized users.

λ = scale parameter
r = shape parameter
γ = correction constant

This chapter is to assess, whether gamma distributions are also helpful for the analysis of medical data, particularly those with outcome scores.

Primary Scientific Question

Is gamma regression a worthwhile analysis model complementary to linear regression, can it elucidate effects unobserved in the linear models.

Example

In 110 patients the effects of age, psychological and social score on health scores was assessed. The first 10 patients are underneath. The entire data file is entitled "gamma.sav", and is in extras.springer.com.

age	psychologic score	social score	health score
3	5	4	8
1	4	8	7
1	5	13	4
1	4	15	6
1	7	4	10
1	8	8	6
1	9	12	8
1	8	16	2
1	12	4	6
1	13	1	8

age = age class 1–7
psychologicscore = psychological score 1–20
socialscore = social score 1–20
healthscore = health score 1–20

Start by opening the data file in SPSS statistical software. We will first perform linear regressions.

Command:
Analyze....Regression....Linear....Dependent: enter healthscore....Independent (s): enter socialscore....click OK.

Example 653

The underneath table gives the result. Social score seems to be a very significant predictor of health score.

Coefficients[a]

Model		Unstandardized Coefficients		Standardized Coefficients	t	Sig.
		B	Std. Error	Beta		
1	(Constant)	9.833	.535		18.388	.000
	social score	-.334	.050	-.541	-6.690	.000

a. Dependent Variable: health score

Similarly psychological score and age class are tested.

Coefficients[a]

Model		Unstandardized Coefficients		Standardized Coefficients	t	Sig.
		B	Std. Error	Beta		
1	(Constant)	5.152	.607		8.484	.000
	psychological score	.140	.054	.241	2.575	.011

a. Dependent Variable: health score

Coefficients[a]

Model		Unstandardized Coefficients		Standardized Coefficients	t	Sig.
		B	Std. Error	Beta		
1	(Constant)	7.162	.588		12.183	.000
	age class	-.149	.133	-.107	-1.118	.266

a. Dependent Variable: health score

Linear regression with the 3 predictors as independent variables and health scores as outcome suggests that both psychological and social scores are significant predictors of health but age is not. In order to assess confounding and interaction a multiple linear regression is performed.

Command:

Analyze....Regression....Linear....Dependent: enter healthscore....Independent (s): enter socialscore, psychologicscore, age....click OK.

Coefficients[a]

Model		Unstandardized Coefficients		Standardized Coefficients	t	Sig.
		B	Std. Error	Beta		
1	(Constant)	9.388	.870		10.788	.000
	social score	-.329	.049	-.533	-6.764	.000
	psychological score	.111	.046	.190	2.418	.017
	age class	-.184	.109	-.132	-1.681	.096

a. Dependent Variable: health score

The above table is shown. Social score is again very significant. Psychological score also, but after Bonferroni adjustment (rejection p-value $= 0.05/4 = 0.0125$) it would be no more so, because $p = 0.017$ is larger than 0.0125. Age is again not significant. Health score is here a continuous variable of nonnegative values, and perhaps better fit of these data could be obtained by a gamma regression. We will use SPSS statistical software again.

Command:

Analyze....click Generalized Linear Models....click once again Generalized Linear Models....mark Custom....Distribution: select Gamma....Link function: select Power....Power: type -1....click Response....Dependent Variable: enter healthscore click Predictors....Factors: enter socialscore, psychologicscore, age.... Model: enter socialscore, psychologicscore, age....Estimation: Scale Parameter Method: select Pearson chi-square....click EM Means: Displays Means for: enter age, psychologicscore, socialscore....click Save....mark Predict value of linear predictor....Standardize deviance residual....click OK.

Tests of Model Effects

Source	Type III		
	Wald Chi-Square	df	Sig.
(Intercept)	216.725	1	.000
ageclass	8.838	6	.183
psychologicscore	18.542	13	.138
socialscore	61.207	13	.000

Dependent Variable: health score
Model: (Intercept), ageclass, psychologicscore, socialscore

The above small table give the overall result. The result is similar to that of the multiple linear regression with only social class as significant independent predictor.

Example   655

Parameter Estimates

Parameter	B	Std. Error	95% Wald Confidence Interval		Hypothesis Test		
			Lower	Upper	Wald Chi-Square	df	Sig.
(Intercept)	.188	.0796	.032	.344	5.566	1	.018
[ageclass=1]	-.017	.0166	-.050	.015	1.105	1	.293
[ageclass=2]	-.002	.0175	-.036	.032	.010	1	.919
[ageclass=3]	-.015	.0162	-.047	.017	.839	1	.360
[ageclass=4]	.014	.0176	-.020	.049	.658	1	.417
[ageclass=5]	.025	.0190	-.012	.062	1.723	1	.189
[ageclass=6]	.005	.0173	-.029	.039	.087	1	.767
[ageclass=7]	0[a]	.	.	.	.	.	.
[psychologicscore=3]	.057	.0409	-.023	.137	1.930	1	.165
[psychologicscore=4]	.057	.0220	.014	.100	6.754	1	.009
[psychologicscore=5]	.066	.0263	.015	.118	6.352	1	.012
[psychologicscore=7]	.060	.0311	-.001	.121	3.684	1	.055
[psychologicscore=8]	.061	.0213	.019	.102	8.119	1	.004
[psychologicscore=9]	.035	.0301	-.024	.094	1.381	1	.240
[psychologicscore=11]	.057	.0325	-.007	.120	3.059	1	.080
[psychologicscore=12]	.060	.0219	.017	.103	7.492	1	.006
[psychologicscore=13]	.040	.0266	-.012	.092	2.267	1	.132
[psychologicscore=14]	.090	.0986	-.103	.283	.835	1	.361
[psychologicscore=15]	.121	.0639	-.004	.247	3.610	1	.057
[psychologicscore=16]	.041	.0212	-.001	.082	3.698	1	.054
[psychologicscore=17]	.022	.0241	-.025	.069	.841	1	.359
[psychologicscore=18]	0[a]	.	.	.	.	.	.
[socialscore=4]	-.120	.0761	-.269	.029	2.492	1	.114
[socialscore=6]	-.028	.0986	-.221	.165	.079	1	.778
[socialscore=8]	-.100	.0761	-.249	.050	1.712	1	.191
[socialscore=9]	.002	.1076	-.209	.213	.000	1	.988
[socialscore=10]	-.123	.0864	-.293	.046	2.042	1	.153
[socialscore=11]	.015	.0870	-.156	.185	.029	1	.865
[socialscore=12]	-.064	.0772	-.215	.088	.682	1	.409
[socialscore=13]	-.065	.0773	-.216	.087	.703	1	.402
[socialscore=14]	.008	.0875	-.163	.180	.009	1	.925
[socialscore=15]	-.051	.0793	-.207	.104	.420	1	.517
[socialscore=16]	.026	.0796	-.130	.182	.107	1	.744
[socialscore=17]	-.109	.0862	-.277	.060	1.587	1	.208
[socialscore=18]	-.053	.0986	-.246	.141	.285	1	.593
[socialscore=19]	0[a]	.	.	.	.	.	.
(Scale)	.088[b]						

Dependent Variable: health score
Model: (Intercept), ageclass, psychologicscore, socialscore

a. Set to zero because this parameter is redundant.
b. Computed based on the Pearson chi-square.

However, as shown in the above large table, gamma regression enables to test various levels of the predictors separately. Age classes were not significant predictors. Of the psychological scores, however, no less than 8 scores produced pretty small p-values, even as small as 0.004 to 0.009. Of the social scores now no one is significant.

In order to better understand what is going on SPSS provides marginal means analysis here.

Estimates

age class	Mean	Std. Error	95% Wald Confidence Interval	
			Lower	Upper
1	5.62	.531	4.58	6.66
2	5.17	.461	4.27	6.07
3	5.54	.489	4.59	6.50
4	4.77	.402	3.98	5.56
5	4.54	.391	3.78	5.31
6	4.99	.439	4.13	5.85
7	5.12	.453	4.23	6.01

The mean health scores of the different age classes were, indeed, hardly different.

Estimates

psychological score	Mean	Std. Error	95% Wald Confidence Interval	
			Lower	Upper
3	5.03	.997	3.08	6.99
4	5.02	.404	4.23	5.81
5	4.80	.541	3.74	5.86
7	4.96	.695	3.60	6.32
8	4.94	.359	4.23	5.64
9	5.64	.809	4.05	7.22
11	5.03	.752	3.56	6.51
12	4.95	.435	4.10	5.81
13	5.49	.586	4.34	6.64
14	4.31	1.752	.88	7.74
15	3.80	.898	2.04	5.56
16	5.48	.493	4.51	6.44
17	6.10	.681	4.76	7.43
18	7.05	1.075	4.94	9.15

However, increasing psychological scores seem to be associated with increasing levels of health.

Estimates

social score	Mean	Std. Error	95% Wald Confidence Interval	
			Lower	Upper
4	8.07	.789	6.52	9.62
6	4.63	1.345	1.99	7.26
8	6.93	.606	5.74	8.11
9	4.07	1.266	1.59	6.55
10	8.29	2.838	2.73	13.86
11	3.87	.634	2.62	5.11
12	5.55	.529	4.51	6.59
13	5.58	.558	4.49	6.68
14	3.96	.711	2.57	5.36
15	5.19	.707	3.81	6.58
16	3.70	.371	2.98	4.43
17	7.39	2.256	2.96	11.81
18	5.23	1.616	2.06	8.40
19	4.10	1.280	1.59	6.61

In contrast, increasing social scores are, obviously, associated with deceasing levels of health, with mean health scores close to 3 in the higher social score patients, and close to 10 in the lower social score patients.

Conclusion

Gamma regression is a worthwhile analysis model complementary to linear regression, and may elucidate effects unobserved in the linear models.

Note

More background, theoretical and mathematical information of linear and nonlinear regression models is given in many chapters of the current book, particularly the chapters in the section entitled (log)linear models.

Index

Printed in the United States
By Bookmasters